Evidence-Based Practice in
Sport and Exercise

A Guide to Using Research

Evidence-Based Practice in
Sport and Exercise

A Guide to Using Research

Brent L. Arnold, PhD, ATC, FNATA

Professor and Chair
Department of Health Sciences
School of Health and Rehabilitation Sciences
Indiana University
Indianapolis, Indiana

Brian K. Schilling, PhD, CSCS

Professor and Chair
Kinesiology and Nutrition Sciences
University of Nevada, Las Vegas
Las Vegas, Nevada

F.A. Davis Company • Philadelphia

F. A. Davis Company
1915 Arch Street
Philadelphia, PA 19103
www.fadavis.com

Copyright © 2017 by F. A. Davis Company

Printed in the United States of America

Last digit indicates print number: 10 9 8 7 6 5 4 3 2 1

Publisher: Quincy McDonald
Director of Content Development: George W. Lang
Developmental Editor: Gary O'Brien
Design and Illustration Manager: Carolyn O'Brien

As new scientific information becomes available through basic and clinical research, recommended treatments and drug therapies undergo changes. The author(s) and publisher have done everything possible to make this book accurate, up to date, and in accord with accepted standards at the time of publication. The author(s), editors, and publisher are not responsible for errors or omissions or for consequences from application of the book, and make no warranty, expressed or implied, in regard to the contents of the book. Any practice described in this book should be applied by the reader in accordance with professional standards of care used in regard to the unique circumstances that may apply in each situation. The reader is advised always to check product information (package inserts) for changes and new information regarding dose and contraindications before administering any drug. Caution is especially urged when using new or infrequently ordered drugs.

Library of Congress Cataloging-in-Publication Data

Names: Arnold, Brent L., author. | Schilling, Brian K., author.
Title: Evidence-based practice in sport and exercise : a guide to using
  research / Brent L. Arnold, Brian K. Schilling.
Description: Philadelphia, PA : F.A. Davis Company, [2017] | Includes
  bibliographical references and index.
Identifiers: LCCN 2016024666 | ISBN 9780803640283
Subjects: | MESH: Sports Medicine | Research | Clinical Trials as Topic |
  Data Accuracy | Evidence-Based Practice
Classification: LCC RC1210 | NLM QT 261 | DDC 617.1/027—dc23 LC record available at
https://lccn.loc.gov/2016024666

Dedication

This book is dedicated to three important groups of people:
my mentors, my colleagues, and my students.

A work of this nature is not solely the author's work but is a compilation of all
the individual people who helped guide him or her.
To that end I would first like to thank my key mentors:
Kip Smith (Indiana University), John Schrader (Indiana University), Gary
Delforge (University of Arizona), Bruce Gansneder (University of Virginia),
and Dave Perrin (University of Virginia).
In particular I want to thank Dave Perrin for his efforts in helping me build
my career and the many hours of mentoring he gave me.

Careers are not built without the help of friends and colleagues.
While there are many and I am grateful for them all, I am especially
grateful to Carl Mattacola, Thomas Kaminski, and Kevin Guskiewicz.
Their friendship and comradery have been and remain
an important part of what I do.

Finally, thanks to all of my students.
I especially want to thank my graduate students.
These are the people who have formed the
foundation of my academic efforts.
Thanks to them for keeping me thinking.

> *Brent L. Arnold*

I would like to dedicate this book to my wife, Leslie, who has whole-heartedly
supported me in my career. Her empathy and kindness astound me,
and I would be truly lost without her.

> *Brian K. Schilling*

Evidence-based practice is a growing influence in exercise science and sports medicine. This is most evident in the profession of athletic training. In athletic training, competencies have been added to accreditation standards that require evidence-based practice to be taught in all accredited curriculums. Similarly, the athletic training Board of Certification has added evidence-based practice as a category required to maintain certification through continuing education. Exercise science programs have less formal mechanisms for including evidence-based practice in their educational structure or credentialing, but the inclusion of scientific principles is implied by its name. Additionally, professional organizations such as the National Strength and Conditioning Association present principles of evidence-based practice in their mission statements.

Regardless of the specific profession with which you identify, extending scientific knowledge into professional practice is becoming increasingly important. It is also becoming the expectation of our clients and patients. Thus, the purpose of this book is to provide you with the tools needed:

- to ask clinically relevant questions
- to understand the different types of research available to practitioners and identify the resources applicable to the needs of specific clients and patients
- to critically evaluate the quality of those resources
- to synthesize those resources into a meaningful outcome for your client or patient.

Several features have been included in the book to help facilitate your understanding of evidence-based practice principles:

Where have you been?

The Where Have You Been? section occurs before the chapters to highlight content that has been previously presented in the book. It is intended to give a summary perspective and set the stage for the upcoming chapter.

Where are you going?

Each chapter starts with an overview called Where Are You Going? This is a continuation of the Where You Have Been? section and sets up the chapter ahead. It is useful for getting the big picture before tackling the details of the chapter.

Connections

Research is an interconnected set of steps that leads to an outcome. Because of its interconnections, it can often be perceived as a maze. The Connections feature is designed to connect topics in one chapter to a related topic in another chapter. The hope is the reader will be able to relate connected ideas more quickly for a greater understanding.

Pros and Cons

Producing research and applying research often involve choices and compromises. Pros and Cons is a feature that points out these choices and addresses the advantages and disadvantages of each.

The Critical Consumer

The Critical Consumer is a feature that points out a critical component on which the consumer of research should focus. The goal is to emphasize research elements that can be easily overlooked as unimportant but should not be. Overlooking these elements often leads to misuse of the information by the practitioner.

Retention Questions

At selected points in each chapter are Retention Questions. These questions are designed to challenge the reader by emphasizing the key components of previously presented material.

Trust and Apply

At the end of each chapter is Trust and Apply. This feature provides a research article to be retrieved and read by the reader. It also includes a set of questions related to the article. The goal is to provide a directed exercise by which the reader can apply the content of the chapter to actual research.

Research Scavenger Hunt

The final feature is the Research Scavenger Hunt. For this feature the reader must follow the instructions and find a research article that meets the criteria. This feature has enough flexibility to allow the reader to select an article that addresses a practice problem of his or her interest.

All these features together are intended to help you learn the principles and applications of evidence-based practice and make you into the best professional you can be. We hope you find this book to be an effective tool in your professional education.

Contributors

Scott E. Ross, PhD, LAT, ATC

Associate Professor
Director, Athletic Training Program
Associate Chair, Kinesiology
School of Health & Human Sciences
Department of Kinesiology
University of North Carolina Greensboro
Greensboro, North Carolina

Gregory W. Heath, DHSc, MPH

Guerry Professor and Assistant Vice Chancellor for Research
University of Tennessee at Chattanooga
Professor of Medicine and Research Director
University of Tennessee College of Medicine
Chattanooga, Tennessee

Christopher R. Harnish, PhD, ACSM EP-C EIM, CSCS, FMSc

Assistant Professor
Department of Health & Human Performance
Ferrum College
Ferrum, Virginia

Reviewers

Brent A. Alvar, Ph.D. CSCS*D, RSCC*D, FNSCA, FACSM
Vice President of University Research
Rocky Mountain University of Health Professions
Provo, Utah

Joseph A. Beckett, EdD, ATC
Director, Athletic Training Program
Marshall University
Huntington, West Virginia

Joe D. Bell, PhD
Associate Professor and Exercise Science Chair
Abilene Christian University
Abilene, Texas

Resa M. Chandler, PhD
Associate Professor of Exercise Science and Exercise Science Degree Coordinator
Brevard College
Brevard, North Carolina

Nicole Chimera, PhD, ATC, CSCS
Assistant Professor
Athletic Training
Daemen College
Amherst, New York

Lisa Chinn, PhD, AT
Assistant Professor
Athletic Training
Department of Health Sciences
Kent State University
Kent, Ohio

Patricia Fehling, PhD
Professor and Chair
Health and Exercise Sciences
Skidmore College
Saratoga Springs, New York

Bradley Floy, PhD, ATC, CSCS
Athletic Trainer
Intercollegiate Athletics
University of Iowa
Iowa City, Iowa

Philip Ford, PhD, ATC, PES, CES

Program Director
Applied Exercise Science, Associate Professor
Azusa Pacific University
Azusa, California

Danny T. Foster, PhD, ATC

Program Director
Athletic Training
University of Iowa
Iowa City, Iowa

Hugh W. Harling, EdD, LAT, ATC

Athletic Training Program Director
Methodist University
Fayetteville, North Carolina

Valerie W. Herzog, EdD, LAT, ATC

Graduate Athletic Training Program Director
Health Promotion and Human Performance
Weber State University
Ogden, Utah

Michael Brian Hudson, PhD, ATC

Associate Professor
Sports Medicine and Athletic Training
Missouri State University
Springfield, Missouri

Erin M Jordan, MS, ATC

Clinical Instructor in Athletic Training
Georgia Southern University
Statesboro, Georgia

Thomas W. Kaminski, PhD, ATC, FNATA, FACSM

Professor
Kinesiology and Applied Physiology
University of Delaware
Newark, Delaware

Ryan Krzyzanowicz, MSEd, ATC

Assistant Professor, Clinical Education Coordinator
Massachusetts College of Liberal Arts
North Adams, Massachusetts

Kim O'Connell-Brock, MS, ATC/L

Assistant Director
Athletic Training Education Program
New Mexico State University
Las Cruces, New Mexico

Rhonda J. Olson, MED, ATC, LAT

Head Athletic Trainer, Assistant Professor
University of Mary
Bismarck, North Dakota

Katy Pietz, MEd, ATC, AT/L

Clinical Education Coordinator, Instructor
Washington State University
Pullman, Washington

Kathy Remsburg, MS, ATC, LAT

Director, Athletic Training Program; Associate Professor
Franklin College
Franklin, Indiana

Tara Tietjen-Smith, DA

Associate Professor, Health & Human Performance
Texas A & M University Commerce
Commerce, Texas

Bonnie Van Lunen, PhD, ATC

Director, Athletic Training and Human Movement Science Programs
Old Dominion University
Norfolk, Virginia

Acknowledgments

I would like to first acknowledge Quincy McDonald. I am grateful that he gave me this opportunity. His vision and encouragement have been greatly appreciated.

Gary O'Brien has been a remarkable help in getting this project completed. This project has sputtered and temporarily stalled at times. His behind-the-scenes efforts have been critical for keeping the project moving forward. His ability to recruit contributors was a great relief. He graciously handled the details that can drive me nuts.

This book was written for two audiences, and I am expert on only one of these. So thanks go to Brian Schilling for joining this project. His perspective has been a great help in keeping the book aligned with the needs of exercise science. He has also been helpful in challenging some of my perspectives and allowing us to produce a more refined product.

Finally, I want to thank our contributors: Scott Ross, Greg Heath, and Chris Harnish. It is difficult to be expert on all topics. Lending their expertise to the book has greatly enhanced the final product.

Brent L. Arnold

I'd like to thank Lawrence W. Weiss, EdD, who is always a trusted advisor for professional endeavors, not the least of which was taking on this book project.

Brian K. Schilling

Contents in Brief

Contents

SECTION 3

Other Methods in Clinical Research

10 Evaluating Research Quality 248

Christopher R. Harnish, PhD, ACSM EP-C EIM, CSCS, FMSc

APPENDICES

Introduction to Applying Research

Evidence-based practice (EBP) is becoming the standard for medicine and allied health, so it is not surprising that athletic training and exercise science are also adopting evidence-based practice. For you to become a professional in these fields, you must understand what constitutes evidence-based practice and to which types of questions it can be applied. These issues form the discussion of Chapters 1 and 2. In Chapter 3, you will learn about outcome measures dealing with disease and disability, along with performance measures more associated with fitness and sports performance. At the close of this section, in Chapter 4, you will learn about statistical methods for compiling outcome measures and how researchers interpret these statistical values. With this information you can then apply their findings to your clinical questions.

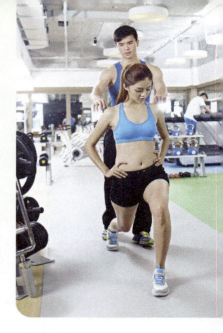

What Is Evidence-Based Practice?

Where Have You Been?

Up to this point in your educational journey, you have probably been focused on learning the scientific and clinical fundamentals of your discipline and profession. You have probably learned clinical and/or laboratory techniques, many of which are directly derived from scientific studies. It is these fundamentals and techniques derived from science that lead to what we know as the "current state of the art." You should have the sense that science *evolves,* and as it evolves, the methods used in the practice setting should evolve to reflect the new state of the art. Unfortunately for the busy practitioner, keeping up with the science can be a challenge. Despite this challenge, there are methods to help you stay on the cutting edge of your profession, and that is what this textbook is about.

Where Are You Going?

Assuming at this stage in your professional preparation that you may not have been introduced to evidence-based practice, your first step is to understand what constitutes *evidence.* Evidence is the keystone to state-of-the-art practice, and it comes in many different forms. Some forms of evidence are very good and can be trusted; other forms are less trustworthy and must be considered with less confidence. Thus, you must be able to recognize and understand the different forms of evidence and the ways in which those forms of evidence are rated in terms of strength. You must also recognize that there is no uniform system for evaluating evidence, and this realization makes your judgment an important part of the process.

To apply the available science to your profession, several steps are necessary. First, you must recognize that you have a clinical or practice question that needs answering. Second, you must ask your question properly. Third, you must find the information needed to answer the question. Fourth, you must correctly interpret the information. Fifth, you must apply what you learned to your client or patient. Finally, you must assess whether your application of what you learned (e.g., a new treatment or training technique) worked. This process may sound daunting, but it is not, as long as it is treated as a systematic process.

Learning Outcomes

After reading this chapter, you should be able to answer these questions:

1. What is evidence-based practice?
2. What are levels of evidence?
3. How is evidence-based practice used in professional decision-making?
4. What is an evidence pyramid?
5. What types of evidence are better than others?

Key Terms

Critically appraised paper (CAP)
Critically appraised topic (CAT)
Disease-oriented evidence (DOE)

Evidence-based medicine (EBM)
Evidence-based practice (EBP)
Levels of evidence
Patient-oriented evidence

Secondary study
Strength of recommendation
Systematic review (SR)

■ EVIDENCE-BASED PRACTICE IN EXERCISE SCIENCE AND HEALTH CARE

Evidence-based practice (EBP) can be defined as the application of research to a profession. The concept originally started in the field of medicine as evidence-based medicine (EBM), but it has since been adopted by other health-care professions and fields such as education. In fact, there is no limit to which fields it can be applied. Although not all exercise scientists work with a patient or client base, many do (e.g., strength coaches, fitness instructors). Thus, for these professionals, understanding evidence-based practice offers added credibility and validity to their work.

One of the primary implications of evidence-based practice is that you, as a practitioner, must become familiar with the research process to the extent that you can evaluate the merits of research findings and determine their applicability to your practice. You will face several challenges in applying research. First, you must understand the different types of research designs. This is a challenging task, but one that need not be intimidating. Second, you must understand the different measurement techniques, methodologies, and analysis techniques used to address different questions. These three aspects may be discipline specific. Third, you must find relevant research. Because of the vast number of journals in exercise and sport science, this is also a challenging step. (See Appendix A for a list of selected journals that apply exercise, sport science, and related health and medical topics.) You may also quickly learn that the research does not yet exist to cover every question you may ask. Furthermore, the research you do find may only *partially* address your question, and you will have to apply your judgment about whether it applies closely enough to you and your client.

As you begin trying to apply evidence-based practice to your practice, you will probably be startled to learn that many of the procedures you are taught are not supported by large amounts of research, if any research at all. For instance, imagine that you are an exercise physiologist working with a marathoner who has type 1 diabetes. Because persons with type 1 diabetes do not produce insulin, they rely on administration of insulin to manage their blood glucose levels. Obviously, this management is difficult in endurance athletes, and much of what is known about blood glucose regulation in nondiabetic athletes does not apply. At the time of this writing, a search of a popular academic database (SPORTdiscus) listed only one research article with the keywords "type 1 diabetes" and "marathon"!

Evidence-based practice (EBP): The practice of applying research findings to professional practice.

Evidence-based medicine (EBM): Medicine that is based on data, rather than anecdote, intuition, or belief.

Role of Evidence in the Practitioner's Decision-Making Process

Evidence has multiple roles in professional practice. The chief purpose is finding answers to unknown questions—more specifically, finding answers to questions that are important to you. Historically, professional practice has been as much "art" as it has been "science." As you begin your career, you will find many instances where you or your colleagues must improvise to solve a problem for a client. However, as science advances, these improvisations can, and should, be replaced by practices that are founded on scientific evidence. Evidence-based practice is about applying that scientific evidence to practice.

One of the most obvious uses—and probably the primary use—of evidence-based practice is identifying the best treatment for a clinical condition. However, finding the best treatment is not limited to medical treatments. It includes all areas of exercise and sport science, such as finding the best strength training protocol, the best flexibility program, the best exercise program for controlling diabetes, the best exercise progression for general fitness, and so on. Furthermore, evidence-based practice can be used to tailor treatment programs to individual clients' needs. By focusing on a particular client's characteristics, evidence-based practice allows you to match evidence to the client. This approach allows you to fine-tune your practice and exclude methods that may not be beneficial to a particular case. One example of evidence-based practice for fine-tuning your practice would be looking at resistance training volume for maximizing strength. A 2004 meta-analysis of strength training studies (Wolfe, LeMura, & Cole, 2004) concluded that the appropriate volume of strength training depends on the training status of your client. An untrained person may see gains with a low-volume program, but the volume would likely need to be increased over time as the person becomes better trained.

A second purpose of evidence-based practice is identifying the best use of available resources, including material and personnel. If your work setting has limited personnel, then it is important to keep personnel focused on activities that truly benefit clients. Similarly, if equipment in your work setting is limited and in high demand, then it is important to make sure that equipment is available for those clients who would benefit the most. For example, a systematic review and meta-analysis in the subdiscipline of athletic training demonstrated that isokinetic strength testing of the ankle cannot adequately detect weakness (Arnold, Linens, de la Motte, & Ross, 2009). Thus, this type of testing has little value in ankle therapy. To take the evidence a step further, the relatively high expense of isokinetic dynamometers means that they are probably not a wise purchase for rehabilitation clinics that focus on foot and ankle conditions.

Evidence-based practice also identifies tests that are appropriate for evaluating and/or diagnosing injury or disease. Many tests can be found in the literature, including tests for blood pressure, strength, joint and muscle flexibility, and ligament stability. However, many of these tests are not sufficiently established as reliable or valid. Using evidence-based practice, you can determine which tests can be trusted and which tests have limited value. For example, evidence-based practice can be used to decide whether the Lachman or anterior drawer test is the better test for anterior cruciate ligament deficiency. Furthermore, you can identify those tests that can improve or change your diagnosis of a condition or injury. One example of a newer test is the Functional Movement Screen. Although it has become a popular test for evaluating movement patterns, narrative reviews have suggested that even though the reliability is high, this test may lack sufficient validity and sensitivity to be highly useful.

● LEVELS OF EVIDENCE

The term **levels of evidence** refers to the strength of the research you may find regarding your question. Based on its specific design, a research study can be categorized into one of several different levels. These levels are often depicted in the form of a pyramid (Fig. 1–1). The goal of this classification is to provide a quick reference for you to assess the strength of the evidence. When making professional practice decisions, you should use the highest level of evidence available.

As a critical consumer of research, you must understand that the level of evidence refers to the strength of the evidence, not the quality of the research. The level of evidence is based on the type of study performed and the strength given to that type, whereas research quality refers to how well a study was done and whether the results of the study can be trusted (see Chapter 5 for more information on study designs). Because of this dichotomy, you may encounter a study high on the pyramid that is of poor quality. Conversely, just because a study belongs to a lower level of evidence does not mean that it is low quality. For example, sometimes lower-level studies are done because the condition being studied does not exist in large enough numbers to conduct a higher-level study.

Levels of evidence: Indicators, by category, of the strength of research.

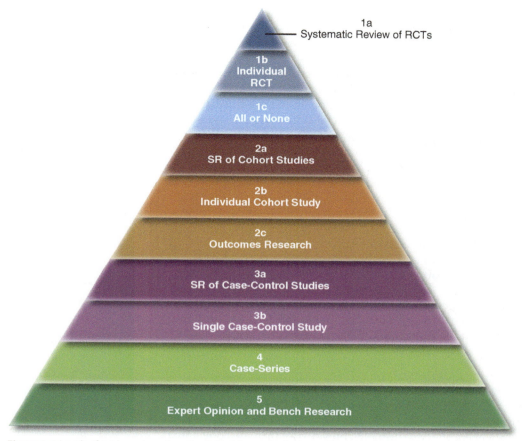

Figure 1–1 Levels of evidence based on the Oxford Centre for Evidence-Based Medicine model.

Centre for Evidence-Based Medicine Hierarchy

Probably the most commonly used evidence pyramids is the University of Oxford's Centre for Evidence-Based Medicine (CEBM) model (Oxford Centre for Evidence-Based Medicine, 2009). Other pyramids or hierarchies are available, but they generally follow a structure similar to the CEBM model (Fig. 1–1).

The CEBM divides types of research into five broad categories, some with two or three subcategories. Conceptually, the hierarchy starts with the form of research that provides the most convincing evidence for decision-making and descends to lower, less-convincing forms. However, learning the levels of the hierarchy is easier when you start at the bottom because each level builds on the next.

Level 5: "First Principles," Physiological Evidence and Bench Research, Expert Opinion

First Principles

First principles are fundamental rules or assumptions that a group accepts as culturally important. In medicine, the most frequently used first principle is "do no harm." There is no scientific basis for this statement, and it cannot be deduced from scientific evidence. Nevertheless, you would probably accept at face value that it is the proper thing to do. First principles frequently form the basis of our ethics systems. For example, if you accept the principle "do no harm," then that belief will help define your ethics regarding research. In other words, you would probably agree that a researcher should not perform research simply for the sake of knowledge if it harms a person.

For example, the National Athletic Trainers' Association (NATA) periodically produces consensus statements. The statements are put together by a group of sports medicine experts to clarify a best practice (e.g., how to treat exertional heat illness). Appendix B provides a list of current published research-based position and consensus statements by both the National Athletic Trainers' Association and the American College of Sports Medicine (ACSM).

Physiological Evidence and Bench Research

Also known as *basic science*, physiological evidence and bench research refer to research done in a laboratory setting on cells, tissues, or nonhuman animals. Although these models may have a physiological corollary to humans, they do not provide conclusive evidence that a treatment will work in human patients. From a scientific perspective, this research is important in that it forms a foundation from which to build future research. However, from a professional practice perspective, little emphasis should be placed on these studies unless no other evidence is available. For example, a great deal about muscle function can be used from examining single fibers taken from human muscle. These studies show that fast-twitch fibers (IIx) are the fastest contracting, followed by the type IIa and type I fibers. However, in vivo analyses show that well-trained persons actually may possess very few IIx fibers.

Expert Opinion

Expert opinion is exactly what it sounds like—an expert or, more typically, a group of experts in a discipline forms an opinion on an issue. Expert opinion is used when the research in an area is preliminary, low quality, or incomplete. That is not to say that these types of opinions themselves are of poor quality. Rather, they may

---

Pros and Cons 1-1

Expert opinions are usually good summaries of the existing state of the art and are commonly associated with current best practices. Thus, they are often perceived as very useful by practitioners. However, you must keep in mind that expert opinions are created when complete or high-quality evidence is lacking. As such, you should be mindful of this shortcoming and be judicious when using expert opinions to inform practice. Also, the definition of "expert" is open to interpretation, and thus sometimes knowledge about the author is important.

---

be the best evidence available when convincing scientific evidence does not yet exist. You should know that some position stands, such as the American College of Sports Medicine position stand on exercise in older adults (American College of Sports Medicine et al., 2009), are actually a type of narrative review; the difference between these types of opinions or reviews is the level of available evidence on which they are based.

Level 4: Case-Series and Poor-Quality Cohort or Case-Control Studies

Level 4 evidence consists of case-series studies, which means simply research involving a series of individual study subjects (i.e., cases) who all received the same treatment (e.g., blood pressure medicine, strength training). Across the series, these persons either improved or did not. If they improved, the researcher concludes that the treatment worked. This type of study is considered to be a very poor scientific design (see Chapter 5) because it does not include experimental controls and violates many principles of research design. Because of its poor design, case-series studies are classified as a lower level of evidence and should be considered only when higher levels are not available. Also at this level are poor-quality cohort or case-control studies. These types of studies are discussed later, but poor-quality examples of these studies are at the same level of evidence as case-series studies.

Level 3b: Individual Case-Control Study

A case-control study (see Chapter 5) involves taking a group of patients with a disease or condition (the cases) and comparing them with a group of healthy or normal persons (the controls). For example, you could compare a group of obese persons with a group of nonobese persons to study differences in exercise patterns—the assumption being that differences in exercise patterns may explain the obesity. Unfortunately, because you are assessing the obese persons *after* the obesity has developed, you cannot determine whether exercise differences between the groups existed before or after the formation of obesity. Thus, you cannot conclude whether the exercise patterns influenced or caused the obesity. Because of this causality disconnect, case-control studies are considered a lower form of evidence.

Level 3a: Systematic Review of Case-Control Studies

Although a case-control study is considered a weak design, its value is improved if several case-control studies are combined. This can be done through the process of a systematic review (SR). A systematic review uses existing research studies, such as case-control studies, and compiles the findings into a single research finding. Also referred to as *research synthesis*, systematic reviews are considered "systematic" because they involve a thorough literature search and the research studies included meet strict, predetermined inclusion criteria that are reported in the paper. By compiling many studies and synthesizing the results into a summary finding, the result of a systematic review is considered stronger than that of any single study alone. (Systematic reviews are more fully discussed in Chapter 9.)

Systematic review: A systematic compilation of existing research studies and a synthesis of those research study results into a single research finding.

Level 2c: Outcomes Research and Ecological Studies

Outcomes Research

Outcomes research refers to the study of the final patient outcome of a treatment (Clancy & Eisenberg, 1998). Its focus is on measures that matter to the patient (such as quality of life) or to other stakeholders such as the government. Examples of outcome measures include death rates, patient treatment preferences, patient function, and patient satisfaction.

Outcomes research is contrasted with clinical trials that focus on measures of disease. In exercise science, a clinical trial of strength training would focus on whether the training produced changes in strength, whereas an outcomes study may focus on the client's change in body image, the client's perception of how easy the training protocol was to follow, or the complexity of administering the program to clients. Because outcomes research is not focused on a person's change in disease or condition, it is given a lower evidence level.

Ecological Research

Ecological research is a form of epidemiological research that focuses on populations rather than individuals. It is commonly used to compare disease rates in different geographic areas, such as different countries or states. The key difference between this and other types of research is the focus on populations, not individual persons. Because of the population focus, it ranks lower in the levels of evidence.

Level 2b: Individual Cohort Study or Low-Quality Randomized Controlled Trial

Cohort studies are a form of observational study. An observational study does not manipulate a treatment. Rather, it studies intact groups (cohorts) across time. Cohort studies identify persons who have been exposed or not exposed to a disease risk factor. These groups of individual persons are followed across time to determine whether they develop the target disease. The classic example of a disease risk factor is cigarette smoking. In a cohort study looking at this risk factor, smokers and nonsmokers would be identified and then followed across time to determine whether they develop lung cancer, for example. If the rate of lung cancer is higher in the smoking group, the evidence suggests that smoking caused the cancer.

Cohort studies can be either prospective or retrospective. In a prospective study, the researcher begins studying persons after they have had an exposure to a suspected disease cause (an unexposed cohort is also identified at this time), and the two cohorts are followed forward in time, as in the previous example on smoking. In a retrospective design, the researcher begins by looking backward in time at preexisting data for disease and an exposure. Retrospective studies are typically faster and have a better way to examine rare occurrences, but they also suffer from disadvantages such as recall bias.

Although cohort studies can provide strong evidence for a causal relationship, they cannot establish a true cause-and-effect relationship. By their nature, cohort studies cannot control extraneous factors that can influence the outcomes of the study. For example, in the smoking study, such extraneous factors as environmental exposure to asbestos or secondhand smoke could affect whether both smokers and nonsmokers develop lung cancer. Thus, the study cannot support cause and effect as much as an experimental study can. Experimental studies provide more rigorous controls on extraneous factors, thus preventing more competing causes for the observed outcome. (Experimental research is described in more detail in Chapter 5.)

Level 2a: Systematic Review of Cohort Studies

Similar to case-control studies, when cohort studies are aggregated into systematic reviews, the strength of the evidence increases.

Connections 1-1

Cohort studies are commonly confused with case-control studies. The distinction is that case-control studies start with disease and then look for exposures. Cohort studies start with exposures and then look for disease.

This is especially true when studies show consistent results in favor (or against) a link between an exposure and a disease.

Level 1c: All-or-None

All-or-none studies are a form of case-series studies, and they are organized in the same way; however, their results are interpreted differently. In a typical case-series study, the treatment is considered to work if the majority (or a previously specified percentage) of cases demonstrated a specified level of improvement or a trend toward improvement. In all-or-none studies, all persons receiving the treatment must respond, or all the persons not receiving the treatment must not have responded. For example, assume that you are placing obese clients on an aerobic exercise program to reduce weight. Each individual client would be a case. For an all-or-none study, every individual client enrolled in the exercise program would have to lose weight. Conversely, an all-or-none study of a human immunodeficiency virus (HIV) vaccine would require that all subjects receiving the vaccine do not contract the infection.

As you may imagine, the all-or-none standard is quite rigorous. It also requires large numbers of individual subjects to be conclusive. Furthermore, individual persons rarely respond consistently. Even if large numbers respond, a minority may not. In this situation, what explains the nonresponders? Because groups of individuals typically do not respond consistently, all-or-none studies are rarely used. Instead, experimental studies known as *randomized controlled trials* (RCTs) are considered the gold standard in determining cause and effect.

Level 1b: Individual Randomized Controlled Trial

Randomized controlled trials are experimental studies. They involve two essential elements: a control group and random assignment of subjects to groups (treatment and control). The purpose of the control group is to have a comparison condition that represents what happens when no treatment occurs. The purpose of random assignment is to create groups that are presumed equal on all factors before the treatments are started. In cases in which the groups must be very similar on one or more traits, stratified randomization may be used. A more detailed explanation of control groups, random assignment, and experimental studies is provided in Chapter 5.

Level 1a: Systematic Reviews of Randomized Controlled Trials

As with case-control and cohort studies, systematic reviews of randomized controlled trials add strength to the evidence. As with

Pros and Cons 1-2

Randomized controlled trials are considered the "gold standard" in medical research. They have the advantage of being able to control for outside influences on the outcomes. However, they typically require many subjects, are often very large scale, usually extend over long periods of time, and can be very expensive.

other types of research, the more studies included in the systematic review, the stronger the result. Whenever available, systematic reviews of randomized controlled trials provide the strongest evidence.

Centre for Evidence-Based Medicine Pyramid for Other Studies

The previous discussion of the Centre for Evidence-Based Medicine pyramid focused on therapeutic trials because applying a treatment is a typical goal of the practitioner. However, the Centre for Evidence-Based Medicine pyramid is not limited to therapeutic trials. With some adjustments, it is equally applicable to prognostic (effects of a particular patient characteristic on an outcome) and diagnostic (evaluation of a particular test) studies (Oxford Centre for Evidence-Based Medicine, 2009).

Alternative Levels of Evidence

The pyramid of evidence provided by the Centre for Evidence-Based Medicine is not the only way to construct an evidence pyramid. Some investigators have proposed that other sources of evidence should be included in the pyramid. One example is presented in Figure 1–2. As you can see, this pyramid looks similar to Figure 1–1; however, some levels have been combined, and two levels have been added: one for **critically appraised individual articles** (or **critically appraised papers [CAPs]**) and one for **critically appraised topics (CATs)**. Critically appraised topics are more commonly reported in the literature.

A critically appraised topic appraises current research on a focused clinical question. It is shorter than a typical systematic review, and it focuses on three to five studies representing the most current research. Critically appraised topics include both a critique of the included studies and a statement of clinical application (Fetters, Figueiredo, Keane-Miller, McSweeney, & Tsao, 2004). The goal is to present the practitioner with a critical summary of the research. One weakness of critically appraised topics is they may not be as rigorously peer reviewed as randomized controlled trials (the level below) or systematic reviews. Their form may make them more useful to a practitioner, but that does not necessarily make them a better level of evidence. Thus, some caution is warranted in relying on the conclusions found in a critically appraised topic.

Despite this concern, Figure 1–2 has another interesting feature. On the right side, the different levels are grouped into filtered and unfiltered evidence. As discussed in Chapter 9, these categories may also be referred to as *secondary* and *primary studies*, respectively.

Critically appraised paper (CAP): A professional summary of a single research study.

Critically appraised topic (CAT): A professional summary, typically focused on a clinical question, of a small number of research studies (three to five). The CAT is typically shorter and less rigorous than the systematic review (SR).

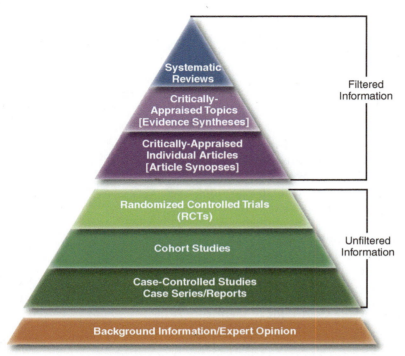

Figure 1–2 An evidence-based pyramid that includes critically appraised papers (i.e., individual articles) and critically appraised topics and distinguishes between filtered and unfiltered evidence. *(From Glover, J., Izzo, D., Odato, K., & Wang, L. [2006]. EBM pyramid and EBM generator. Trustees of Dartmouth College and Yale University.)*

Secondary studies are reviews and syntheses of existing primary studies. As previously discussed, because secondary studies synthesize existing studies, they are given a higher rank on an evidence pyramid. Primary studies are original research, meaning that the researchers recruited and collected data on subjects.

Base and Shape of the Evidence Pyramid

When you examine Figures 1–1 and 1–2, you probably tend to focus on the levels of the pyramid. However, the shape of the pyramid also has meaning. First, you should understand that the lower levels of the pyramid serve as the base of support for the upper levels. These lower levels are either foundational or precursory for the upper levels. For example, bench research is at the very bottom of the pyramid. Although bench research tends to have less direct clinical impact, these studies are foundational to finding promising treatments (e.g., medicines, exercises) that could be subsequently applied to human studies. Similarly, case-control studies can be viewed as precursory to randomized controlled trials. In other

Secondary study: Reviews and syntheses of existing primary studies.

Retention Questions 1-2

1. What is the difference between a critically appraised paper and a critically appraised topic?
2. Which type of study is considered to provide better evidence, and why?
3. What is a shortcoming of a critically appraised topic?
4. What is the distinction between filtered and unfiltered information?

words, case-control studies are useful in identifying potential causes of disease to which treatments can be applied using a randomized controlled trial. For example, a case-control study may find that subjects with low back pain may have weak abdominal muscles. From this finding, a randomized controlled trial could be designed to determine whether improved abdominal strength reduces low back pain.

The other obvious but overlooked feature of evidence pyramids is that they narrow as you move from the bottom to the top. This feature may be coincidental, but it represents a typical problem with the current status of health-care and exercise science research. Specifically, as you move from the bottom to the top, fewer studies exist. A quick literature search using any library search engine reveals that most research is at the bottom half of the pyramid. Furthermore, many fewer critically appraised topics and systematic reviews exist. Because of this, as a practitioner you may find it difficult to locate applicable studies near the top of the pyramid.

Strength of Recommendation Taxonomy

The Centre for Evidence-Based Medicine pyramid and other evidence pyramids are essential to understanding which individual studies should be given more or less weight in decision-making. However, one limitation of evidence pyramids is that some levels categorize one study at a time and offer no summary statement about the strength of evidence when multiple studies exist. In fact, evidence gleaned from multiple sources is ideal. However, these multiple studies may produce inconsistent or varied results. One available solution is the Strength of Recommendation Taxonomy, or SORT (Ebell et al., 2004). Through a systematic process, the Strength of Recommendation Taxonomy assigns a letter grade to groups of existing studies that address an important clinical problem. The letter grade for the group of studies determines how much emphasis a practitioner should place on the overall evidence.

A unique feature of the Strength of Recommendation Taxonomy is it focuses on patient-oriented measures rather than disease-oriented measures. **Patient-oriented information** are measures that assess qualities related to the whole patient and include such factors as mortality and quality of life. Thus, the goal is to emphasize changes patients easily understand. This is contrasted with disease-oriented measures (also known as **disease-oriented evidence [DOE]**), which assess qualities related to the disease such as decreased blood pressure and increased bone density.

The Strength of Recommendation Taxonomy also emphasizes that groups of studies are graded on three criteria: quality, quantity, and consistency. *Quality* refers to a study's minimization of bias and is synonymous with validity (see Chapter 5). *Quantity* refers

Patient-oriented information: Measures that assess qualities that are related to the whole patient, such as mortality and quality of life, with the goal of emphasizing changes that patients easily understand.

Disease-oriented evidence (DOE): Measures that focus on the qualities or aspects of the disease and are collected by the clinician and help with the understanding of the current state of the disease.

Strength of Recommendation Based on a Body of Evidence

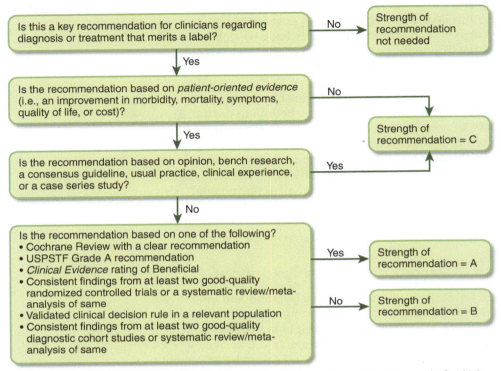

Figure 1–3 Strength of Recommendation Taxonomy (SORT) algorithm for determining the strength of multiple sources of evidence. USPSTF = United States Preventive Services Task Force. (*From Ebell, M. H., Siwek, J., Weiss, B. D., Woolf, S. H., Susman, J., Ewigman, B., et al. [2004]. Strength of Recommendation Taxonomy [SORT]: A patient-centered approach to grading evidence in the medical literature.* American Family Physician, 69[3], 548-556.)

to the number of studies addressing the clinical question and the number of subjects in those studies. Topics with more studies and studies with larger numbers of subjects provide stronger evidence. *Consistency* refers to whether the studies have consistent or differing results among themselves. Several studies with consistent findings provide greater strength (see Chapter 9). Figure 1–3 provides an algorithm for determining the **strength of recommendation** using the Strength of Recommendation Taxonomy.

■ SUMMARY

The purpose of evidence-based practice is to help you select the best treatments and techniques, to serve your clients most effectively. Evidence-based practice provides an approach by which science is applied to practice to develop best practices. All original research (or evidence) can be divided into hierarchical categories

Strength of recommendation: A letter grade assigned to groups of existing studies that address an important clinical problem by using patient-oriented measures. Grades are assigned based on the quality, quantity, and consistency of available data by using the Strength of Recommendation Taxonomy (SORT).

of an evidence pyramid. At the base of the pyramid are items of evidence such as expert opinion and bench research. At the top of the pyramid is synthesized research, such as systematic reviews. Although original research can be categorized and subsequently weighted, this practice is often cumbersome for the practitioner. Thus, alternatives such as critically appraised topics can provide useful critiques of existing research. Finally, when multiple pieces of evidence are available, grading systems such as the Strength of Recommendation Taxonomy are useful. The Strength of Recommendation Taxonomy assigns a letter grade to a group of studies based on the validity of each study, the number of studies, participants included, and the consistency of findings across studies.

CRITICAL THINKING QUESTIONS

1. How are evidence-based medicine and evidence-based practice similar and different?

2. Within each level of evidence (for levels 1, 2, and 3) in the Centre for Evidence-Based Medicine's evidence pyramid, what is the highest sublevel and why?

3. Why are animal studies at the bottom of an evidence pyramid?

TRUST AND APPLY

Arnold, B. L., Linens, S. W., de la Motte, S. J., & Ross, S. E. (2009). Concentric evertor strength differences and functional ankle instability: A meta-analysis. *Journal of Athletic Training, 44*(6), 653-662.

Locate the article above and, using this article, address the following questions.

1. What kind of research does this study employ? Is this a primary or a secondary study?

2. What kinds of studies were reviewed? What levels of evidence would you assign to the included studies?

3. What level of evidence would you assign to this study?

4. Were the variables studied disease oriented or patient oriented?

RESEARCH SCAVENGER HUNT

Using a topic of your choice, find journal articles on one systematic review, one randomized controlled trial, and one critically appraised topic.

1. Which of these studies would be given the highest level of evidence?

2. Given a choice among the three, which study would you use to make a clinical decision?
3. Which of the three studies provides filtered evidence?

REFERENCES

American College of Sports Medicine, Chodzko-Zajko, W. J., Proctor, D. N., Fiatarone Singh, M. A., Minson, C. T., Nigg, C. R., et al. (2009). American College of Sports Medicine position stand: Exercise and physical activity for older adults. *Medicine and Science in Sports and Exercise, 41*(7), 1510-1530.

Arnold, B. L., Linens, S. W., de la Motte, S. J., & Ross, S. E. (2009). Concentric evertor strength differences and functional ankle instability: A meta-analysis. *Journal of Athletic Training, 44*(6), 653-662.

Centre for Evidence-Based Medicine. (2009). Oxford Centre for Evidence-Based Medicine: Levels of Evidence. Retrieved from http://www.cebm.net/index.aspx?o=1025

Clancy, C. M., & Eisenberg, J. M. (1998). Outcomes research: Measuring the end results of health care. *Science, 282*(9), 245-246.

Ebell, M. H., Siwek, J., Weiss, B. D., Woolf, S. H., Susman, J., Ewigman, B., et al. (2004). Strength of Recommendation Taxonomy (SORT): A patient-centered approach to grading evidence in the medical literature. *American Family Physician, 69*(3), 548-556.

Fetters, L., Figueiredo, E. M., Keane-Miller, D., McSweeney, D. J., & Tsao, C. C. (2004). Critically appraised topics. *Pediatric Physical Therapy: The Official Publication of the Section on Pediatrics of the American Physical Therapy Association, 16*(1), 19-21.

Glover, J., Izzo, D., Odato, K., & Wang, L. (2006). EBM pyramid and EBM generator: Trustees of Dartmouth College and Yale University.

Wolfe, B. L., LeMura, L. M, Cole, P. J. (2004). Quantitative analysis of single- vs. multiple- set programs in resistance training. *Journal of Strength and Conditioning Research, 18*, 35-47.

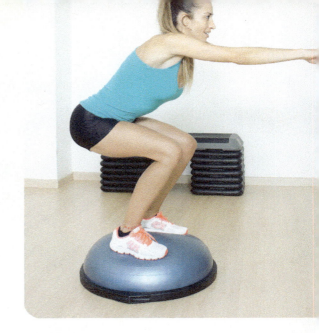

2

Answering a Clinically Relevant Question

Where Have You Been?

In Chapter 1, you learned what role evidence-based practice plays in being a sport and exercise science professional. You also learned that evidence could be divided into five primary levels. These levels represent the varying strength that can be assigned to the available evidence. The levels range from expert opinion and basic research on the lower end to randomized controlled trials and systematic reviews of randomized controlled trials on the upper end. This ranking system should not be used to ignore some evidence or suggest that it is unimportant; rather, it is a method by which you can sort evidence to ensure that you are making decisions based on the strongest evidence available.

You also learned that ranking evidence does not create a complete picture. Other sources of evidence, including clinical appraised topics and critically appraised papers, should also be included as part of your decision-making process. Finally, by using the *Strength of Recommendation Taxonomy*, you can assess groups of studies to determine whether the overall results of several studies provide strong enough evidence to recommend a change in practice.

Where Are You Going?

To find evidence to support your evidence-based practice, a five-step process is recommended. In this chapter, you will learn that process. The first step involves asking a focused clinical question that includes defining the following:

1. The patient of interest
2. The intervention or treatment of interest

3. The comparison among treatments defined as the new treatment versus the standard treatment
4. The clinical result or outcome

Once the question is defined, evidence must be found to address that question by searching electronic databases to locate potentially relevant published research. After that, the articles must be assessed for their validity and relevance to your patient or client.

Once the evidence has been found and assessed, it must be applied to your patient. Not all patients have the same set of goals or values or are at the same developmental or clinical stage. Thus, you will need to consider their priorities, so you can choose an effective treatment plan. You will learn that the cultural context of a patient's life affects the value of potential treatment options. Finally, you will learn that the last step in the process is evaluating yourself as an evidence-based practitioner. If evidence-based practice is to be effective, you must be good at implementing it. That requires self-assessment. In other words, you need to ask yourself how well you are implementing the evidence into your practice and daily workflow.

Learning Outcomes

After reading this chapter you will be able to answer the following questions:

1. What five steps are necessary to be an effective evidence-based practitioner?
2. What are some different types of electronic databases you can use to search for evidence?
3. How can literature searches be made more efficient using Boolean operators, filters, and medical subject headings?
4. How can a question be crafted using the Patients, Intervention, Comparison, Outcome (PICO) format?
5. What factors should be considered in assessing your effectiveness as a professional?

Key Terms

Applicability
Boolean operator
Clinical relevance
Cochrane Library
Comparison
Database of Abstracts of
   Reviews of Effects (DARE)

Intervention
Number needed to harm
   (NNH)
Number needed to treat
   (NNT)
Outcome
Patients

Physiotherapy Evidence
   Database (PEDro)
PubMed
Science Citation Index
Turning Research into Practice
   (TRIP)
Validity

Engaging in evidence-based practice requires a systematic approach to problem-solving. Simply finding evidence to support your question is not evidence-based practice. To engage in true evidence-based practice requires a multistep process, including critically appraising the literature, applying the results, and evaluating the outcomes.

■ THE FIVE-STEP APPROACH

The five-step approach is the most common approach used in evidence-based practice (Straus, Richardson, Glasziou, & Haynes, 2005a). It outlines the systematic process from defining the question through assessing the evidence-based decision. The five-step approach can be summed up as follows:

1. Ask.
2. Acquire.
3. Appraise.
4. Act.
5. Analyze and adjust.

The purpose of this approach is to provide a problem-solving framework for assessing your patient, or population, and identifying where new information is needed to pursue the best quality care through the application of evidence.

1. Asking Focused Questions: Translating Uncertainty to an Answerable Question (Ask)

Finding appropriate evidence to answer a clinical question requires that the question be very specific. To accomplish this, it is best to use a specified format. A common format, PICO, directs you to ask your question by addressing four specific elements: **P**atients, **I**ntervention, **C**omparison, and **O**utcome.

Patients

The first element of a question, **patients**, refers to the person or group you are trying to treat or serve. Keep in mind that for many professions in exercise science, the question of interest may not be clinical. For you to have an effective question, the patient or group should be defined as specifically as possible. For example, if you are working with a patient with a meniscal tear, appropriate treatment may depend on the location of the tear. Thus, identifying the meniscus (i.e., medial or lateral) and the type of tear or tear location (i.e., peripheral or central) are essential for ensuring that your question is focused correctly. Alternatively, if you are developing

Patients: Patients comprise one element of the Patients, Intervention, Comparison, and Outcome (PICO) format that is used to create a specific clinical question before beginning research. The term patients refers to the person or group you are trying to treat or serve in the clinical question.

a strength training program for a client, your question should reflect whether your client is a collegiate athlete, a high school athlete, an adolescent, a baby boomer, and so forth. What may be effective for a baby boomer may not be effective for a collegiate athlete. Thus, the point of defining patients as specifically as possible is twofold. First, you want to make sure you are searching for research that applies as closely to your patient as possible. Second, when you begin searching the literature, it is likely you will find a large volume of articles, most of which will not apply to your question. Focusing your question to a specific group will narrow your literature to a more manageable size.

Intervention

The next element of a good clinical question is defining the intervention. Typically, the intervention represents treatments applied to patients (e.g., compression to reduce extremity swelling) or to clients (e.g., strength training). As with defining subjects, it is important to define the treatment as specifically as possible. For the example of extremity compression to reduce swelling, variations could include compression garments versus pneumatic compression devices. A strength training intervention could refer to training with free weights, weight machines, or manual resistance, and it could include variations of training prescription such as using three sets of 10 versus three sets of eight. As before, the purpose is to narrow your search to evidence that most closely matches your clinical question.

Interventions do not necessarily have to be treatments. Sometimes you may be interested in diagnostic and screening tests. For example, how accurate are skinfold calipers in measuring skinfold thickness to estimate the percentage of body fat in adolescents? In this case, you are not interested in a treatment as an intervention, but you want to know whether a diagnostic test is supported by evidence. Another example could be how accurate the *McMurray's meniscal test* is in detecting a meniscal tear. Thus, intervention does not have to be limited to a treatment. It could be a prognostic factor, an environmental factor, or other disease cause. You should think of it broadly as the thing that is affecting your patient or client. Diagnostic tests are discussed in more detail in Chapter 7.

Comparison

The next level of the clinical question is the comparison. Comparison simply refers to what is being compared in the question. For example, you were told above to be specific in terms of prescription

Intervention: Intervention is one element of the Patients, Intervention, Comparison, and Outcome (PICO) format that is used to create a specific clinical question before beginning to search research literature. Intervention refers to treatments that are applied to patients or clients in the clinical question.

Comparison: Comparison is one element of the Patients, Intervention, Comparison, and Outcome (PICO) format that is used to create a specific clinical question before beginning to search research literature. Comparison refers to what is being compared in the clinical question.

for a strength training intervention. However, you might want to compare higher versus lower-volume strength programs. In this case, you want to be specific in what your intervention is, and to what you are comparing it. Similarly, the McMurray's meniscal test could be compared to the Apley's compression test for diagnostic accuracy.

Comparison in a clinical question is optional. Some items may not have alternatives. When no alternatives exist, it is impossible to define the comparison. However, even when no *explicit* alternative exists there is always an *implied* alternative. The implied alternative is the status quo.

Outcome

Outcome is an aspect of a patient's health or fitness that is expected to change in response to an intervention. The broad range of these measures is discussed in more detail in Chapter 3. Outcomes exist in a variety of forms. On one end of the spectrum are measures such as death rate. It may be important to know whether exercise reduces the death rate from heart disease. Another outcome of interest could be the presence of disease. For example, does exercise reduce the *occurrence* of heart disease? You may also want to know whether regular exercise improves the patient's quality of life. On the other end of the scale, you may be interested in the intervention's effect on pathophysiology (functional changes that accompany a disease); for example, has a specific type of exercise been shown to reduce arterial plaque?

At a glance, each of the foregoing outcomes may strike you as equally relevant, as if you are asking the same fundamental question. After all, arterial plaque leads to heart disease, which interferes with quality of life and potentially leads to death. However, the relevance of each of these outcomes depends on your purpose or your clients. As a clinician, you may be interested in discovering whether exercise will reduce arterial plaque. This is important to you because you know that the accumulation of plaque leads to heart disease, but this probably has little meaning to the client. Instead, the client is more likely to be interested in knowing whether exercise will make him or her feel better, make it easier to be active with family, or simply allow pursuit of a "healthy lifestyle." These are elements of quality of life. Your client will place value on knowing that exercise will extend his or her life span.

Consider how client-centered outcomes have affected the field of orthopedics. Historically, the focus of orthopedic surgery has been on restoration of normal joint mechanics. If normal joint mechanics were reestablished, then the operation was a success. This

Connections 2-1

In experimental terminology, the intervention is given to the treatment group, and the comparison is made with the control (or standard treatment) group. The treatment group and the control group are described as being two different levels of the independent variable. If there are multiple interventions, then there are more than two levels of the independent variable.

Outcome: Outcome is one element of the Patients, Intervention, Comparison, and Outcome (PICO) format that is used to create a specific clinical question before beginning research. Outcome refers to aspects of a patient's health or fitness that are expected to change in response to an intervention in the clinical question.

Connections 2-2

In experimental terminology, the outcome is known as the dependent variable.

reflects an outcome on the pathophysiology end of the spectrum. Until recently, what had been ignored is whether the client felt better after rehabilitating from the surgical procedure. Answering this question necessitates outcome measures such as pain and quality of life. Clients may also be interested in the frequency of needing multiple joint replacements (one joint replacement often leads to a second one later in life) and the amount of time between the first and second joint replacements. The key component to selecting an outcome is your goal or your client's goal for the service being provided. As an exercise science professional, it may be important to you that a treatment or exercise improves strength. However, does that increase in strength correspond with an improvement in the client's function and/or performance? If the client's goal is simply to be stronger, then strength and performance are the same thing. If the client's goal is improved performance or better quality of life, then strength outcomes alone may not be a good choice. In summary, you need to give careful thought to the outcome of interest and make sure that it matches the clinical goal of your client.

2. Finding the Evidence: Systematic Retrieval of Best Evidence Available (Acquire)

After defining your question, the next step is to find literature to answer the question. There are several different types of literature you may use and several different sources. The sources for the literature are the focus here.

To be efficient in retrieving useful information, you will need to become familiar with electronic search engines or databases that aid in finding original articles in primary literature (journals). Several search engines and databases are very useful, and as a strategy, you may want to use more than one. Different databases specialize in different types of literature (e.g., exercise science research versus medicine), but these databases often include overlapping content. Using more than one database maximizes your ability to find relevant research. Eventually, you will discover which databases work best for you and come to rely predominantly on them. However, you must always be aware that finding the best answer may require searching more than one database. The different databases most commonly used in health care and exercise science are described here. However, these are not the only databases available, and you should spend time exploring multiple databases to find those that best suit your needs. The Cochrane Collaboration provides a periodically updated list of common databases (Cochrane Collaboration, 2014). Other databases that you may find useful are also provided by EBSCO Information Services (EBSCO, 2014; Table 2–1).

Electronic Databases

PubMed

PubMed is an electronic database operated by the National Center for Biotechnology Information, which is part of the U.S. National Library of Medicine. Articles are indexed from a broad range of medical and nursing journals, life science journals, and textbooks. The articles indexed range across all levels of the evidence pyramid.

Figure 2–1 is an example of a search for ankle instability. At the top of the figure, you will note that the results produced 2,245 sources for the search term "ankle instability." This total includes all sources across the evidence pyramid, and as such, some may not be particularly helpful. To improve the results, you may want to limit the search to the top of the pyramid by searching for systematic reviews. This is easily done by using the filter in the left-hand column. Under article types, you will see "systematic reviews." Selecting that choice limits the search to 70 sources (Fig. 2–2). Several other limiting options are also available, such as a publication date in the last 5 years. Selecting this limit allows you to be certain that you are looking at the most current reviews.

An alternative method of filtering results for clinical studies is to use the PubMed Clinical Queries feature that can be found under PubMed Tools on the home page. Figure 2–3 is an example of a clinical query. In this format, PubMed divides the search into clinical studies, systematic reviews, and medical genetics. Of these three, the systematic review section should be your primary focus,

PubMed: This database includes MEDLINE as its primary subset. It contains articles indexed from a broad range of medical and nursing journals, life science journals, and textbooks. The database is maintained by the National Center for Biotechnology Information (NCBI), part of the U.S. National Library of Medicine.

Table 2–1 Additional Databases From EBSCO Host	
Database	**Description (EBSCO, 2014)**
CINAHL Plus	Database of nursing and allied health journals that provides full text articles for more than 770 journals
Health Source: Nursing/ Academic Edition	Database of more than 500 scholarly journals focusing on many medical disciplines
SPORTDiscus with full text	Database for sports and sports medicine journals, providing full text for 550 journals indexed in SPORTDiscus

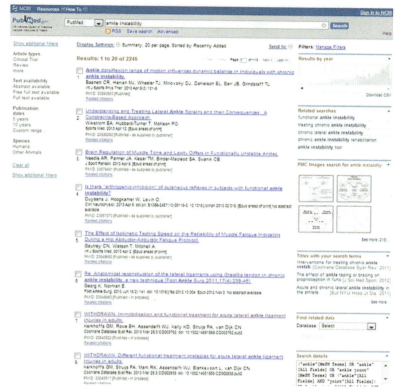

Figure 2–1 An example of a PubMed search for ankle instability. *(From National Library of Medicine.)*

with clinical studies as a second option if nothing relevant exists in the systematic reviews. The clinical studies presented are therapy studies by default. However, the drop-down menu at the top of the column allows you to change the search focus (e.g., to diagnostic trials).

Medical Subject Headings (MeSH) is another useful feature of PubMed. Medical Subject Headings are tags given to articles that allow them to be sorted into content areas. Staff members at the National Library of Medicine review every indexed manuscript, categorize it into subject categories, and tag it with as many medical subject headings as appropriate. You can then use these headings to locate articles related to the subject heading. The headings are useful in finding the best terms to use in your search. For example, the word "strength" brings up articles on bone strength, tissue strength, muscle strength, and so forth. In contrast, using a Medical Subject Headings search brings up all the medical headings associated with strength. As part of that list you will find "muscle strength." Thus, using "muscle

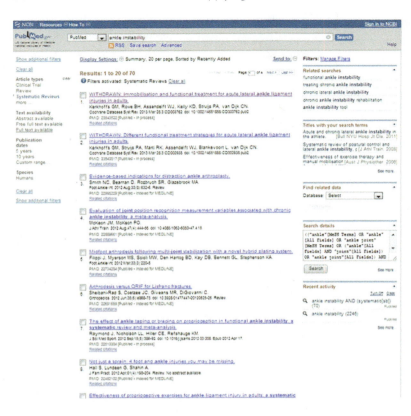

Figure 2–2 The ankle instability search filtered to include only systematic reviews. *(From National Library of Medicine.)*

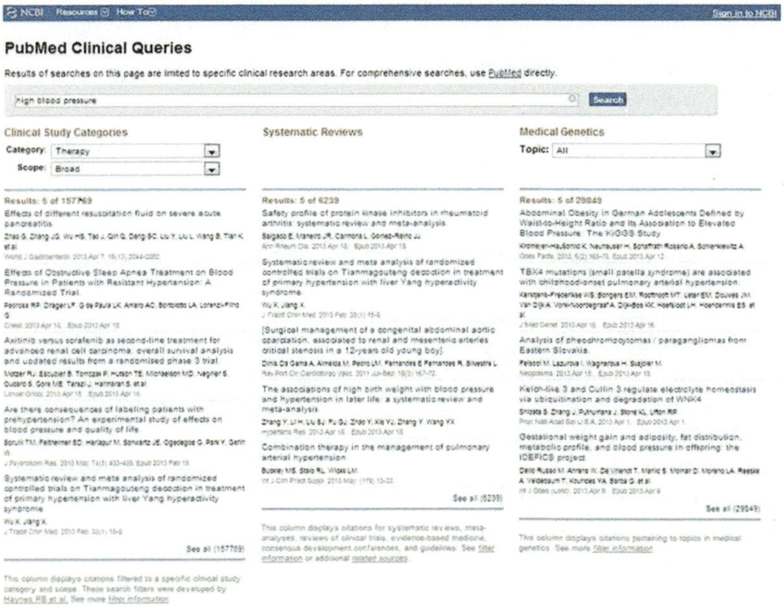

Figure 2–3 An example of a PubMed Clinical Query search. *(From National Library of Medicine.)*

strength" rather than just "strength" will give you sources that are more relevant. A Medical Subject Headings search can be performed by selecting MeSH in the drop-down box to the left of the search box in PubMed.

Cochrane Library

The Cochrane Collaboration is an organization devoted to producing systematic reviews on all topics in clinical medicine. One of the key advantages of Cochrane Reviews is that they are periodically reviewed to determine whether they represent the current state of the art. If new information has become available since the time these reviews were originally published, the reviews are updated and reissued or withdrawn for being out of date. The Cochrane Library collects both systematic reviews produced by the Cochrane Collaboration and clinical trials and other types of relevant research. For the purpose of evidence-based practice, you should focus on the systematic reviews when available. If a systematic review is not available, moving down to the clinical trials listed would be appropriate.

In the Cochrane Library, distinguishing between clinical trials and systematic reviews is easy by using their filter options. Figure 2–4 is an example of a search done on high blood pressure. Looking at the

Cochrane Library: This collection of databases contains Cochrane Reviews, clinical trials, and other types of relevant research. The collection is maintained by the Cochrane Collaboration and is updated regularly.

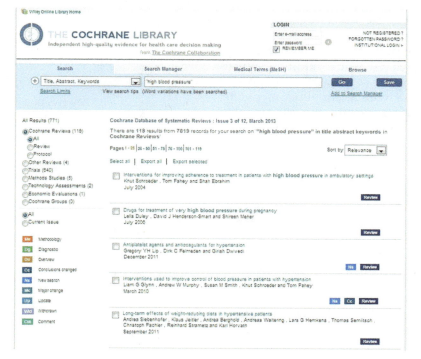

Figure 2–4 Example of a search for high blood pressure using the Cochrane Library. *(From Cochrane Collaboration, with permission.)*

left-hand column, you can see that 771 sources were found. Below that, you see that there were 119 Cochrane Reviews (this is what they call their systematic reviews). You can also see that there were 640 clinical trials (listed as Trials) found with this search. Only the Cochrane Reviews are selected and thus displayed. If you wanted to examine the trials, you would simply select Trials, and those 640 sources would be displayed. As a strategy, you should start with the reviews to determine whether anything useful was available. If not, moving to the clinical trials would be appropriate.

Another useful feature of the Cochrane Library is the color coding of articles. Under each article on the right-hand side is a color-coded tag that identifies the article. In the left-hand column, you can see the key that explains the coding. This coding permits a quick and easy identification of reviews and other important qualities such as whether they have been recently updated or withdrawn.

Turning Research Into Practice (TRIP)

Turning Research Into Practice (TRIP) is a search engine available on the Internet that is similar to others, but with some unique features. This search engine uses a sorting process to identify sources of evidence that rank higher on the evidence pyramid and thus are presented higher on the search page. For example, Cochrane Reviews appear higher in the search because they are classified as systematic reviews, but articles in the journal *Medicine and Science in Sport and Exercise* appear lower on the search page because they are considered original research. In addition, sources whose title includes the terms you are searching for are given a higher rating, as are sources with a more recent publication date. The purpose of this rating system is to organize the results so that stronger, more relevant, and more recent sources are presented near the top of the search results.

An example of a Turning Research into Practice (TRIP) search is shown in Figure 2–5. As with the other databases, a filter function is located on the right side in this search engine. As you can see, it is sorted by levels of evidence. Selecting one of these options will narrow your search to sources in that category (e.g., evidence-based synopses or systematic reviews). The color coding of the filters matches the color coding of the sources (on the left margin), so the type of sources can be quickly identified. Other features include a Patients, Intervention, Comparison, and Outcome search feature that allows you to search based on the elements of the Patients, Intervention, Comparison, and Outcome format. A Rapid Review is also available that allows you to identify the patients and the intervention of interest. These features can expedite your

Turning Research Into Practice (TRIP): Turning Research Into Practice (TRIP) is a search engine that organizes results so that stronger, more relevant, and more recent sources, based on their rank on the evidence pyramid, are presented near the top of the search results.

The Critical Consumer 2-1

Because Cochrane Reviews publishes *only* systematic reviews, you can trust that these articles are indeed systematic reviews. However, other journals also publish systematic reviews, in addition to other types of evidence. For example, *Medicine and Science in Sport and Exercise* publishes predominantly original research but also publishes systematic reviews. Thus, to be an effective user of the literature, you will need to look for relevant evidence in multiple sources.

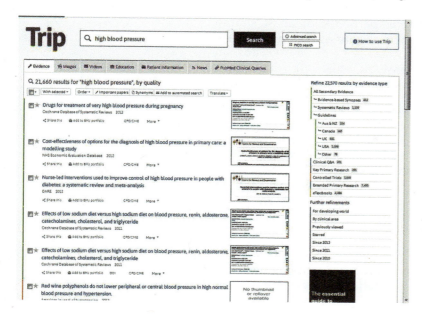

Figure 2–5 Example of a search for high blood pressure using the Turning Research Into Practice (TRIP) database. *(From Tripdatabase.com, with permission.)*

search, but beware that too many filters may limit search results and may unintentionally exclude relevant sources.

Database of Abstracts of Reviews of Effects (DARE)

Another alternative is **Database of Abstracts of Reviews of Effects (DARE)**, originally produced by the Centre for Reviews Dissemination in the United Kingdom (Centre for Reviews and Dissemination, 2013) and now managed by PubMed of the U.S. National Library of Medicine. (The Centre for Reviews and Dissemination is part of the U.K. National Health Service's National Institute of Health Research.) The focus of this database is on cataloging systematic reviews, and it is updated weekly. To be included, the following three criteria must be met (Centre for Reviews and Dissemination, 2013):

1. Were inclusion and exclusion criteria reported?
2. Was the search adequate?
3. Were the included studies synthesized?

Additionally, at least one of the following two criteria must also be met:

1. Was the quality of the included studies assessed?
2. Are sufficient details about the individual included studies presented?

Because these criteria must be met, some level of minimal quality is ensured. This is not to say that all the sources in other

Database of Abstracts of Reviews of Effects (DARE): This database contains abstracts of systematic reviews that have been assessed for quality, by using a specific set of criteria. The database was originally maintained and regularly updated by the Centre for Reviews Dissemination in the United Kingdom and since 2015 has been managed by PubMed of the U.S. National Library of Medicine.

databases are of lower quality. This particular database simply uses a specific set of criteria to help ensure a minimum quality for sources to be included.

Physiotherapy Evidence Database (PEDro)

The **Physiotherapy Evidence Database (PEDro)** is another database that catalogs systematic reviews and clinical trials in the field of physical therapy. It is maintained by the Centre for Evidence-Based Physiotherapy at the George Institute for Global Health at the University of Sydney, Australia. As the name suggests, this is a database focused on rehabilitation and can be searched as with the previous databases. It is most useful if you are in one of the physical rehabilitation fields.

Science Citation Index

One unique database that can be helpful in identifying literature that is more current is the **Science Citation Index**. The databases previously described are retrospective databases (i.e., they look backward in time). For example, you can see from Figure 2–1 that the references listed start in 2013. If you progressed through the search, you would see that the dates run backward to earlier years. This is because the search starts from the current point in time and looks backward.

A Science Citation Index search works differently. Instead of looking for a topic, (e.g., ankle instability), you look for a known article or author. For example, maybe you know that the author Arnold has completed a systematic review on ankle strength. Figure 2–6 shows a two-step search looking for meta-analysis (a type of systematic review; see Chapter 9) and for the author Arnold. From the results, you can see that the author has published three meta-analyses. On the last line of each item, you can see how many times it was cited. Each item has been cited zero, 10, and 18 times, respectively. This is the number of other journal articles that cited each of the meta-analyses. The number of times an item has been cited partially depends on the item's age. The first item, Michener et al., was published in 2012, whereas the last item, Arnold et al., was published in 2009. The number of citations for each item is also a link to those other journal articles that cited the meta-analysis. Selecting the "18" of the third item launches a new search that includes the 18 articles that cited that meta-analysis. The first seven of these articles are shown in Figure 2–7. Note that the articles in the new search were published after 2009 (i.e., 2012). This is what is meant by a "forward" search. The search looked forward in time from an article's publication date, in this case 2009 for the meta-analysis, and found only articles published since 2009.

Physiotherapy Evidence Database (PEDro): This database catalogs systematic reviews and clinical trials in the field of physical therapy and are focused on rehabilitation. It is maintained by the Centre for Evidence-Based Physiotherapy at the George Institute for Global Health at the University of Sydney, Australia.

Science Citation Index: This database of articles allows a researcher to identify which later articles cite any particular earlier article, or the articles of any particular author, or which articles are cited most frequently.

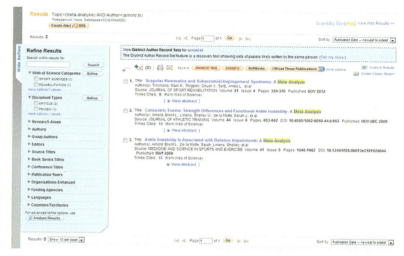

Figure 2–6 Example of a search using the Science Citation Index. *(From Science Citation Index, with permission.)*

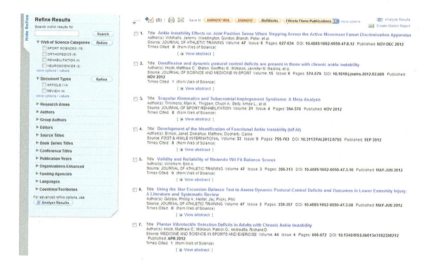

Figure 2–7 Example of a forward search's results using the initial search in Figure 2–6. *(From Science Citation Index, with permission.)*

This type of search can be very useful in keeping up to date. Assume you found a systematic review or clinical trial that you have based your practice on, but now that item is 5 years old. It may be time to try to find evidence that is more current. The forward search can be a quick way of finding newer material that was based on the first article you used. Keep in mind that a forward search looks only for items that cited the original work. Other sources may also exist that were not cited by the first article. Thus, you should not solely rely on the forward search to update your original article.

Search Strategies

Now that you know where to search, knowing some strategies for finding material is necessary. A variety of search strategies can be employed, but the two most common are subject and author searches.

Subject Searches

Subject searches, the most common search type, focus on searching for a specific word or set of words. All the previous examples were subject searches. This type of search typically produces the most results, but it can also generate too many results if the subject is too general. Subject searches often have to be narrowed by conducting Boolean searches (described later). Unfortunately, narrowing a search risks eliminating items that may be useful.

One of the important elements in generating a successful search is understanding that several different words may be used to describe the idea or concept of interest. When trying to search for a concept, you need to think about what words would be used to describe it. For example, "muscular strength" may be a useful search term. However, other terms such as "maximal voluntary contraction" or "10-repetition maximum" may also be used to convey the concept of muscular strength. Thus, you need to think about which words the author may have used to describe muscular strength.

Balance is another concept that can be of interest to clinicians helping a client rehabilitate the lower extremity. However, postural sway and time to stabilization are also words used to convey the concept of balance. For an efficient search, it is often useful to retrieve a few initial articles and identify the terms used to describe your topic.

Author Searches

Another search method is to use an author's name rather than a subject. Author searches are useful when you know that an author has written something in which you are interested, especially if that person is considered an expert in that area. These searches can also be useful in tracking updates or additional research conducted by an author.

Refining Searches

It is also possible to combine or exclude search terms to improve results. To combine search terms, special **Boolean operators** are used. The two most commonly used commands are AND and OR. These two operators have opposite effects. The AND operator requires that all search terms be present to produce a result. For

Boolean operator: A connecting symbol or word, such as AND or OR, that allows a computer user to include or exclude items from a text search.

example, Figure 2–8 is a three-step search. The first step searched for "ankle" and produced 3,742 results. The second step searched for "instability" and produced 2,397 results. Step 3 used AND to combine the first and second searches. At first, you could think that this would increase the result because you are adding the two searches. However, when search terms are combined with AND, both terms must be present for an item to be found in the search. In this case, the third search produced only 207 results because those were the only items that contained both the term "ankle" and the term "instability."

The operator OR has the effect of combining the searches so that any item that contains either "ankle" or "instability" is included in the results. Figure 2–9 shows the same search as before, except in the third step OR has been used. This combination produced 5,932 results. All the results contain at least the words "ankle" or "instability," and, as we know from the previous search, exactly 207 of these results contain both words. You will note that the final result (5,932) is not the sum of the first two steps (i.e., 3,742 + 2,397 = 6,139). This is because the combination of step 1 and step 2 included duplicates, and those duplicates are eliminated in step 3.

The final common operator is NOT. NOT is used to exclude a specific search term. In the previous AND search, the ankle instability article results included items for both chronic and acute ankle sprains. However, maybe you are interested only in acute injuries. To eliminate the chronic ankle instability items, NOT "chronic" could be added as a fourth step.

The Critical Consumer 2-2
Boolean searches are a convenient way to manage your search strategy. However, it is impossible always to predict the results when combining Boolean operators. Thus, every time terms are combined in a Boolean search, check the result to confirm that you are obtaining the desired effect. Many times, you think you will be improving your strategy but in fact may be harming it.

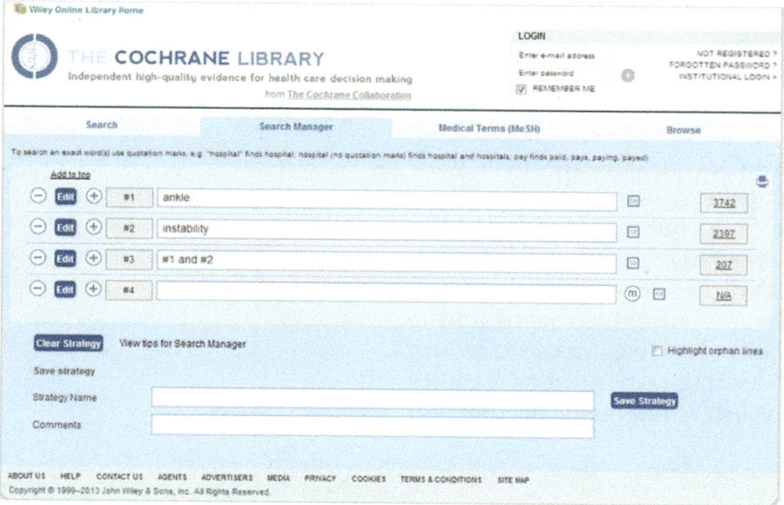

Figure 2–8 Example of a Boolean AND search. *(From Cochrane Library, with permission.)*

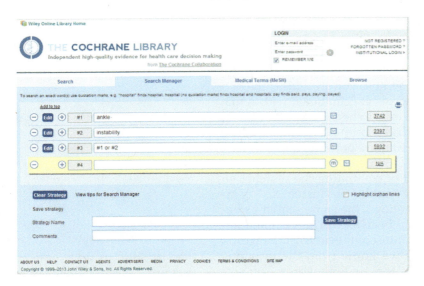

Figure 2–9 Example of a Boolean OR search. *(From Cochrane Library, with permission.)*

3. Critical Appraisal: Testing Evidence for Validity, Clinical Relevance, and Applicability (Appraise)

The next step in the process is appraising the evidence that you have found. Not everything that you find in an electronic search is relevant. Thus, the next step is eliminating or ignoring sources that are unrelated or not applicable to your topic. Every search identifies articles that are off topic because it is impossible for you to anticipate every way your search words will be used. If multiple irrelevant items of the same topic appear frequently in your search, then using the NOT operator may help you eliminate these items and narrow your search.

Assessing Validity

Once you have identified articles that potentially meet your needs and your client's needs, the next step is to assess the article for validity. **Validity** is a complex topic, but in general, validity refers to a study's ability to establish what it intended to establish (validity is addressed in more detail in subsequent chapters). For treatment studies, validity is very straightforward and is known as the cause-and-effect relationship (e.g., does ice reduce swelling?). For other studies, such as diagnostic studies, validity refers to the study's ability to establish a diagnostic accuracy in detecting disease.

Validity: The degree to which data or results of a study are correct or true; a measure of a study's ability to establish what it intended to establish.

Regardless of the type of study, validity must be established before moving to the next step. If the study is not valid, then the results have little value. In that case, proceeding further is a waste of effort because the results cannot be expected to be attainable in the clinical setting or with your clients.

Assessing Clinical Relevance

Assuming you have determined that the evidence you have found is valid, your next step is to determine whether it is clinically relevant. Clinical relevance means that the results apply to your typical circumstances. In other words, do the results apply to:

> Your clients?
> Your setting?
> Your available treatments?
> Qualities that matter to your client or clients (e.g., pain, quality of life, playing basketball)?

Not all articles you find on a given topic will be relevant to you and your clients. Thus, you need to spend some time carefully considering who the subjects of the study were and what type of experiment was conducted. If it was a laboratory experiment, the results may be interesting and demonstrate promise for the future. However, if the subjects were not part of a real clinical population, or were not studied under real clinical conditions, then the results may not carry over to your circumstances. For example, assume you are interested in the latest form of balance training to prevent falls. In looking for evidence, you find a laboratory study using simple one-legged standing as the treatment, and the results showed significant improvement in balance. However, the research was conducted with university-age, physically active participants. The question that you must address is whether these research subjects are substantially similar to the clients you are treating. If you are a therapist working with clients in assisted living facilities, then this study is probably not relevant to your practice, and you should keep looking. Another question that you should ask is whether the results will matter to your client. Does improved balance really matter to your client? If improved balance directly translates to fewer falls and injury, then it probably does matter to your client. However, if there is no evidence that it does reduce falls, except theoretically, then it may have questionable value to your client. Ideally, your goal should be to find evidence that most closely matches your circumstances. Otherwise, implementation of the evidence may not produce the desired result for your clients.

Clinical relevance: How well results from clinical evidence apply to your typical circumstances, such as your clients, setting, and available treatments.

Connections 2-3

As you will see later, validity may refer to four types of validity: internal validity, external validity, construct validity, and measurement validity. Validity as described previously refers to the internal validity and construct validity of the study. Clinical relevance refers to external validity. Measurement reliability refers to the reliability of the outcomes measured.

Assessing Applicability

Because of the varied clinically relevant evidence, you must next address its applicability. Applicability is the relevance of the results, not to your typical population of clients, but to the specific client you are treating. Whereas clinical relevance applies to groups of clients, applicability applies to the single client. Each client has his or her own unique medical history, and that history may alter or negate treatment results for the individual person. For example, assume you want to know whether knee braces prevent knee injury. You have located a clinical research study that followed recreational athletes across time. Some of those study subjects were required to wear knee braces, whereas the others were not. The results showed that knee braces reduced the risk of knee ligament injury in recreational athletes with an existing knee injury, but not in those with no history of injury. Based on this information, you now know that, as a group, recreational athletes with a history of knee injury benefit from wearing braces. However, your client has a cartilage injury, not a ligament injury. Thus, this study is clinically relevant in that it establishes that braces prevent further ligament injuries, but it is not applicable because your client has a cartilage injury.

Applicability: Applicability refers to how relevant the clinical evidence is to the specific client you are treating.

> **Retention Questions 2-2**
> 1. How do validity and clinical relevance differ?
> 2. How do clinical relevance and applicability differ?
> 3. Of validity, clinical relevance, and applicability, which must come first and why?

4. Making a Decision: Application of Results in Practice (Act)

The final step in the process is to act on what you have learned. At first, this may seem simple. However, other factors can intervene. For example, the client may have priorities that affect the use of a treatment. A client may prioritize quality of life over a long life. Other factors could include whether the research included meaningful outcomes, whether the treatment frequently or occasionally produced a meaningful result, or whether the treatment had a risk of producing harm. You will see that all these factors may alter the decision you make with your client or clients.

Client Values and Priorities

Just finding and evaluating the scientific evidence, albeit a critical step, is not evidence-based practice. Once you have established the scientific facts and determined that the known science is applicable to your client, the question arises whether it should be applied to your client. In deciding to apply a therapy or diagnostic test, factors other than science should be considered. Chief among these are the concerns and priorities of the client and the client's family. For example, pancreatic cancer is an especially difficult cancer to treat because it is often diagnosed too late for curative care. Rather, it is often likely that treatments such as chemotherapy will, at most, extend life from a few months to a year. However, chemotherapy has considerable side effects that can significantly degrade a client's quality of life. Therefore, the client and family, because of their value system, may decide that an aggressive course of chemotherapy is too arduous.

In the exercise and rehabilitation sciences, these types of concerns arise when treatments are especially complex or time consuming. For example, fitness programs that require an hour or two of effort several days per week may simply not fit into individual priorities. Family obligations, career concerns, and other competing factors affect the appropriateness of a treatment.

Different cultures place different values on different entities, and thus, culture must be considered in the clinical context. Cultural impact is demonstrated in American football. Evidence has accumulated showing that significant brain injury can result from football. This includes injuries that occur at a level that is challenging to detect with standard neurological examinations. Based on this, there is clear evidence that could be used to argue for the elimination of football. However, considering how embedded football is in U.S. culture, it is not likely to be eliminated. Thus, alternative strategies such as better education, better equipment, and better injury detection methods will be the likely culturally acceptable solution.

Family history also plays a role in clinical decision-making. As we know, high cholesterol is a risk factor for heart disease. We also know that high cholesterol can be the result of genetic factors. Thus, a client with high cholesterol and a family history of high cholesterol who is otherwise healthy with a healthy lifestyle may not be a strong candidate for cholesterol-lowering drugs. Alternatively, a family history of high cholesterol and high blood pressure may indicate that a more aggressive approach to treatment is needed.

Finally, you and your client may want to consider disease trajectory. Disease trajectory refers to the disease's progression, whether the disease condition is improving or worsening, and the rapidity of that change. For example, advanced-stage knee arthritis will most likely require joint replacement. In an overweight client with severe osteoarthritis, discussing weight reduction as a solution is probably inappropriate because the benefits are not likely to reduce the osteoarthritis. (Keep in mind that a person with severe osteoarthritis is not likely to be able to exercise because of pain.) Conversely, an overweight person with mild osteoarthritis may benefit greatly from weight reduction. Weight reduction would reduce the load on the joint, and the load reduction would slow the trajectory of the disease.

Were Clinically Meaningful Outcomes Studied?

Not all outcomes that are measured as part of research are clinically relevant. For example, assume you are interested in the benefit of a new fitness program to your client, and you found a valid research study that demonstrates that the fitness program improves lactate threshold. Is this information valuable to your client? The answer depends on the goal of the client. If the client hopes to run a marathon, then the answer would be yes. However, if the goal is improved strength development, then the wrong outcome was assessed. Similarly, if your client were interested in fitness for a better quality of life, then a quality of life measure would have been more appropriate. This does not mean that lactate threshold is a poor outcome for the research that was done, just that it was simply not the best measure for your and your client's needs.

One of the challenges you will face as you search the literature is finding research that is very close to meeting your need but falls short in the outcome measure. The researchers' goals may have been very different, and, as such, they did not measure what you needed them to measure. The research may not be clinically relevant to you, but it may be relevant to others with different goals. The ideal solution is for the research to be repeated with outcomes that are relevant to you and your client.

Proxy measures, or outcomes, are alternative ways to finding research that is clinically relevant to your question. Proxy measures are substitutes for the outcome of interest. For example, lactate threshold may be a useful measure to show physiological change, especially as it relates to fitness. In other words, people with higher lactate thresholds tend to be fitter. As such, lactate threshold may be used as a proxy measure for fitness. In addition, if evidence shows that quality of life is related to fitness, then lactate threshold could be a proxy for quality of life. To attain the quality of life outcome, two steps were needed: (1) lactate threshold is a proxy for fitness; and (2) fitness is a proxy for quality of life. It is important to understand that taking these steps is not equivalent to directly assessing the fitness program's impact on quality of life. Furthermore, the more steps there are in the proxy variable chain, the less certain you can be about the connection between intervention and outcome.

Number Needed to Treat

Another factor to be considered in clinical applicability is a measure known as **number needed to treat (NNT)**. A fuller description is provided in Chapter 6, but basically, it is the number of persons who would have to be treated before a single person

Number needed to treat (NNT): The number of people needed to be treated so that one person experiences a benefit.

benefited. Ideally, the number needed to treat would equal 1 (for every treatment there is a benefit); however, that is rare. For example, previous research has shown that for patients with a previous ankle sprain, ankle bracing can prevent additional sprains, but 26 patients would have to be braced to prevent one ankle sprain (Olmsted, Vela, Denegar, & Hertel, 2004). Furthermore, in uninjured persons, 143 would have to be braced to prevent one ankle sprain. Based on this, it is probably not reasonable to expect an uninjured person to benefit greatly from bracing the ankle. This is especially true when considering the cost and effort needed to apply the brace consistently. Considering these additional factors, it may not be worthwhile even for injured persons. The main point is that even when an intervention (ankle bracing) produces a desired outcome (fewer ankle sprains), this outcome may not be substantial enough in the context of cost and effort of the treatment. The number needed to treat should be considered when discussing a treatment option with a client.

Number Needed to Harm

Number needed to harm (NNH) is opposite to number needed to treat, and it refers to the number of people needed to be treated to produce one harm. If the number needed to harm equals one, it means that every person treated is harmed. A number needed to harm of 100 would mean that for 100 people treated, one harm was produced. This does not mean that the one client received no benefit. That person may have received a benefit and a harm. It is also important to understand that harm does not have a uniform definition. Harm could mean any side effect such as death, limb loss, or an upset stomach. Almost anything adverse could be defined as a harm, but the term usually refers to something with a large impact on your patient or client. Number needed to harm and number needed to treat can be used together to assess the value of a treatment. If the number needed to harm and the number needed to treat are equal, then the value of the treatment is questionable. For example, if a treatment designed to reduce heart attacks requires five people to be treated to prevent one heart attack, and for every five people treated the treatment causes one death, then the value of the treatment is questionable. Keep in mind that this needs to be considered in the context of the disease and the disease trajectory. If the current state of disease or its trajectory suggests that death is imminent, then a treatment with a higher number needed to harm may be justified. It is also possible that the harm may be less harmful than the possible benefit is beneficial. For example, assume the benefit is

Number needed to harm (NNH): The number of people needed to be treated so that one person experiences an adverse effect, or harm.

prolonged life and the harm is severe nausea (e.g., in the case of cancer chemotherapy). In this case, even if the number needed to harm equals or is greater than the number needed to treat, the degree of the benefit outweighs the harm. Generally, the number needed to harm should be higher than the number needed to treat. When this is the case, on balance, the treatment favors a benefit rather than a harm. Balancing benefit and harm can be complex and should include the client and consider the client's values.

Dealing With Inadequate Science

One of your greatest challenges will be finding evidence for every clinical decision you need to make. You will most likely have more clinical questions than the evidence can answer, so you will have to make do with the best evidence available. Sometimes that will mean relying on the lower levels of evidence. It also means that sometimes all you will have is your own clinical judgment. The lack of evidence does not indicate that you should not treat. Rather, the point of evidence-based practice is to base as much of your treatment as possible on the highest levels of available evidence, use scientifically supported rather than hypothetical treatments, and be watchful for new evidence that suggests that a change in treatment strategy is appropriate.

5. Evaluating Performance: Auditing Evidence-Based Decisions (Analyze and Adjust)

The final step in the process is auditing the decision you have made. When auditing yourself and the decisions you have made, at least two broad levels of assessment should be considered. First is an assessment of your progress. Second is an assessment of the client's progress as an indicator of effectiveness.

Self-Assessment

Self-assessment refers to the effectiveness of your ability to use the evidence-based process. Straus et al. (Straus, Richardson, Glasziou, & Haynes, 2005b) suggest five areas critical to clinical practice that should be assessed. The first four of these directly relate to the first four steps of evidence-based practice.

The first area is asking answerable questions. More specifically, are you answering questions at all? If you are asking questions, are they following the Patients, Intervention, Comparison, and Outcome format? When presented with a clinical problem, you may not be able to answer the question immediately. Thus, you should develop a strategy for writing down and storing the question, so that you can address it at a more appropriate time.

The second area is an assessment of your searches for evidence. The first question to assess is this: Are you doing searches? Do you have access to electronic databases that will allow you to search for evidence? If you do have access to electronic databases you should assess whether your searching is becoming more efficient (i.e., are you finding results and finding them more quickly?). If you have access to reference librarians, it is worth comparing your strategy with theirs. Often they can help you refine your search strategies for a more effective search.

The third area Straus et al. suggest is assessing your critical appraisal of the literature (Straus, Richardson, Glasziou, & Haynes, 2005b). Similar to the foregoing, your first question is this: Are you appraising the literature? Of the evidence you have collected, you should be assessing the evidence for validity (see Chapter 5). You should also determine whether you are getting better at using the clinical measures noted in each of the studies you locate (e.g., number needed to treat, likelihood ratios; see Chapter 7). Finally, are you writing summaries of the evidence that you can refer to later?

The fourth area you should evaluate is your inclusion of evidence into your clinical practice. Are you using evidence in your treatment of clients? If so, are you able to adjust clinical measures such as number needed to treat to meet your client's needs? Also, you should be able to justify for decisions based on the evidence to colleagues and clients, especially when discrepancies in the evidence exist.

Finally, you should assess whether your clinical practice is improving. One of the key components to assess is barriers to your implementation of changes. One barrier could be new skills. It may be that the evidence suggests a new type of exercise device or therapeutic modality for which you have no training. Thus, you may need both training and acquisition of equipment to carry out the new treatment plan. You should also consider carrying out client assessment of new treatment strategies. Implementing new strategies without assessing their effectiveness is basically guessing at whether the strategy worked, and it results in a significant waste of time and resources.

Client Assessment

Assessing a client's progress is one of the best tools to determine the effectiveness of your evidence-based practice. Other methods are also available (e.g., assessment at the hospital level); however, for the typical clinician, the client sitting in front of you is your best tool for assessment. At the client level, the best method of assessment is by using an n-of-one research design or single-subject research design (see Chapter 5). The n in the name simply refers to the number of subjects in the research. Most studies use several subjects in the research and may range up to thousands. This is not feasible for the typical clinician. However, the single-subject design permits very effective assessment of a client's progress. Chapter 5 provides a further description of this method.

Experimenting on clients without following appropriate approval procedures is unethical, and to use experimental procedures with clients is not being advocated. What is being advocated is the use of research techniques such as the n-of-one design to monitor the progress of your client on a recognized treatment program. To do so will provide the most objective assessment of your treatment plan's value for your client.

Finally, in considering your approach to assessing your client's progress you should consider measures other than the typical physiological measures. As discussed previously, measures such as blood pressure and strength are often of value to you, but they may have limited meaning to the client. Other more practical measures that the client can assess and value should also be included. These may include measures of pain, mobility, or even happiness.

SUMMARY

Evidence-based practice is a five-step process that includes defining a question, finding evidence, appraising the evidence, making a decision, and evaluating performance. Effective practitioners use all five of these steps while keeping in mind that evidence may not be available for every clinical question. Practitioners must be mindful that evidence is constantly being added and changed. Thus, the effective practitioner is in continuous pursuit of updated information on which to base decisions.

CRITICAL THINKING QUESTIONS

1. How does using a Boolean search strategy improve the efficiency of your search?
2. What would be the benefit of using a filter as part of your search strategy, and would you apply the filter before or after a Boolean search?

3. After performing a literature search for the best treatment for patellar tendonitis (or some other condition of interest), you find studies examining interventions in collegiate age recreational athletes. However, your client is a 50-year-old U.S. Marine officer. Does the treatment of these athletes apply to your client?

4. You have a client who has recently been complaining of not being able to keep up with his grandchildren. His physician has determined that there is no medical reason for this and has approved him for a fitness program. As his personal trainer, you look for research on fitness programs directed at older populations. You find a research study that fits your client. However, the outcomes measured were muscular strength and maximal oxygen consumption (i.e., VO_{2max}). Do these outcomes apply to your client's stated need? How would you apply these data to your client?

■ TRUST AND APPLY

Lepley, L. K., & Palmieri-Smith, R. M. (2013). Effect of eccentric strengthening after anterior cruciate ligament reconstruction on quadriceps strength. *Journal of Sport Rehabilitation, 22*(2), 150-156.

Locate the foregoing article, and using this article, address the following questions.

1. Identify the clinical question appraised by the authors.

2. Was the Patients, Intervention, Comparison, and Outcome format used? If yes, identify each of the components.

3. What were the characteristics of the defined clients? Were these characteristics specific or general? Were they too specific or general?

4. What comparison was defined? Was this comparison appropriate? What comparison would you have selected?

5. How was the outcome defined? Was this outcome appropriate for the goal?

■ RESEARCH SCAVENGER HUNT

1. State a clinical question in the Patients, Intervention, Comparison, and Outcome format.
2. Using PubMed, conduct a search for a topic of interest.
3. Use the AND function to narrow the search.
4. Use the filters to narrow the search to clinical trials.

5. Using your chosen clinical trial, apply your clinical question to the clinical trial.

   A. Did all elements of the Patients, Intervention, Comparison, and Outcome format fit?

   B. Were elements missing?

   C. Was the clinical trial both clinically relevant and applicable to a patient or client?

6. Using the Turning Research Into Practice (TRIP) database, repeat your search.

   A. Did you obtain the same result?

   B. Did you find better articles?

REFERENCES

Cochrane Collaboration. (2014). Databases offering online access to medical evidence. (Online). Available: from http://www.cochrane.org/about-us/evidence-based-health-care/webliography/databases

EBSCO. (2014). Medical databases. (Online). Available: http://www.ebscohost.com/academic/subjects/category/medical-databases

Olmsted, L. C., Vela, L. I., Denegar, C. R., & Hertel, J. (2004). Prophylactic ankle taping and bracing: A numbers-needed-to-treat and cost-benefit analysis. *Journal of Athletic Training, 39*(1), 95-100.

PubMed Health. Centre for Reviews and Dissemination. (2013). Database of Abstracts of Reviews of Effects (DARE). (Online). Available: http://www.crd.york.ac.uk/crdweb/AboutDare.asp

Straus, S. E., Richardson, W. S., Glasziou, P., & Haynes, R. B. (2005a). Asking answerable clinical questions. In *Evidence-based medicine* (3rd ed., pp. 13-30). Edinburgh: Elsevier.

Straus, S. E., Richardson, W. S., Glasziou, P., & Haynes, R. B. (2005b). Evaluation. In *Evidence-based medicine* (3rd ed., pp. 247-261). Edinburgh: Elsevier.

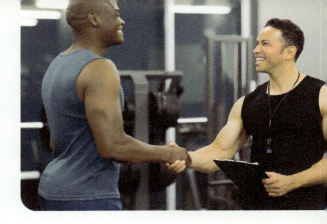

3

Outcome Measures in Health and Exercise Science

Where Have You Been?

In the previous chapter, you learned that the first step in evidence-based practice is to ask a meaningful question. You also learned to ask this question in a format that identifies the patient of interest, the intervention of interest, the treatments compared, and the target outcome. Once you had framed your question, the next step was to identify and assess articles to determine whether they could answer your question, including assessing these articles for validity, relevance, and applicability to your patients or clients.

You also learned that people have different sets of goals or values. These may differ widely from your values and goals as a professional. The goals and values may also differ among the clients you serve. When asking questions and determining the needs of your clients, these factors have to be considered. Thus, you learned that the patient's priorities are important for an effective intervention. You learned that the cultural context of a person's life affects the value of potential treatment options. Finally, you have been encouraged to consider the disease's stage and trajectory when framing a question, if it applies.

Where Are You Going?

Now that you can frame the question, much of what is left relates to the research process. You will learn how research is conducted and how evidence is sorted. This knowledge is essential to understand if the answer to your question is to have meaning. Measurement and research are both multifaceted, and subsequent chapters explore the topics in more depth.

This chapter focuses on the measurement of health and performance outcomes. Health is a complex idea, and models of disablement were developed to address this complexity. These models help the practitioner and the patient or client think about what is important to the patient's health. Several models exist, each with advantages and disadvantages. The models imply that the different facets of health can be measured but that no single measure can capture all aspects of health. You will then learn that a variety of outcomes should be used simultaneously to capture as many health dimensions as possible. Included are measures that capture information important to both the patient (or client) and the practitioner and that consider the patient's or client's values. It will become apparent that research that uses measures focused on a single facet of health provides an incomplete picture of a treatment's value.

In contrast, performance-related outcomes are less structured. They can be across all the domains of exercise and sport science, and they are specific to the individual goals of the client. Because these outcomes are less structured, there is increased burden on practitioners to make sure that the outcomes examined are applicable to their clients. We will discover that norms exist for many of these outcomes so that a proper evaluation can be made.

Learning Outcomes

After reading this chapter, you will be able to answer the following questions:

1. What are the common disablement models?
2. What is the difference between disease-oriented evidence and patient-oriented evidence that matters?
3. What is the difference between clinician-based and patient-based outcomes?
4. What are the different types of patient-based outcomes?
5. What are the domains of physical fitness that are often tested?

Key Terms

Administration burden
Administration time
Clinician-based outcomes
Dimension-specific outcomes
Disablement continuum

Disablement models
Disease-specific outcomes
Disease-oriented outcomes
Generic outcomes
Global rating of change
Patient-based outcome

Patient-oriented evidence that matters (POEM)
Readability
Region-specific outcomes
Summary scales

In Chapter 2, you learned about the Patients, Intervention, Comparison, Outcome (PICO) model for asking clinical questions. One part of that model is the outcome, which is the *dependent measure* in experimental terminology. The challenge with outcomes is that they come in a variety of forms. For clinical research, outcomes represent one or more aspects of the disablement continuum. The disablement continuum is the range of factors that contribute to or detract from health and normal function of the individual. A disablement continuum is represented by a disablement model. Disablement models are structured representations or frameworks of the disablement continuum that identify the components of disablement and the interactions among them.

Fitness- and sport-related outcomes, conversely, are less structured in the literature. They usually involve one or more physiological or biomechanical traits. This chapter focuses on outcomes typically used to measure range of outcomes in clinical or exercise populations.

Disablement continuum: The range of factors that contribute to or detract from health and normal function of the individual.

Disablement models: Structured representations or frameworks of the disablement continuum that identify the components of disablement and the interactions among them.

◼ DISABLEMENT CONTINUUM

Saad Nagi proposed the original disablement model in 1965 (Nagi, 1965). The purpose of this model was to better characterize disease across a continuum of dysfunction, rather than limit it to a description of the disease process. Being interested in exercise science and/or sports medicine, you will recognize that an injury affects multiple aspects of life. It is not limited to the injury itself, but also includes how the injury can affect performance of tasks in our daily life such as doing laundry, shopping, and yard work (Fig. 3–1).

World Health Organization Model

A more current disablement model, produced by the World Health Organization, is known as the International Classification of Functioning, Disability, and Health (World Health Organization, 2002). This model is a two-part model rather than a continuum (Fig. 3–2). The first part of the model focuses on the four levels of the Nagi model, but with different names. *Pathophysiology, impairment, functional limitations,* and *disability* of the Nagi model become *health condition, body functions and structure, activity,* and *participation* in the International Classification of Functioning, Disability, and Health, respectively. The second part of the International Classification of Functioning, Disability, and Health model focuses on personal and environmental aspects of disablement. It recognizes that individual personal experiences also affect a person's level of disablement. The advantage of this model is that it structurally separates those factors

Connections 3-1
Models play a fundamental role in science because they provide the basis of experimentation. The best experiments are based on models, and the goal of experiments is to support or fail to support the components of the model. In the case of experiments involving treatments (e.g., strength training or rehabilitation in general), using one of the disablement models as a guide increases the validity of the experiment and establishes (or refutes) the value of the treatment.

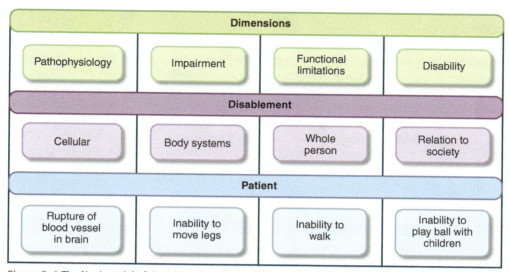

Figure 3–1 The Nagi model of disability. *(From Snyder, A. R., Parsons, J. T., Valovich McLeod, T. C., Bay, R. C., Michener, L. A., & Sauers, E. L. [2008]. Using disablement models and clinical outcomes assessment to enable evidence-based athletic training practice, part I: Disablement models.* Journal of Athletic Training, 43[3], 428-436.)

that the practitioner can influence from those that the individual person and the environment influence. However, that does not mean that the clinician cannot or should not try to influence aspects of the model's second part. Appendix C contains an expanded discussion of disablement.

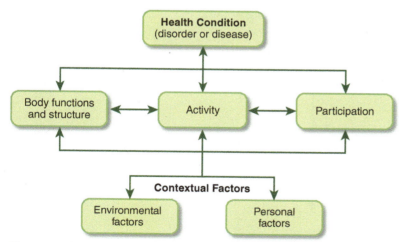

Figure 3–2 The World Health Organization model of disability. *(From World Health Organization. [2002]. Towards a common language for functioning, disability, and health: ICF the International Classification Of Functioning, Disability, and Health. Geneva: World Health Organization.)*

Pros and Cons 3-1

Disablement models are valuable in helping us focus on multiple levels of a person's disability in clinical settings. However, they should be reviewed critically. Not all the dimensions of each model may apply to your setting. For example, a physical therapist or athletic trainer may not have a great deal of control over the environmental limitations placed on their patients. However, a personal trainer or fitness club manager may have a great deal of control in selecting equipment that would meet the access needs of disabled clients. Thus, not all dimensions of a given model may apply to your circumstances. You will need to be judicious in selecting the best model and then fitting its dimensions to your setting.

◼ TYPES OF MEASURES OR OUTCOMES

Measures used in evidence-based practice can be divided into four broad types: disease oriented, patient oriented, clinician based, and patient based (McLeod et al., 2008). These types of measures overlap to some degree, and Figure 3–3 shows the relationship among the four types.

Disease-Oriented Evidence

A disease-oriented outcome is defined as a measure that focuses on the qualities or aspects of the disease. These measures may be of great interest to the clinician but often have little intuitive meaning to the patient (Snyder et al., 2008). This type of evidence is collected by the clinician and helps with the understanding of the

Retention Questions 3-1

1. Assessing the function of tissue (e.g., a ligament's laxity) would belong to which dimension?
2. Assessing someone's ability to participate on a basketball team would belong to which dimension?
3. Assessing someone's ability to walk on a treadmill without chest pain or shortness of breath would belong to which dimension?
4. Assessing someone's ability to walk around the block would belong to which dimension?

Disease-oriented outcome: Measures that assess qualities that are related to a disease, such as blood pressure and bone density.

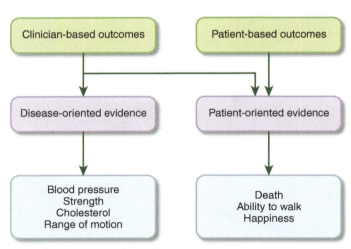

Figure 3–3 The relationship of clinician-based and patient-based outcomes with disease-oriented and patient-oriented evidence.

current state of the disease. Typical disease-oriented evidence would include x-ray studies for an orthopedic examination. Blood pressure is another example of disease-oriented evidence. Other examples would include muscle strength, joint range of motion, and swelling.

Based on the examples given previously, it should be obvious that disease-related evidence is mostly focused on the health condition, body function, and activity dimensions of the International Classification of Functioning, Disability, and Health model. For example, an x-ray study assesses the status of the bone (i.e., tissue) for normalcy. Blood pressure and strength assess the function of the cardiovascular and neuromuscular systems, respectively. By their nature, these measures tend to be more objective and/or quantifiable with numbers.

Patient-Oriented Evidence that Matters

A patient-oriented measure is defined as measure that directly assesses the patient's health status (Snyder et al., 2008). Sometimes these measures are called **patient-oriented evidence that matters (POEM)**. Measures that fall into this category include risk of dying, quality of life, loss of function, life span, and so forth. One of the challenges with this category of outcome is that it is somewhat subjective. For example, blood sugar levels are not particularly relevant to a normal, healthy person. However, to the diabetic patient, they are critically important. Blood sugar levels relate to the diabetic patient's mortality, as well as to quality of life. Thus, they are important to the diabetic patient across multiple levels of the disablement continuum.

Blood sugar levels are an interesting exception to a general rule about POEM measure. Blood sugar levels relate directly to the health condition and body function components of the International Classification of Functioning, Disability, and Health model. This is atypical. Most POEM measures relate to the upper levels of the continuum (i.e., activity and participation). Most patients and clients are more concerned about being able to perform than about the components that make it possible. In other words, they want to be able to complete meaningful tasks and participate in normal life activities. Because of this, POEM measures tend to be patient-based outcomes, as described in more detail later.

Clinician-Based Outcomes Measures

Clinician-based outcomes are defined as measures that are collected by the clinician (McLeod et al., 2008), such as range of motion or strength. As you can see from Figure 3–3, clinician-based measures may include disease-oriented and patient-oriented

Connections 3-2
Clinician-based evidence and disease-oriented outcomes are the typical forms of evidence collected as part of experiments because this type of outcome is considered more valid and reliable. However, as is shown, clinician-based measures often provide little information that is of intuitive value to the patient.

Patient-oriented evidence that matters (POEM): Measures that directly assess the patient's health status, including risk of dying, quality of life, loss of function, life span, etc.

Clinician-based outcomes: Measures that are collected by a clinician; data and information that cannot be provided by the patient without the involvement of the clinician.

measures. These measures may occur across the disablement continuum, but what is implied is that the information cannot be provided by the patient without the involvement of the clinician. Therefore, these measures typically include measures of health condition, body function, and activity. In the areas of rehabilitation and exercise science, this is usually further restricted to measures of body function and activity because of the expertise of the practitioners.

As you may have guessed, clinician-based outcomes are typically diseased-oriented measures. This is because a clinician often needs to understand the progression of a disease or injury to prescribe treatment. For example, an athletic trainer may assess cognition as part of a concussion assessment. To do so would inform the athletic trainer of the progression of the concussion and aid in the decision of returning the athlete to competition. Similarly, an exercise physiologist may perform a cardiac stress test on a patient to determine heart function in preparation for more strenuous exercise.

Clinician-based outcomes may include measures of body function and activity. For example, following an ankle sprain the clinician would be interested in ankle strength, a measure of musculoskeletal function. In later stages of ankle rehabilitation, the clinician may be interested in how well a patient can bear weight, hop, run, and climb stairs. These factors would be representative of the patient's activity. In the case of cardiac rehabilitation, the clinician may want to know the patient's maximal oxygen consumption as a measure of body function or the patient's ability to walk for extended distances as a measure of activity.

As suggested earlier, which clinician-based measures are measured and collected may depend on the phase of a patient's recovery. In the early stages of rehabilitation, the clinician is likely to focus on measures of health condition and body function (e.g., strength, swelling, and range of motion). This is expected because the earlier phases are focused on restoring normal tissue and body system physiology. As the patient progresses through rehabilitation, the focus often changes to restoring the patient's activity, such as normal gait, the ability to throw a ball, or the ability to climb a ladder. Thus, it is normal for the measures important to the clinician to change as the patient makes progress during rehabilitation.

To summarize, clinician-based outcomes are those measures that the clinician measures. As such, they tend to be measures that focus on the needs of the clinician. They also tend to be associated with health condition, body function, activity, and occasionally participation. Participation is typically not included because participation usually relates to the patient's perspective of how he or she is functioning and as such requires the patient's input. To achieve this input, patient-based outcomes are needed.

Patient-Based Outcomes Measures

Patient-based outcomes are defined as those measures that patients complete for themselves. This type of measure tends to comprise pencil-and-paper measures such as surveys or questionnaires (McLeod et al., 2008). It is also true that patient-based measures tend to be patient oriented. Patient-based outcomes fall into six broad categories (disease specific, region specific, dimension specific, generic, global rating of change, and summary scales), which are defined next.

Patient-based outcomes: Measures that the patients complete for themselves. This type of measure tends to be surveys or questionnaires.

Disease-Specific Outcomes

As the name suggests, **disease-specific outcomes** measure patients' function in relation to a specific disease (Fitzpatrick, Davey, Buxton, & Jones, 1998). One such measure is the Knee Injury and Osteoarthritis Outcome Score (KOOS) (Fig. 3–4). This 42-item questionnaire assesses knee symptoms, pain, stiffness, and functional activities (Roos, Roos, Lohmander, Ekdahl, & Beynnon, 1998). It is

Disease-specific outcomes: Measures of patient function in relation to a specific disease.

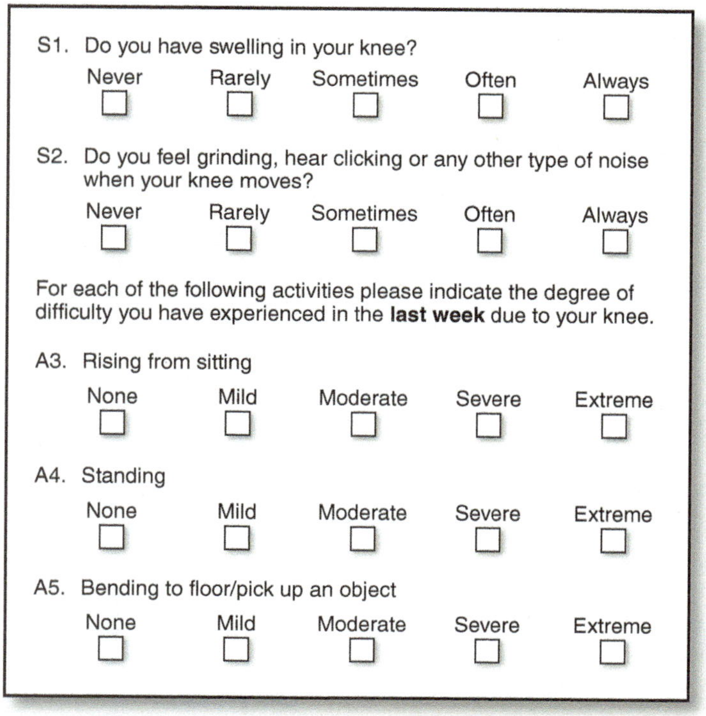

S1. Do you have swelling in your knee?

Never ☐ Rarely ☐ Sometimes ☐ Often ☐ Always ☐

S2. Do you feel grinding, hear clicking or any other type of noise when your knee moves?

Never ☐ Rarely ☐ Sometimes ☐ Often ☐ Always ☐

For each of the following activities please indicate the degree of difficulty you have experienced in the **last week** due to your knee.

A3. Rising from sitting

None ☐ Mild ☐ Moderate ☐ Severe ☐ Extreme ☐

A4. Standing

None ☐ Mild ☐ Moderate ☐ Severe ☐ Extreme ☐

A5. Bending to floor/pick up an object

None ☐ Mild ☐ Moderate ☐ Severe ☐ Extreme ☐

Figure 3–4 The Knee Injury and Osteoarthritis Outcome Score. *(From Roos, E. M., Roos, H. P., Lohmander, L. S., Ekdahl, C., & Beynnon, B. D. [1998]. Knee Injury and Osteoarthritis Outcome Score [KOOS]: Development of a self-administered outcome measure.* Journal of Orthopaedic and Sports Physical Therapy, *28[2], 88-96.)*

classified as disease specific because it focuses on one joint. A more obvious example of a disease-specific outcome is the Arthritis Impact Measurement Scale (AIMS) (Fig. 3–5). This is a 58-item questionnaire that addresses function in patients with arthritis (Meenan, Mason, Anderson, Guccione, & Kazis, 1992). In this case, the Arthritis Impact Measurement Scale is not joint specific and can be used with arthritis that is either localized to a joint or present across all or part of the body.

When using disease-specific outcomes, the focus of the measure must be considered. As in the foregoing examples, you should decide whether you want information on the specific joint or more systemically across the body. Thus, the selection of the outcome measure should match the model dimensions that are important to you and your patients. It is also the case that scores on one measure (e.g., the Knee Injury and Osteoarthritis Outcome Score), cannot be compared with similar measures for different diseases. If multiple diseases are to be assessed, then separate measures are needed for each disease.

Region-Specific Outcomes

As the name suggests, region-specific outcomes are limited to a specific area of the body (Fitzpatrick et al., 1998). Common

Region-specific outcomes: Measures that are limited to a specific area of the body.

During the past month...	All Days (1)	Most Days (2)	Some Days (3)	Few Days (4)	No Days (5)
6. Did you have trouble doing vigorous activities such as running, lifting heavy objects, or participating in strenuous sports?	____	____	____	____	____
7. Did you have trouble either walking several blocks or climbing a few flights of stairs?	____	____	____	____	____
8. Did you have trouble bending, lifting or stooping?	____	____	____	____	____
9. Did you have trouble either walking one block or climbing one flight of stairs?	____	____	____	____	____
10. Where you unable to walk unless assisted by another person or by a cane, crutches, or walker?	____	____	____	____	____

Figure 3–5 The Arthritis Impact Measurement Scale. *(From Meenan, R. F., Mason, J. H., Anderson, J. J., Guccione, A. A., & Kazis, L. E. [1992]. AIMS2: The content and properties of a revised and expanded Arthritis Impact Measurement Scales Health Status Questionnaire. Arthritis and Rheumatism, 35[1], 1-10.)*

examples include the Foot and Ankle Ability Measure (FAAM) (Fig. 3–6), the Disabilities of the Arm, Shoulder, and Hand Scoring System (DASH) (Fig. 3–7), and the Oswestry Low Back Pain Disability Questionnaire (Fairbank, Couper, Davies, & O'Brien, 1980; Hudak, Amadio, Bombardier, & Upper Extremity Collaborative Group, 1996; Martin, Irrgang, Burdett, Conti, & Van Swearingen, 2005). As you can see from the names, the regions can be narrow, as in the Foot and Ankle Ability Measure, or include large regions such as the upper extremity as assessed by the Disabilities of the Arm, Shoulder, and Hand Scoring System (see Fig. 3–6). Region-specific measures are useful for documenting dysfunction across large areas of the body. However, the broader the region covered, the less detail the measure will give you on specific body parts. For example, the Lower Extremity Function Scale (Fig. 3–8) is useful for documenting dysfunction in the entire lower quarter (Binkley, Stratford, Lott,

	Not at all	Slightly	Moderately	Quite a bit	Extremely
22. During the past week, *to what extent* has your arm, shoulder or hand problem interfered with your normal social activities with family, friends, neighbors or groups? *(circle number)*	1	2	3	4	5

	Not limited at all	Slightly limited	Moderately limited	Very limited	Unable
23. During the past week, were you limited in your work or other regular daily activities as a result of your arm, shoulder or hand problem? *(circle number)*	1	2	3	4	5

Please rate the severity of the following symptoms in the last week. *(circle number)*

	None	Mild	Moderate	Severe	Extreme
24. Arm, shoulder or hand pain.	1	2	3	4	5
25. Arm, shoulder or hand pain when you performed any specific activity.	1	2	3	4	5
26. Tingling (pins and needles) in your arm, shoulder or hand.	1	2	3	4	5
27. Weakness in your arm, shoulder or hand.	1	2	3	4	5
28. Stiffness in your arm, shoulder or hand.	1	2	3	4	5

Figure 3–6 Foot and Ankle Ability Measure (FAAM). *(From Martin, R. L., Irrgang, J. J., Burdett, R. G., Conti, S. F., & Van Swearingen, J. M. [2005]. Evidence of validity for the Foot and Ankle Ability Measure [FAAM]. Foot and Ankle International, 26[11], 968-983.)*

Section 1 – Pain intensity

☐ I have no pain at the moment

☐ The pain is very mild at the moment

☐ The pain is moderate at the moment

☐ The pain is fairly severe at the moment

☐ The pain is the worst imaginable at the moment

Section 3 – Lifting

☐ I can lift heavy weights without extra pain

☐ I can lift heavy weights but it gives extra pain

☐ Pain prevents me from lifting heavy weights off the floor, but I can manage if they are conveniently placed eg. on a table

☐ Pain prevents me from lifting heavy weights, but I can manage light to medium weights if they are conveniently positioned

☐ I can lift light weights

☐ I cannot lift or carry anything at all

Figure 3–7 The Disabilities of the Arm, Shoulder, and Hand Scoring System. *(From Hudak, P., Amadio, P. C., Bombardier, C., & Upper Extremity Collaborative Group. [1996]. Development of an Upper Extremity Outcome Measure: The DASH [Disabilities of the Arm, Shoulder, and Hand]. American Journal of Industrial Medicine, 29, 602-608.)*

& Riddle, 1999). However, if you were interested in foot and ankle function, the Foot and Ankle Ability Measure would be a better choice. As with disease-specific outcomes, region-specific scores cannot be compared across regions. In other words, Foot and Ankle Ability Measure scores are not comparable to Disabilities of the Arm, Shoulder, and Hand Scoring System scores, and multiple regions would need to be assessed with different outcomes.

Dimension-Specific Outcomes

The **dimension-specific outcomes** are outcomes that assess "one specific aspect of health status" (Fitzpatrick et al., 1998). One such aspect could be a symptom. Measures of pain fit into this group, and the most common of these is the McGill Pain Questionnaire (Melzack, 1975). It assesses pain across three dimensions: quality (e.g., pulsing, throbbing, pounding), time (e.g., continuous versus rhythmic), and strength (e.g., mild versus excruciating; Fig. 3–9). Another dimension-specific outcome could include cognition, which is often used to assess concussion. Nausea, appetite, social

Dimension-specific outcomes: Outcomes that assess one specific aspect of health status.

Activities (circle one number on each line)	Extreme Difficulty or Unable to Perform Activity	Quite a Bit of Difficulty	Moderate Difficulty	A Little Bit of Difficulty	No Difficulty
a. Any of your usual work, housework, or school activities.	0	1	2	3	4
b. Your usual hobbies, recreational or Sporting activities.	0	1	2	3	4
c. Getting into or out of the bath.	0	1	2	3	4
d. Walking between rooms.	0	1	2	3	4
e. Putting on your shoes or socks.	0	1	2	3	4
f. Squatting.	0	1	2	3	4
g. Lifting an object, like a bag of groceries from the floor.	0	1	2	3	4
h. Performing light activities around your home.	0	1	2	3	4
i. Performing heavy activities around your home.	0	1	2	3	4
j. Getting into or out of a car.	0	1	2	3	4
k. Walking 2 blocks.	0	1	2	3	4
l. Walking a mile.	0	1	2	3	4
m. Going up or down 10 stairs (about 1 flight of stairs).	0	1	2	3	4
n. Standing for 1 hour.	0	1	2	3	4
o. Sitting for 1 hour.	0	1	2	3	4
p. Running on even ground.	0	1	2	3	4
q. Running on uneven ground.	0	1	2	3	4
r. Making sharp turns while running fast.	0	1	2	3	4
s. Hopping.	0	1	2	3	4
t. Rolling over in bed.	0	1	2	3	4
Column Totals:					

Figure 3–8 The Lower Extremity Function Scale. *(From Binkley, J. M., Stratford, P. W., Lott, S. A., & Riddle, D. L. [1999]. The Lower Extremity Functional Scale [LEFS]: Scale development, measurement properties, and clinical application.* North American Orthopaedic Rehabilitation Research Network. Physical Therapy, 79[4], 371-383.)

contact, and fatigue, are other examples of facets measured by dimension-specific scales.

Although they are useful, dimension-specific scales often do not distinguish among different potential sources for the health feature being measured. For example, the McGill Pain Questionnaire does not ask the patient to locate or focus on a specific source of pain (e.g., at the knee). Although the measure is typically used to address pain from a particular location, it may be possible for the patient to sum the pain across the entire body. Thus, the final score may represent a bodily pain score rather

3 (punctate pressure)	pricking	1
	boring	2
	drilling	3
	stabbing	4
	lancinating	5
4 (incisive pressure)	sharp	1
	cutting	2
	lacerating	3

Question	Response	Points
Which word describes your pain right now?	mild	1
	discomforting	2
	distressing	3
	horrible	4
	excruciating	5

Figure 3–9 Selections from the McGill Pain Questionnaire. *(From Melzack, R. [1975]. The McGill Pain Questionnaire: Major properties and scoring methods. Pain, 1[2], 277-299.)*

than joint-specific pain. You should consider this possibility when evaluating the patient's responses.

Generic Outcomes

As indicated in discussing the previous measures, among the disadvantages are that region-specific measures do not apply to multiple regions, dimension-specific measures can measure only one dimension, and disease-specific measures cannot be used to compare different diseases. One solution to this limitation is to use generic outcomes. Generic outcomes are measures that assess a "very broad range of aspects of health status" (Fitzpatrick et al., 1998). One of the most common generic measures is the Short Form 36 (SF-36). This measure is a 36-item questionnaire that measures eight dimensions of general health: physical functioning, social functioning, role limitations from physical problems, role limitations from emotional problems, mental health, vitality, pain, and general health perceptions (Ware et al., 2007). These eight dimensions are then combined into two summary scores for physical health and mental health.

One of the clear advantages of the Short Form 36 is that different diseases and conditions can be compared. Because the different dimensions are referenced across many populations (e.g., young, old, kidney disease, arthritis), it is possible to compare among them. For example, it is possible to assess the general health of an individual patient with knee arthritis and compare it with other

Generic outcomes: Measures that assess a very broad range of aspects of health status.

diseases. Thus, it is possible to determine whether knee arthritis is as disabling as cancer. It is also possible to compare a patient with arthritis with the normal healthy population and determine how much the arthritis has affected the patient relative to the normal population.

Although infrequently used, generic measures are increasing in popularity. This is likely because generic measures may be the most appropriate of the patient-based outcomes for exercise science. These types of measures have potential for assessing the benefit of physical activity programs on general health. For example, resistance training in older adults has been shown to improve not only strength but also cognitive function and general health (as measured by the Short Form 36) (Cassilhas et al., 2007). As with therapeutic treatments, documenting exercise's impact on quality of life greatly enhances the value of the exercise and extends the understanding of the value of exercise to the upper levels of the disability continuum.

The main disadvantage of generic measures is that they do not provide details specific to the disease that may be affecting quality of life. These measures also capture quality of life relative to all the diseases or conditions present in the individual patient. In other words, if a patient has multiple conditions (e.g., knee arthritis and low back pain), it is not possible to associate any specific condition with the quality of life level.

Global Rating of Change

Another measure that may be used to assess a patient's progress is the **global rating of change (GRC)**. The global rating of change is a measure that asks the patient whether he or she is better, is about the same, or is worse across some period of time (e.g., from the last visit). Global ratings of change are used when you are interested in assessing changes across time. For example, does a cardiac rehabilitation patient's stamina improve across time? Thus, the clinician may assess the patient weekly to determine progress of the patient and the effectiveness of the treatment. One version of the global rating of change (Fig. 3–10) is a simple 15-point scale with "a great deal worse" scored as –7 and "a great deal better" scored as 7, with "about the same" scored as 0 (Jaeschke, Singer, & Guyatt, 1989). An alternative global rating of change is known as the Global Quality of Life Scale (Hyland & Sodergren, 1996). This is a 100-point scale divided into 5-point increments ranging from "perfect quality of life" (100) to "rather be dead" (0), with several other qualifiers (e.g., "good quality of life" and "very bad quality of life") listed at points in between.

As with the Short Form 36, global ratings of change have potential use in assessing the effectiveness of physical activity

The Critical Consumer 3-1

Questionnaire measures such as the Short Form 36 are often perceived as less rigorous than laboratory measures. They are also perceived as providing less valuable information because they seek the patient's or client's opinion. In fact, because these measures are often measuring psychological dimensions that can be assessed only indirectly, the process of establishing their rigor is as demanding as that of measures commonly used in the laboratory.

Global rating of change: Measures that ask patients whether they are better, are about the same, or are worse across some period of time.

Please rate the overall condition of your injured body part or region *FROM THE TIME THAT YOU BEGAN TREATMENT UNTIL NOW* (Check only one)

A very great deal better	7.00
A great deal better	6.00
Quite a bit better	5.00
Moderately better	4.00
Somewhat better	3.00
A little bit better	2.00
A tiny bit better	1.00
About the same	0.00
A tiny bit worse	-1.00
A little bit worse	-2.00
Somewhat worse	-3.00
Moderately worse	-4.00
Quite a bit worse	-5.00
A great deal worse	-6.00
A very great deal worse	-7.00

Figure 3–10 An example of a global rating of change. *(From Jaeschke, R., Singer, J., & Guyatt, G. H. [1989]. Measurement of health status: Ascertaining the minimal clinically important difference.* Controlled Clinical Trials, 10[4], 407-415.)

programs. These measures are especially useful in determining whether a fitness program is having an effect on overall health. Whereas traditional measures of fitness have focused on body function and activity, use of a global rating of change expands the assessment to the participation level.

The key advantage of these scales is that the client or patient gives a single measure. All the previous outcomes require combining multiple items into a single value. This means the client or patient must answer multiple items, and the clinician must combine the items into a summary value. Sometimes this is simply adding up points, but depending on the outcome, more complicated formulas are required. For global ratings of change, clients provide one response to their overall quality of life, and that value is the indicator of their health.

Compared with generic outcomes, global ratings of change are even more limited in the amount of detail that they can provide. Because a single measure is made, the root causes of poor quality of life cannot be determined. Thus, to understand why a client rates his or her health as poor, other questions or outcomes measures are required. In other words, all the diseases or conditions present in the individual patient contribute to the global rating.

Pros and Cons 3-2

The global rating of change is a valuable measure for assessing patients from one time to the next. It can give you a quick snapshot of whether your patient is progressing or regressing. However, as with generic measures, the reason for the change cannot be captured by the global rating of change, and thus, other measures may be necessary. It is also the case that the global rating of change must be used to compare two time points (e.g., one clinic visit to the next). If this is your patient's or client's first visit, then you can begin using the global rating of change on the second or some subsequent visit.

Summary Scales

The final type of patient-oriented measures is summary scales. **Summary scales** consist of one or two questions about general health or disability that assess a person's overall health. The General Household Survey (Haynes, 1991) is a questionnaire used in the United Kingdom to assess multiple aspects of a household, including health. Because this is a survey of all British households, similar to a census, brevity becomes necessary to allow the collection of a broad spectrum of data. Thus, only two health questions are asked: (1) "Do you have a long-standing illness or disability?" and (2) "Does this illness or disability limit your activities in any way?" As you can see, these questions are very broad and give no information about the type of disability or its severity. However, these types of questions can be efficient in identifying disabilities within a large population.

Properties of Patient-Based Outcomes

When considering which patient-oriented measure to use, several things must be considered. Obviously, the patient's needs are important. Is the outcome going to measure something relevant to the patient's view of his or her health? In addition, you should consider which level of the disability continuum you are trying to measure. The measurement properties of the questionnaire should also be considered. Measurement properties related to all outcomes are presented in Chapter 4.

When using a questionnaire, three other issues should be considered (Table 3–1) (Eechaute, Vaes, VanAerschot, Asman, & Duquet, 2007). The first is **readability**, referring to the reading level of the questionnaire or the ease with which it is understood. Different questionnaires can be written at different reading levels. If they are written at too high a level, your patient may not understand the question. If they are written at too low a level, the questions may not be sophisticated enough to capture the information you want. In this case, the reading level needs to be adjusted for the population. If you are working with children, different questions with lower reading levels are needed. Therefore, some outcome measures may not be appropriate for your client group.

The second property is **administration time**. Administration time refers to the time it takes the client or patient to complete the questionnaire. Patients or clients tend to become bored if a questionnaire is too long. They then tend to be less attentive when answering questions because they become tired. This situation decreases the accuracy of their responses. This problem can also arise when you ask someone to answer multiple questionnaires.

Summary scales: One or two questions about general health or disability that assess the overall health of an individual.

Retention Questions 3-2

1. Which type of outcome would you use if you were interested in assessing spine function?
2. Which type of outcome would you use if you were interested in assessing quality of life?
3. Which type of outcome would you use if you were interested in assessing progress during cardiac rehabilitation?

Readability: The reading level of a questionnaire, or the ease with which it is understood.

Administration time: The time it takes the client or patient to complete a questionnaire.

Table 3–1 **Properties of Questionnaires**	
Property	**Definition and Consideration**
Readability	The reading level of the questionnaire. Is it appropriate for your patient group?
Administration time	The time it takes for the patient or client to complete the questionnaire. Is the length of the questionnaire so long that the patient or client will lose interest?
Administration burden	The time it takes you to score the questionnaire. Is the scoring so complicated that you are unlikely to score it?

From Eechaute, C., Vaes, P., VanAerschot, L., Asman, S., & Duquet, W. (2007). The clinimetric qualities of patient-assessed instruments for measuring chronic ankle instability: A systematic review. *BMC Musculoskeletal Disorders, 8:6.*

Even if the questionnaires are short, the total number of questionnaires completed can greatly increase the administration time and affect the accuracy of all the questionnaires.

The final property to consider is **administration burden**. Administration burden refers to the time, complexity, work force needed, and cost of scoring a questionnaire (Lohr et al., 1996). A questionnaire with multiple questions must be scored to derive a measure of the outcome. Some of these scoring systems can be elaborate and require computer assistance, and others require simply adding up the total number of affirmative answers. Most questionnaires fall somewhere in between. For example, the Foot and Ankle Ability Measure is scored by summing the items' values (Martin et al., 2005). Each item has a value range of 0 to 4, with 4 equal to "no difficulty" and 0 equal to "cannot do." These values are then summed, and the percentage score is calculated. This is a straightforward scoring system. However, it does take time. The more time it takes a questionnaire to be scored, the less likely it is to be consistently used.

Administration burden: The time, complexity, work force needed, and cost required to score a questionnaire.

Performance-Based Assessments

In nonclinical populations, assessments tend to focus on a physiological or biomechanical trait that can be improved by training. These traits have been broadly categorized into health-based and skill-based aspects of fitness (Hoeger and Hoeger, 2013). You could even consider these aspects as "dimension specific," focusing on one aspect of health or skill. The health-related aspects include *cardiovascular endurance, muscular strength and local muscular endurance, flexibility,* and *body composition.* The skill-based aspects include *agility, balance, coordination, power, reaction time,* and *speed.*

Although a discussion of all the potential tests that could be used for evaluating these traits is beyond the scope of this book, practitioners should be aware that these measures are somewhat "dimension specific," as well as "region specific." For instance, someone who scores well on a test of upper body local muscular endurance may not also do well on a test of lower body local muscular endurance. The level in specificity of training will determine how well the test can assess the particular trait that is the focus of the exercise program.

Although these health- and skill-related categories are helpful to sort different traits, several shortcomings should be addressed. For instance, the trait of anaerobic capacity (commonly assessed with the Wingate test) is not included in either category. Anaerobic capacity is important for intermittent sports such as ice hockey. Another problem is that muscular strength and muscular endurance are not a single trait, but rather two traits that are somewhat overlapping. Yet another shortcoming is that some of the categories and traits overlap. Power can be considered a composite of both speed of movement and strength. Agility tests may also include an aspect of speed.

SUMMARY

Measuring patients' progress requires consideration of many factors. The first is what is to be measured. One way to address this is by following one of the disability models and to determine which or how many of the levels of disability you want to consider. Once you have established the levels of disability you will measure, the next step is to identify the measures. The measures you select will depend on your interests, and some decisions need to be made about whether disease-specific, region-specific, or other types of measures are to be included. In any case, you should consider including patient-based measures in addition to your standard clinician-based measures. For performance-based outcomes, consider the specific adaptations the client is seeking, in addition to the region specificity.

CRITICAL THINKING QUESTIONS

1. Of the disablement models presented, which of the models best fits your purposes as a clinician and why?

2. Which dimensions of the disablement model would be most useful for you in improving your patient's or client's health and why?

3. Given the choice between disease-*oriented* and patient-*oriented* evidence, which would best capture the dimensions of health condition, body function, activity, and participation? Explain your answers.

4. Given the choice between clinician-*based* and patient-*based* evidence, which would best capture the dimensions of health condition, body function, activity, and participation? Explain your answers.

5. Which category of performance-based outcomes best fits the population with which you work?

◼ TRUST AND APPLY

Silva, F., Ribeiro, F., & Oliveira, J. (2012). Effect of an accelerated ACL rehabilitation protocol on knee proprioception and muscle strength after anterior cruciate ligament reconstruction. *Archives of Exercise in Health and Disease*, 3(1/2), 139-144.

Using the foregoing article, answer the following questions:
1. Were the outcomes used patient-based or clinician-based?

2. If clinician-based outcomes were assessed, were they patient oriented? Explain why or why not.

3. Using the International Classification of Function, identify which levels of the model were included in the research.

4. Based on the foregoing answers, does this research adequately address whether this treatment benefits the patient?

◼ RESEARCH SCAVENGER HUNT

1. Using the original World Health Organization model:
   A. Find an article that assesses health condition.
   B. Find an article that assesses body function.
   C. Find an article that assesses activity.
   D. Find an article that assesses participation.
2. Identify all the measures that belong in each of the foregoing categories.
3. Is each of the measures disease oriented or patient oriented?
4. Is each of the measures clinician based or patient based?
5. How many of the articles include more than two dimensions of the National Center for Medical Rehabilitation Research model?

◼ REFERENCES

Binkley, J. M., Stratford, P. W., Lott, S. A., & Riddle, D. L. (1999). The Lower Extremity Functional Scale (LEFS): Scale development, measurement properties, and clinical application. North American Orthopaedic Rehabilitation Research Network. *Physical Therapy, 79*(4), 371-383.

Cassilhas, R. C., Viana, V. A., Grassmann, V., Santos, R. T., Santos, R. F., Tufik, S., & Mello, M. T. (2007). The impact of resistance exercise on the cognitive function of the elderly. *Medicine and Science in Sports and Exercise, 39*(8), 1401-1407.

Eechaute, C., Vaes, P., VanAerschot, L., Asman, S., & Duquet, W. (2007). The clinimetric qualities of patient-assessed instruments for measuring chronic ankle instability: A systematic review. *BMC Musculoskeletal Disorders, 8:6.*

Fairbank, J. C., Couper, J., Davies, J. B., & O'Brien, J. P. (1980). The Oswestry low back pain disability questionnaire. *Physiotherapy, 66*(8), 271-273.

Fitzpatrick, R., Davey, C., Buxton, M. J., & Jones, D. R. (1998). Evaluating patient-based outcome measures for use in clinical trials. *Health Technology Assessment, 2*(14), i-iv, 1-74.

Haynes, R. (1991). Inequalities in health and health service use: Evidence from the General Household Survey. *Social Science and Medicine, 33*(4), 361-368

Hoeger, W.W.K., & Hoeger, S.A. (2013) *Fitness and wellness* (10th ed.). Independence, KY: Cengage Learning.

Hudak, P., Amadio, P. C., Bombardier, C., & Upper Extremity Collaborative Group. (1996). Development of an upper extremity outcome measure: The DASH (Disabilities of the Arm, Shoulder, and Hand). *American Journal of Industrial Medicine, 29,* 602-608.

Hyland, M. E., & Sodergren, S. C. (1996). Development of a new type of global quality of life scale, and comparison of performance and preference for 12 global scales. *Quality of Life Research, 5*(5), 469-480.

Jaeschke, R., Singer, J., & Guyatt, G. H. (1989). Measurement of health status: Ascertaining the minimal clinically important difference. *Controlled Clinical Trials, 10*(4), 407-415.

Lohr, K. N., Aaronson, N. K., Alonso, J., Burnam, M. A., Patrick, D. L., Perrin, E. B., & Roberts, J. S. (1996). Evaluating quality-of-life and health status instruments: Development of scientific review criteria. *Clinical Therapeutics, 18*(5), 979-992.

Martin, R. L., Irrgang, J. J., Burdett, R. G., Conti, S. F., & Van Swearingen, J. M. (2005). Evidence of validity for the Foot and Ankle Ability Measure (FAAM). *Foot and Ankle International, 26*(11), 968-983.

McLeod, T. C. V., Snyder, A. R., Parsons, J. T., Bay, R. C., Michener, L. A., & Sauers, E. L. (2008). Using disablement models and clinical outcomes assessment to enable evidence-based athletic training practice, part II: Clinical outcomes assessment. *Journal of Athletic Training, 43*(4), 437-445.

Meenan, R. F., Mason, J. H., Anderson, J. J., Guccione, A. A., & Kazis, L. E. (1992). AIMS2: The content and properties of a revised and expanded Arthritis Impact Measurement Scales Health Status Questionnaire. *Arthritis and Rheumatism, 35*(1), 1-10.

Melzack, R. (1975). The McGill Pain Questionnaire: Major properties and scoring methods. *Pain, 1*(2), 277-299.

Nagi, S. (1965). Some conceptual issues in disability and rehabilitation. In M. Sussman (Ed.), *Sociology and rehabilitation* (pp. 100-113). Washington, DC: American Sociological Association.

Roos, E. M., Roos, H. P., Lohmander, L. S., Ekdahl, C., & Beynnon, B. D. (1998). Knee Injury and Osteoarthritis Outcome Score (KOOS): Development of a self-administered outcome measure. *Journal of Orthopaedic and Sports Physical Therapy, 28*(2), 88-96.

Snyder, A. R., Parsons, J. T., Valovich McLeod, T. C., Bay, R. C., Michener, L. A., & Sauers, E. L. (2008). Using disablement models and clinical outcomes assessment to enable evidence-based athletic training practice, part I: Disablement models. *Journal of Athletic Training, 43*(4), 428-436.

Ware, J. E., Kosinski, M., Bjorner, J. B., Turner-Bowker, D. M., Gandek, B., & Maruish, M. E. (2007). *User's manual for the SF-36v2 health survey* (Vol. 2). Lincoln, RI: QualityMetric.

World Health Organization. (2002). *Towards a common language for functioning, disability, and health: ICF the International Classification of Functioning, Disability, and Health.* Geneva: World Health Organization.

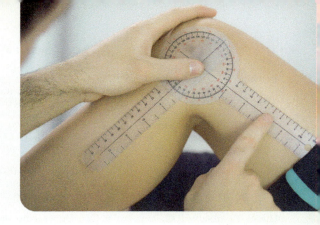

4

Outcome Properties

Where Have You Been

In Chapter 3, you learned that outcomes cannot be simply focused on the disease or physical condition of an individual person. Rather, outcomes exist along a disability continuum that ranges from the pathophysiology of a condition to societal limitations put on the individual person by the disease or physical condition. Within this context, you also learned that different types of outcomes exist for assessing different points along this continuum. These included outcomes that are focused on the disease, as well as outcomes that are meaningful to the clinician and to the patient or client. However, for any of these outcomes to be useful, they must do more than simply make sense at face value. Rather, they must have certain fundamental properties that address their quality as outcomes. These properties tell us that the outcomes are consistent, quantify what they are purported to measure, and behave in meaningful ways as the status of the patient or client changes.

Where Are You Going

In this chapter, you will learn about the properties needed for an outcome to be meaningful. You will start by learning how outcomes of individual clients are compiled into summary indices that quantify the data's central tendency (e.g., the mean). You will also learn how the standard deviation is used to quantify the variability of the data. The four fundamental categories that differentiate all data are described. For an outcome to be meaningful, it must be reliable (consistent). You will learn about the different types of reliability and how they apply to your given question. An outcome must also be valid by measuring what it claims to measure. Like reliability, validity comes in a variety of forms, and knowing the differences is important in selecting the best outcomes. Finally, for outcomes to be meaningful in clinical cases, other properties such as important differences, responsiveness, and interpretability are also required. You will be introduced to these different concepts and how the properties are determined.

Learning Outcomes

After reading this chapter, you should be able to answer these questions:

1. When is it best to use the mean, median, or mode?
2. What is the difference between a standard deviation and a standard error?
3. How is a confidence interval used?
4. What is the difference between standard error of the measure, minimal detectable change, minimal clinical important difference and global rating of change?
5. How are reliability and validity related?
6. What is the difference between interpretability and responsiveness?

Key Terms

Accuracy
Bias
Ceiling effect
Concurrent validity
Confidence interval (CI)
Construct validity
Convergent validity
Criterion validity
Divergent validity
Face validity
Floor effect
Internal consistency
Interpretability

Intersession reliability
Interval data
Intrasession reliability
Mean
Measurement error
Median
Minimal detectable change
Minimal important difference
Minimal clinical important
    difference (MCID)
Mode
Nominal data
Ordinal data

Precision
Predictive validity
Random error
Ratio data
Responsiveness
Sampling error
Standard deviation (SD)
Standard error of the mean
Standard error of the measure
    (SEM)
Test-retest reliability
Variance

Interpreting research requires an understanding of outcomes. Different outcomes have different qualities, and not all outcomes are equal to each another. The purpose of this chapter is to introduce different types of outcomes and the principles used to identify their quality. Table 4-1 contains a general list of terms commonly associated with measurement.

■ TYPES OF DATA

When considering outcome properties, one must first understand the types of data. There are four basic types of data: nominal, ordinal, interval, and ratio. Nominal data simply categorize something. Common examples are male versus female, left versus right, Republican versus Democrat versus Independent. In each of these cases, the order of the items has no meaning, and none of the categories is of greater value than the next. Because nominal data only categorize, mathematical functions (e.g., calculating a mean) cannot be used to combine or manipulate the

Nominal data: Categorically discrete data. One of the four basic types of data, which include nominal, ordinal, interval, and ratio.

Table 4-1 Statistical Terms Associated with Measurement	
Statistical Term	**Definition**
Accuracy	The degree to which a set of measures is centered on the true score
Bias	The magnitude of inaccuracy
Confidence interval	The interval around a measure, often a sample mean, that has a specified chance of containing the true measure (e.g., the population mean); confidence intervals usually specified at the 95% or 99% levels
Measurement error	The difference between the true score and an observed score.
Precision	A measurement's variability resulting from random error, measured by the standard error of the measure
Random error	Measurement error resulting from inconsistent values between measures
Sampling error	The difference between two sample means of the same population
Standard deviation	The average deviation of scores around a group mean; also, the square root of variance
Standard error of the mean	The mathematical estimate of the sampling error
Standard error of the measure	The mathematical estimate of random (measurement) error
Variance	A measure of variability of a group of scores around the group mean; also, the average squared deviation of scores around a group mean

data. However, the frequency of members in each category can be counted.

The second type of data is ordinal data, which represent the rank order among the data. Examples include place in a race (first, second, third) and degree of ankle sprain (first, second, third). Although in these cases the data have an order, there is no assumption that the distance between ranks is equal. In the case of a race finishing position, the distance between the first place and second place runners may be very close, or the runners may be separated by several seconds. Because the intervals are not necessarily equal, mathematical functions such as calculating the mean cannot be performed. However, the members of each group can be counted and sorted based on rank.

The third type of data is interval data. It has the same properties as ordinal data, except the intervals between categories are fixed and equal. Temperatures on the Celsius or Fahrenheit scales are examples. Because the intervals are fixed, the mean can be calculated and other mathematical functions are allowed.

The final category of data is ratio data. It has the same properties as interval data, with the addition of an absolute zero point. Blood pressure is an example. Because of the zero point, it is now possible to calculate mathematical comparisons. For example, a ratio of right to left leg strength could be calculated. The Kelvin temperature scale is a ratio scale because it has an absolute zero point.

Ordinal data: Data that have a rank order, but that order is arbitrary. One of the four basic types of data, which include nominal, ordinal, interval, and ratio.

Interval data: Data on a scale of measurement in which the intervals between points on the scale are fixed and equal. One of the four basic types of data, which include nominal, ordinal, interval, and ratio.

Ratio data: Interval data with an absolute zero point. One of the four basic types of data, which include nominal, ordinal, interval, and ratio.

MEASURES OF CENTRAL TENDENCY

One of the most common ways to summarize a data set is through measures of central tendency. The purpose of central tendency is to reduce a set of outcomes (e.g., the height of students in a class) to a single value that summarizes the midpoint of the entire group. There are three common measures of central tendency: the mode, the median, and the mean. Each of these is appropriate under different conditions, so it is important to understand when to use each.

Mode

The mode is the simplest measure of central tendency. It is the value that occurs most often in a data set. Figure 4–1 depicts the types of ankle sprain collected during a sport season. Each bar represents the number (i.e., frequency) of each type of sprain. Because each data point is a category, calculating a mean across the categories does not make sense. When nominal (i.e., categorical)

Mode: The measure of central tendency representing the value that occurs most frequently.

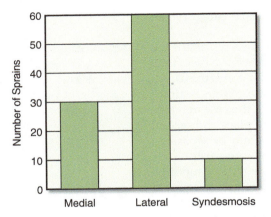

Figure 4–1 The mode is the most frequently occurring value in a set of data. The numbers above the bar represent the actual number of ankle sprains in each category. In this case, the mode "60" is associated with the category lateral ankle sprains.

data are collected, the mode is the appropriate measure of central tendency. In this data set, the mode is 60 and represents lateral ankle sprains.

Median

The **median** represents the value that occurs in the middle, where 50% of the scores are higher and 50% are lower than the median score. Assume you are interested in the frequency with which runners experience pain. Rather than asking runners for a specific number of times they experience pain, you ask runners to rank the frequency as *never, yearly, monthly, weekly,* or *daily.* In this case, the data are ordinal, and the increment from one data point to the next does not have to be equal. For example, *daily* is seven times more often than *weekly,* but *weekly* is only four times more often than *monthly.* To have monthly pain, the pain would have to occur 1 day in 30; weekly pain needs to occur only 1 day in 7. Figure 4–2 represents pain data collected from these runners. From the column on the right side, you should be able to see that the mode is weekly pain, and the median is monthly pain. The column represents the 20 runners in rank order based on their pain rating. By counting down the first 10 runners, the rating is monthly pain. Thus, 50% of the runners (i.e., 10 runners) have monthly pain or less frequent pain and 50% of the runners have weekly pain or more frequent pain.

When the data are ordinal, both the median and mode may be used. However, the median is considered the better measure of

Median: A measure of central tendency that is the middle number in a sorted list.

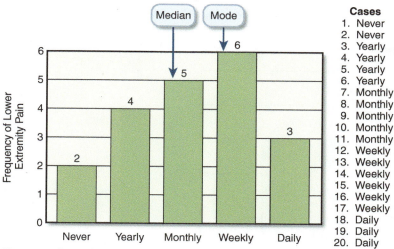

Figure 4–2 The median is the value that divides the data or cases into the upper and lower 50%. In this case, the median is "Monthly" because the 10th and 11th patients are in the category. The mode is "Weekly" with six patients.

central tendency. There are cases in which both measures may be used simultaneously, because each provides slightly different information.

Mean

The most common measure of central tendency is the **mean**, or average. This may be because most of the data collected in health care and exercise science are interval and ratio data. Figure 4–3 illustrates data for maximal oxygen consumption across a normal spectrum of athletes. In this figure, the mean is 37 ml kg^{-1} min^{-1}. Based on the frequency count, the mode is also 37 mL/kg/min, and less obviously, the median is also 37 mL/kg/min. This is an unusual case because the data are uniformly distributed, normal, or symmetrical. In data that are not uniformly distributed, the mean, median, and mode are not identical, but they are often very close. Thus, when data are uniformly distributed, the mean, median, and mode are similar, and the mean is preferred because measures of dispersion (explained later) can be applied to it.

Although the mean is the most common measures of central tendency, it has one weakness. It is susceptible to *outliers*, which are extreme scores in the data set that can influence the measure of central tendency. Figure 4–4 has the same data as in Figure 4–3, except two scores have been added at 94. Because of these extreme scores, the mean is now 41, the median is 37, and the mode is still 37. The

Mean: A measure of central tendency that is the average of all the scores.

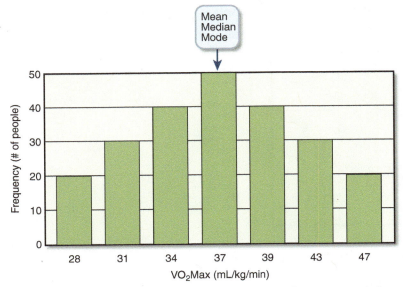

Figure 4–3 The mean is the average value of the data. When the data are symmetrical (i.e., normally distributed) the mode, median, and mean are the same value. VO$_{2max}$, maximal oxygen consumption.

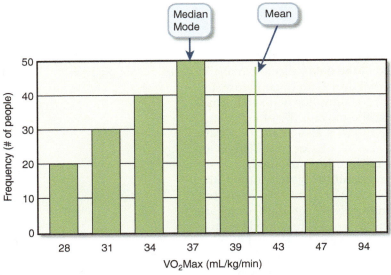

Figure 4–4 These data are skewed or have an asymmetrical distribution. When this happens, the median and mode do not coincide. VO$_{2max}$, maximal oxygen consumption.

influential outliers shift, or skew, the data away from symmetry. In this case, the mean may not be the best measure of central tendency, and the median may be more appropriate.

■ MEASURES OF DISPERSION

Measures of central tendency characterize the midpoint in a set of data, but it is also important to have measures of dispersion to understand how varied the data are. Measures of dispersion inform us about the extent of the spread of the data.

Standard Deviation

The most common measure of dispersion is the standard deviation (SD). It is derived from a measure's variance. Variance is variability of a group of scores around the group mean. The purpose of the standard deviation is to provide a measure of how much, on average, the individual scores differ around the mean. Large standard deviations in relation to the mean indicate large variability of individual scores around the mean. Scores differ around the mean for two reasons: real differences and differences caused by error. First, subjects in the group have real differences from each other. For example, if we collected the weight of everybody at your school, we would expect large differences among the individual students. However, if we collected weights on only the athletes, we would expect the differences to be much smaller because of the fitness level of the athletes. Thus, when measuring the whole school the standard deviation would be large, whereas when measuring the athletes the standard deviation would be smaller. Second, individual scores differ because of error in the measurement. This type of difference among scores is related to the measure's reliability, as discussed later in this chapter.

Figure 4–5 presents the same data as Figure 4–3, but in a different format. In addition to the mean, median, and mode, the figure also includes +1 and –1 standard deviations (SD = 5). As can be seen, ±1 standard deviation identifies a range of scores. This is important because this range captures 68% of the scores around the mean in a normal distribution. If this range is doubled to ±2 standard deviations, then approximately 95% of the scores are captured. The advantage of this is that it provides some perspective. We know that 68% of the subjects have a maximal oxygen consumption between 32 and 42 mL/kg/min or 95% of the subjects have a maximal oxygen consumption between 42 and 52 mL/kg/min.

Standard deviation (SD): The average deviation of scores around a group mean. Also, the square root of variance.

Variance: A measure of variability of a group of scores around the group mean. Also, the average squared deviation of scores around a group mean.

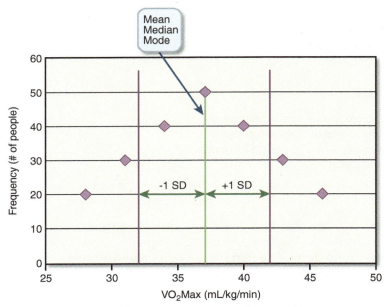

Figure 4–5 A symmetrical data distribution showing the mean at the center and ±1 standard deviation (SD). In a symmetrical distribution, 68% of the scores will be between –1 and +1 standard deviations. VO$_{2max}$, maximal oxygen consumption.

Standard Error and Confidence Intervals

One of the important properties of the mean is that it not only represents the mean of the studied sample, but also it is an estimate of the mean of the population from which the sample is derived. In research, it is usually impossible to study an entire population of interest (e.g., obese persons). Thus, it is rarely possible to know the population's mean on a measure (e.g., percentage of body fat). Instead, we sample people from the population and study the sample. Means reported in the research literature therefore represent the sample studied and are estimates of the population mean.

Unfortunately, the sample mean is never a perfect estimate of the population mean. For example, if we measure the vertical jump of the juniors and seniors from the population of students at your school, we can calculate their vertical jump displacement. If we draw a second sample from the student population, the mean vertical jump displacement of this second sample will not be exactly the same as the first sample's mean. However, both are estimates of the population's vertical jump displacement. The difference between these two means is caused by **sampling error**, which is the difference between a sample mean and the population mean.

Sampling error: The difference between two sample means of the same population.

Because of this error, we know that the sample mean is an imperfect estimate of the population mean. The next question is how imperfect. The sampling error can be estimated by calculating the standard error (SE) of the mean.

Figure 4–6 is the same as Figure 4–5, except the standard error has been added. The small size of this band indicates that the sampling error associated with the mean is relatively small. The mean in this example therefore is a very good estimate of the population mean. What should be apparent is that the standard error band is much smaller than that of the standard deviation. The standard error is always smaller than the SD because it is derived by dividing the SD by the square root of the sample size. Sample size (n) is simply the number of individual subjects used to calculate the mean. You should also note that as the sample size becomes larger, the standard error becomes smaller and is thus a better estimator of the population mean. For example, the standard error bar in Figure 4–6 ranges from 36.7 to 37.3mL/kg/min for n = 230. If the sample were reduced to n = 10, then the standard error bar would range from 35.4 to 38.6 mL/kg/min or be nearly five times wider. In the latter case, the mean would be a poorer estimate of the population mean.

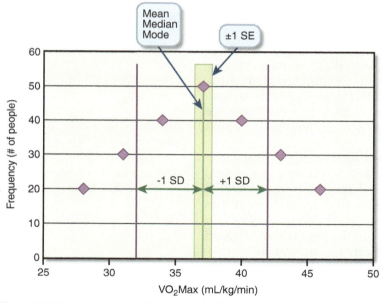

Figure 4–6 The standard error (SE) is overlaid with the sample standard deviation (SD). Note that the standard error is considerably smaller than the standard deviation. The standard error estimates the error of the mean. VO_{2max}, maximal oxygen consumption.

In the research literature, you will see either the standard deviation or the standard error reported. Thus, it is important to know which is being reported and the meaning of each. Fortunately, the sample size (n) is always reported in a research manuscript, and that makes it relatively easy for the reader to convert between the two. The formula for the standard error is as follows:

$$SE = \frac{\text{Sample standard deviation}}{\sqrt{\text{Number of subjects in the sample}}}$$

Or

$$SE = \frac{s}{\sqrt{n}}$$

Although the standard error is an important statistic to understand, it is not the preferred measure. The standard deviation should be reported because most statistical analyses are examining the sample and not making mathematical inferences of the whole population. In addition, some indices such as the standardized mean difference (a form of effect size) are in units of standard deviation, and thus the standard deviation must be reported so that this measure of effect can be contextualized.

Sometimes research reports a **confidence interval (CI)** for the mean instead of the standard error or standard deviation. The confidence interval is a range of values in which there is a level of confidence, expressed as a percentage, that it contains the true value. The confidence interval has the advantage of showing whether results are statistically significant, as well as the magnitude of **measurement error**. Measurement error is the difference between the true score and the observed score (i.e., the measured score).

The typically reported confidence interval is the 95% confidence interval.(CI$_{95}$). Like the standard deviation and standard error, the 95% confidence interval is a range of scores centered on the mean. Figure 4–7 shows the 95% confidence interval with the standard deviation and standard error, and it is clear that the confidence interval is about twice the size as the standard error. This is because the standard error is multiplied by 1.96. For the standard deviation, it was explained that ±2 standard deviations account for approximately 95% of the data. In fact 1.96 standard deviation accounts for exactly 95% of the data. The same is true for the standard error. Keeping in mind that the standard error is an estimate of sampling error, the 95% confidence interval gives us a range of scores that the sample mean is

Confidence interval (CI): The range of values within which the true value of a parameter is expected to lie. The confidence interval shows whether results are statistically significant and the magnitude of measurement error.

Measurement error: The difference between the true value of something that is being measured and the value that is actually obtained by measurement.

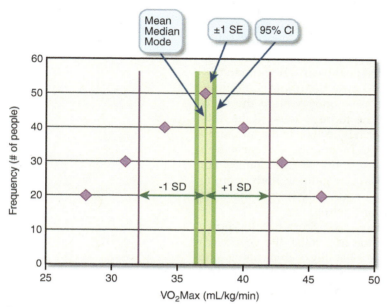

Figure 4–7 The 95% confidence interval (95% CI) is overlaid with the standard deviation (SD) and standard error (SE). Note that the 95% confidence interval is wider that the standard error because it captures 95% of the estimated error, whereas the standard error captures only 68%. VO_{2max}, maximal oxygen consumption.

expected to fluctuate within 95% of the time. In other words, we could say with 95% confidence the mean will fluctuate in this range. Some fluctuation is always expected because of sampling error.

It can be said that the 95% confidence interval has a 95% chance of containing the population mean. Because we know that a sample mean is only an estimate of the population mean, the confidence interval is considered a better method of estimating the value of the population mean. The formula for the 95% confidence interval is as follows:

$$CI_{95} = \text{Mean} \pm SE \cdot 1.96$$

Or

$$CI_{95} = \bar{x} \pm \frac{s}{\sqrt{n}} \cdot 1.96$$

Finally, although the 95% is the most common confidence interval used, the 90% confidence interval and 99% confidence interval are also occasionally used.

Connections 4-1

The 95% confidence interval is commonly used because it is directly related to the common statistical threshold. In most research, statistical tests are required to meet a threshold of 0.05 to be statistically significant. This will be reported as alpha ≤ 0.05 or $P = 0.05$ or less. Mathematically, $1 - 0.05 = 0.95$ or 95% (see Chapter 9).

Retention Questions 4-1

1. When is the median more appropriate than the mean?
2. When is the mode more appropriate than the median and mean?
3. What is the preferred measure for reporting sampling error?
4. What is the difference between the standard error and the confidence interval?

◼ MEASUREMENT RELIABILITY

One of the most important qualities of an outcome is reliability. Reliability simply refers to the outcome's repeatability, and it is an important quality of outcomes used in health care and human performance. For example, if you stand on a bathroom scale three times in a row, it should measure your body weight the same (or very close to the same) each time to be reliable. Reliability comes in different forms, and each form is specific to the measure's purpose (Table 4-2). Repeatability can be defined as a measure's ability to remain unchanged in the absence of real change. For example, assuming you are not losing or gaining body weight, your bathroom scale should measure your body weight the same each day, with the exception of minor fluctuation.

The reliability of an outcome is determined using a statistic known as the reliability coefficient. The value of a reliability coefficient ranges from 0 to 1. Measures that have reliability coefficients close to 1 are very reliable, whereas those close to zero are unreliable. Two statistical measures are frequently used as reliability coefficients: the Pearson product moment correlation coefficient and the intraclass correlation coefficient (ICC). The Pearson correlation coefficient has the disadvantage of being unable to detect systematic error, so the intraclass correlation coefficient is preferred and better estimates the repeatability of a measure. Different methods are used to gather data for establishing reliability. The most common types of reliability encountered in health and exercise science are described here.

Table 4-2 Types of Measurement Reliability	
Reliability	*Definition*
Test-retest	Sequential measures at the same point in time (or in close time proximity) that produce the same value (e.g., blood measured twice in a row or on sequential days)
Intrarater	The typical form of test-retest reliability involving multiple measures by the same tester (e.g., blood pressure measured by the same clinician)
Interrater	An alternative form of test-retest reliability in which two (or more) different testers collects measures (e.g., blood pressure measured by two different clinicians)
Intersession	An alternative form of test-retest reliability in which measures are collected at two different time points (e.g., blood pressure measured 6 months apart)
Intrasession	An alternative form of test-retest reliability with relatively little time between each measure
Internal consistency	A form of reliability typically used to determine the consistency of individual items within a questionnaire

Test-Retest

The most common type of reliability encountered is **test-retest reliability**. Test-retest reliability is defined as sequential measures of an outcome at the same point in time (or in close time proximity), such as hematocrit measured twice in a row or on sequential days. When the time points of test-retest reliability are close, the reliability can be described as **intrasession reliability**. For another example of test-retest reliability, assume we are interested in estimating an adolescent's percentage of body fat by using bioelectrical impedance. Assume we do this 12 times in a row to examine test-retest reliability. Those 12 trials are plotted in Figure 4–8, and the square in the figure represents the person's percentage of body fat as estimated by bioelectrical impedance (i.e., 10%). Each of the diamonds represents the value for each of the 12 trials. As you can see, most of the trials are not exactly 10%, but vary around 10%. The variability of the measures around the true score is caused by **random error**. The size of this variability is measured using the **standard error of the measure** (SEM) and is called the measure's **precision**. The standard error of the measure is similar to the **standard error of the mean** in that both estimate error. In the case of the standard error of the mean, the error is the sampling error associated with the sample mean's precision. In the case of the standard error of the measure, the error is the random error associated with the outcome's precision, which is related to reliability. In the previous example, an adolescent is measured 12 times and receives 12 different percentage of body fat scores. The differences among the scores result from the outcome's error. This error is quantified by the standard error of the measure. In contrast, if we randomly sampled two groups of 100 adolescents from the local community and measured their bioelectrical impedance, two things would be true. First, the mean of both groups would estimate the mean bioelectrical impedance for the population of adolescents in the community. Second, the two means would not be exactly equal. This discrepancy is the result of sampling error, which is estimated by the standard error of the mean.

All outcomes have some amount of random error. In Figure 4–8, the random error causes wide variability and suggests that the measure is not reliable. By comparison, Figure 4–9 shows a similar set of data, but all the scores are much closer to the true value of 10. In this case, the outcome is much more reliable.

In health and exercise science, the preferred test-retest reliability coefficient is the intraclass correlation coefficient. One of the reasons the intraclass correlation coefficient is preferred is because it accounts for both precision and bias in a single measure. If the precision is poor or the bias is high, or both, the intraclass correlation coefficient will be low. Other reliability coefficients account only for

Test-retest reliability: The measure of the ability of a test to produce consistent results when it is used multiple times under nearly identical conditions.

Intrasession reliability: An alternative form of test-retest reliability with relatively little time passing between each measure.

Random error: Errors in measurement caused by factors that vary from one measurement to another.

Standard error of the measure (SEM): The mathematical estimate of random (measurement) error.

Precision: A measurement's variability as a result of random error, measured by the standard error of the measure.

Standard error of the mean: The mathematical estimate of the sampling error.

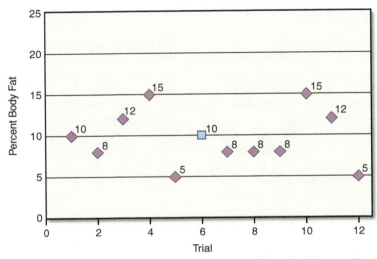

Figure 4–8 Multiple estimates of adolescent percentage of body fat. The true value is 10 (square). The diamonds represent 12 separate measures with random error included in each. The spread of the individual points suggests that the outcome is unreliable.

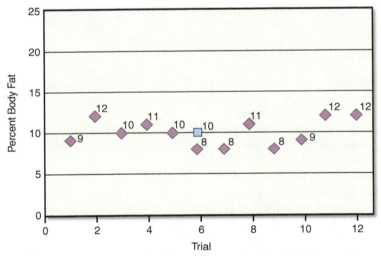

Figure 4–9 Multiple estimates of adolescent percentage of body fat. The true value is 10 (square). The diamonds represent 12 separate measures with random error included in each. Compared with Figure 4–8, the relatively narrower spread of the individual points suggests that the outcome is more reliable.

precision. The percentage of body fat example given earlier is loosely based on the study by Lubans et al. (2011), and it correctly represents the principle of random error and reliability. However, in practice, reliability and precision are determined using different methods. Instead of taking multiple measures of a single person, multiple persons are measured at least twice. For example, Lubans et al. studied 68 adolescents and measured them twice, 7 days apart. By using these 136 data points, the intraclass correlation coefficient was calculated. For bioelectrical impedance, the intraclass correlation coefficient was 0.95 for boys and 0.93 for girls. Because these values are close to 1, the measure is considered very reliable. However, because the intraclass correlation coefficient is a composite of both precision and bias, the intraclass correlation coefficient does not tell us the magnitude of the imprecision by itself. To do that, the standard error of the measure must be calculated. Most reliability studies calculate the standard error of the measure and report it with the reliability coefficient. In this example, it was not reported, but a simple formula can be used to calculate the standard error of the measure from the intraclass correlation coefficient. The formula is included here and conceptually represents the proportion of the group's standard deviation that results from error (i.e., $\sqrt{1 - ICC}$):

$$Standard\ error\ of\ the\ measure = SD\sqrt{1 - ICC}$$

Using the data of Lubans et al. for boys, the formula would be:

$$Standard\ error\ of\ the\ measure = 6.7\sqrt{1 - 0.95}$$

The 6.7 is the standard deviation from the first measure of the boys' bioelectrical impedance data, and the 0.95 is the intraclass correlation coefficient value for the boys. Thus, the standard error of the measure is equal to 1.5% body fat. The standard error of the measure is interpreted similar to a standard deviation of a mean. As with the standard deviation, we would expect 68% of the error in a score to occur between ±1.5% body fat. For example, if the person had a 12% body fat as estimated by bioelectrical impedance, we could say with 68% confidence that the range of 10.5% to 13.5% body fat contains the person's true measure. Like the standard deviation of the mean, the 95% confidence interval of the standard error of the measure is preferred to the standard error of the measure. The 95% confidence interval for the standard error of the measure (SEM_{95}) is calculated as follows:

$$95\%\ confidence\ interval\ for\ the\ standard\ error\ of\ the\ measure$$
$$= standard\ error\ of\ the\ measure \cdot 1.96$$

Using the data of Lubans et al. for boys, the formula would be:

$$95\%\ confidence\ interval\ for\ the\ standard\ error\ of\ the\ measure = 1.5 \cdot 1.96$$

For this example, the 95% confidence interval for the standard error of the measure is 2.9. Using the 95% confidence interval for the standard error of the measure, if the person had 12% body fat as estimated by bioelectrical impedance, we could say with 95% confidence that the range of 9.1% to 14.9% body fat contains the person's measure. Figure 4–10 illustrates the relationship between the standard error of the measure and the 95% confidence interval for the standard error of the measure.

Pros and Cons

The reliability coefficient (e.g., the intraclass correlation coefficient) is a useful summary measure for understanding whether a measure is repeatable. However, by itself it does not tell you how precise the measure is. Thus, you also need to know the standard error of the measure. This value represents the actual amount of random error and is in the original units of the measure, thereby making it more useful to the practitioner.

Interrater

The previous example is the typical form of test-retest reliability in which a single person (i.e., rater) performs the measure to determine the reliability of the measure. This is known as *intrarater reliability*. Intrarater reliability is the typical form of test-retest reliability involving multiple measures by the same person (e.g., blood pressure measured by the same person). Sometimes, it is of interest to know whether the measure is reliable across different

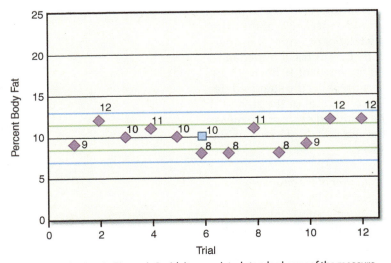

Figure 4–10 The data in Figure 4–9 with its associated standard error of the measure (green lines) and 95% confidence interval of the standard error of the measure (blue lines).

practitioners (i.e., raters). This is known as *interrater reliability,* which is an alternative form of test-retest reliability in which two (or more) different testers collect outcomes (e.g., blood pressure measured by two different people). In this case, each subject is measured more than once, each time by a different rater. From these data the intraclass correlation coefficient and standard error of the outcome are calculated exactly the same as before. However, with interrater reliability the interpretation is different. Instead of interpreting the data in terms of whether the test was reliable, the data are now interpreted in terms of whether the testers are reliable. This type of reliability is important when trying to determine whether an outcome measured by different people will produce the same result. For example, it may be important to know whether therapists in the same clinic who are using a goniometer to measure knee range of motion can obtain the same value for the same patient. Alternatively, it may be worth knowing whether two clinicians will measure the same blood pressure in the same patient.

Intersession

Intersession reliability is a form of test-retest reliability in which measures are collected at two different time points that are not close together (e.g., blood pressure measured 6 months apart). Intersession reliability usually has at least 1 day between the test and retest measure, but there is no specific requirement for the length of the time interval between the test and the retest. The length of time should match the interval typically used in practice. For example, if it is typical for joint range of motion to be measured weekly to assess therapeutic progress after a knee operation, then a reliability study should be designed so that the test and retest measures are 1 week apart. Thus, the reliability study would match the needs of actual practice.

Intersession reliability: An alternative form of test-retest reliability in which measures are collected at two different time points.

Caveats of Test-Retest Reliability

Any true assessment of an outcome's test-retest reliability depends on at least one important principle: from test to retest, there should be no expectation that the measure will change. The purpose of test-retest reliability is to establish the stability or consistency of the measure. If there is a reasonable expectation that the measure will change from test to retest, reliability cannot be established. As a general rule, the more time that elapses between measures, the more likely the true score will be to have changed. For example, if a person's weight is measured today, and again tomorrow, there is no reasonable expectation that the true weight would be different.

Any difference between today and tomorrow would be the result of random error. However, if the two weight measures occurred 6 months apart, there is a reasonable expectation that the person's true weight may have changed. Thus, researchers must apply some judgment about what length of time between measures is appropriate. For body weight, waiting a week may be acceptable, but a month between tests may be questionable.

It is also the case that a measure's reliability is lower for interrater than for intrarater reliability. When more than one rater is used, each rater's error is added to the random error. A decrease in reliability is also expected with intersession reliability. Even if the same rater is used for both sessions, some additional random error will be added when there is some time between tests.

Each type of reliability is used to address a specific need or purpose: error of a rater (intrarater), error among raters (intrarater), or error among sessions (intersession). As a consumer of research, you should look for studies that address the reliability that is relevant to your purpose. Usually, that will be intrarater reliability.

Internal Consistency

A less common form of reliability found in exercise science and health care is **internal consistency**. Internal consistency is a form of reliability typically used to determine the consistency of individual items within a questionnaire or test. The purpose is to determine whether items within a questionnaire measure the same thing. Often this is something that is not directly observable, such as pain or quality of life. Internal consistency is used for questionnaire data when there is a concern that subjects may remember their answers. If subjects can remember their answers, then reliability using other repeated test methods will artificially inflate the reliability. This is because subjects tend to repeat answers they can remember. For example, Janz, Lutuchy, Wenthe, and Levy (2008) assessed the internal consistency of the Physical Activity Questionnaire for older children and adolescents. Although not directly stated, because both questionnaires are relatively short (i.e., eight to nine questions), it is likely the participants could have remembered many of their answers. Thus, test-retest reliability would not have been appropriate.

Internal consistency: A form of reliability typically used to determine the consistency of individual items within a questionnaire.

Retention Questions 4-2
1. What does the standard error of the measure tell us about the measure?
2. What are the distinctions among interrater, intrarater, intersession, and intrasession reliability?
3. What is the difference between test-retest reliability and internal consistency?

◾ VALIDITY

The second important quality of a measurement is its validity. Validity refers to an outcome's ability to measure what it purports to measure accurately. Just because an outcome is reliable, that does not make it valid. Thus, validity must be established separately. There are several types of validity that are highly applicable to exercise and sport science (Table 4-3). Each is described here.

Criterion Validity

In exercise science and health care, the most common form of validity is criterion validity. Criterion validity refers to an outcome's ability to estimate a target value or "gold standard" outcome (i.e., the criterion outcome). Traditionally, criterion validity is assessed with the Pearson correlation coefficient. This correlation coefficient measures the strength of the relationship between any two variables. In the case of validity assessment, it is the relationship between the measure of interest and the gold standard.

Criterion validity: A measure of how well an outcome estimates a target value or gold standard measure.

Concurrent Validity

The most common type of criterion validity is concurrent validity. Concurrent validity is defined as a measures ability to estimate a target value at the same point in time. The challenge in establishing concurrent validity is identifying the gold standard or target outcome. For example in clinical orthopedics, you may want to know

Concurrent validity: A form of criterion validity: the degree to which two measuring devices or methods agree with each other.

Table 4-3	Types of Measurement Validity
Validity	**Definition**
Criterion	Criterion validity refers to an outcome's ability to estimate a target value or gold standard measure (i.e., the criterion measure).
Concurrent	A form of criterion validity. It is defined as an outcome's ability to estimate a target value at the same point in time (e.g., percentage of body fat with skin fold measures predicts percentage of body fat measured with dual-energy x-ray absorptiometry).
Predictive	A form of criterion validity. It is defined as an outcome's ability to predict an event in the future (e.g., blood pressure predicts future heart attacks).
Construct	Construct validity refers to an outcome's ability to quantify the construct of interest (e.g., quality of life).
Convergent	A form of construct validity. It is defined as the new outcome being well correlated with (i.e., related to) other outcomes that measure similar attributes or qualities (e.g., a one-repetition maximum strength test related to a three-repetition maximum strength test).
Divergent	A form of construct validity. It is defined as the new instrument's being poorly correlated with another instrument with dissimilar attributes or qualities (e.g., a physical health questionnaire poorly correlated with a mental health questionnaire).
Face	Face validity is defined as an outcome appearing to measure what it is intended to measure (e.g., does a pain scale contain questions about pain?).

whether a magnetic resonance imaging scan is capable of detecting an anterior cruciate ligament tear. To do this, you would correlate the magnetic resonance imaging findings with what the orthopedist found during an arthroscopic examination. If the Pearson correlation coefficient is high, then the magnetic resonance imaging scan would be considered valid. You may also want to know whether a tympanic membrane thermometer is valid for measuring body temperature. In this case, body temperature could be measured with the tympanic membrane thermometer and compared with the reading from a rectal thermometer (the scientifically accepted gold standard for core body temperature). If the two results had a high Pearson correlation coefficient, then the tympanic membrane temperature would be considered valid for body temperature.

The higher the correlation coefficient is between the tested outcome and the gold standard, the more valid the measure is considered to be. For example, Figure 4–11 shows the same data as in Figure 4–9, except all the data points are 10 points higher than the true score. Because the data points are not centered on the true score, the measure would not be considered accurate. **Accuracy** refers to how well a set of measures are centered on the true score, or how much systematic error is in the assessment. When measures do not center on the true score, this is the result of *systematic error*, and the magnitude of the systematic error is known as **bias**. If an outcome is biased, it will consistently overestimate or underestimate the true value, and the patient's result will look better or worse than it really is. If the size of the bias is known, then the score on a measure can be adjusted appropriately.

Accuracy: A measure of how much systematic error is in an assessment or how well a set of measures is centered on the true score.

Bias: A measure of inaccuracy or any effect or interference that produces results that systematically depart from the true value.

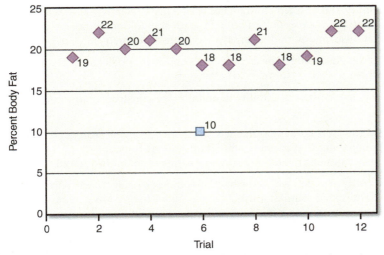

Figure 4–11 The data in Figure 4–9 with a bias of 10. The true score is 10 (square).

Predictive Validity

Predictive validity is the ability of an outcome to predict a future event, and it is another subtype of criterion validity. For example, does performance on a balance test, such as the balance error scoring system, predict future falls in aging populations? The key component of predictive validity is that the predicted event (i.e., falls) must occur in the future. This implies that the study is prospective. In other words, a group of subjects must be identified and then followed across time. One value of establishing predictive validity is that it allows researchers and clinicians to identify subjects at risk of a future event. Knowing this, an intervention could be applied to prevent that event.

Alternatively, predictive validity may be used to predict future performance. For example, the Scholastic Aptitude Test could be used to predict college grade point average. This type of information could be used to identify potential students for academic programs. A somewhat more controversial example of predictive validity is using genetic testing to predict future athletic performance (Roth, 2012).

Construct Validity

Construct validity refers to a measure's ability to quantify the construct of interest. To understand construct validity, it is necessary to understand a construct first. A construct is an idea or concept that cannot be measured directly. One of the common constructs measured in health care is quality of life. Quality of life cannot be measured directly, but it can be assessed using measures such as happiness, depression, and work productivity, among others. In exercise science, muscular fitness would be an important construct that could be assessed by using a battery of tests such as the Resistance Training Skills Battery (Lubans et al., 2014). Construct validity applies to measures, treatments, and populations. A detailed examination of construct validity is provided in Chapter 5. For now, the focus is on how construct validity is established for outcomes.

There is no one method for establishing the construct validity of an outcome. One common method is a complex statistical procedure called factor analysis. Factor analysis is used to determine whether items on the questionnaire are related to each other and form groups of questions (i.e., factors) that are logically meaningful. Factor analysis is particularly appropriate for outcomes that include multiple items (e.g., questionnaires) to establish them as measuring meaningful constructs.

Alternatively, a new questionnaire may be compared to established questionnaires by using a correlation coefficient. If the new

Predictive validity: A form of criterion validity: the degree to which a test measurement accurately predicts a future event.

The Critical Consumer 4-1
Many articles in the exercise science literature use the term predictive validity. However, in reality these studies are usually studies of concurrent validity because they are not predicting a future event. Thus, when reading a study, do not accept the authors' name for the validity at face value. Rather, you need to look at the methods and determine whether the outcome measure occurred in the future. If both the predictor and outcome are measured at the same point in time, it is concurrent validity by definition.

Construct validity: A form of criterion validity: the degree to which a test accurately measures or quantifies the intended construct.

questionnaire is well correlated with (i.e., related to) other questionnaires that measure similar attributes or qualities, this is known as **convergent validity**. Conversely, if the new questionnaire correlates poorly with another questionnaire that measures dissimilar attributes or qualities, this is known as **divergent validity**. Divergent validity is defined as the new measure's being poorly correlated with another measure with dissimilar attributes or qualities. The hope is that a new questionnaire would demonstrate both convergent and divergent validity. For example, Grotle, Garratt, Jenssen, and Stuge (2012) established the construct validity of several questionnaires used for pelvic girdle pain by correlating them with questionnaires or subparts of questionnaires by using both convergent and divergent validity.

Ideally, a new questionnaire's construct validity would be assessed using factor analysis, convergent validity, and divergent validity. This strategy would ensure that the internal structure of the questionnaire logically assessed the intended construct. If this was confirmed with factor analysis, then a follow-up assessment of the questionnaire's convergent and divergent validity could be completed.

Convergent validity: A form of construct validity: the degree to which two measures of constructs that theoretically should be related are actually related.

Divergent validity: A form of construct validity: the degree to which the new instrument is correlated to another instrument with dissimilar attributes or qualities.

Face Validity

The final form of validity frequently encountered is **face validity**. This type of validity simply means that the outcome appears to measure what it is intended to measure. For example, does 40-yard dash time measure running speed? Such outcomes could include measures of strength, speed, endurance, or flexibility. We would probably agree that, at face value, 40-yard dash time does indeed measure running speed. Conversely, if vertical jump is measured, we would probably say this does not assess running speed.

As you may guess, face validity is the weakest form of validity and, by itself, is of little value. However, it is a reasonable starting point for developing a new measure or assessment. For the new measure to have value, face validity should be followed by other forms of validity assessment.

Face validity: A form of criterion validity: the degree to which an outcome measures what it is intended to measure; the degree to which a measurement is logical, reasonable, or acceptable.

◼ CLINIMETRIC PROPERTIES OF MEASUREMENT

Reliability and validity are hallmarks for all outcomes. However, just because an outcome is reliable and valid does not mean that it is useful. To determine whether a measure has actual value, its clinimetric properties must be known. Clinimetric properties refer to an outcome's ability to be translated into meaningful value. Definitions for different clinimetric properties are provided in Table 4-4 and are explained in detail here.

Minimal Detectable Change

The simplest clinimetric property reported in the literature is a statistical measure known as the **minimal detectable change**. It is the minimal amount of change in an individual subject's score that must be detected to ensure that the change was not the result of random error. The minimal detectable change does not necessarily indicate importance from the perspective of the patient or client. Rather, the importance is for the practitioner to know that real change has occurred on the measure.

Minimal detectable change: The minimum amount of change between data points that must exist to ensure the change was not the result of measurement error.

The minimal detectable change is closely related to the standard error of the measure. In fact, the minimal detectable change is an adjusted form of the standard error of the measure. The formula for the minimal detectable change (MDC) is as follows:

$$MDC = \sqrt{2} \cdot \text{Standard error of the measure}$$

Although related, the minimal detectable change and standard error of the measure tell us different things about the same outcome. As described earlier, the standard error of the measure is the precision of an outcome. Using the percentage of body fat example, the standard error of the measure tells you how much error is associated with the outcome. For example, if the percentage of body fat was estimated at 11%, using the 95% confidence interval for the

Table 4-4 Clinimetric Properties of Measures	
Clinimetric Property	**Definition**
Minimal detectable change	The minimal amount of change in a subject's score that must exist to ensure that the change was not the result of measurement error
Minimal important difference	The amount of change in an outcome that represents an important change to the patient
Minimal clinical important difference	The amount of change in an outcome that represents an important change to the clinician and maybe the patient
Responsiveness	An outcome's ability to change when it is expected to change
Interpretability	The ability to assign qualitative meaning to a quantitative score
Floor and ceiling effects	An outcome's inability to distinguish among subjects at the extreme ends of the scale

standard error of the measure, we would have 95% confidence that the range from 7.9% to 14.1% contains the adolescent's percentage of body fat. In contrast, the minimal detectable change tells us how much change is needed for the difference to be the result of more than just error.

Assume you are a practitioner and have placed a group of adolescents on a combination of diet and exercise with the intent of decreasing their percentage of body fat. Your first step in assessing the program is to identify reliable outcomes published in the literature that can be used to estimate body fat. Your second step is to determine how much change on your selected measure is real change (i.e., the minimal detectable change.) Now assume that for this program the bioelectrical impedance measures assessed by Lubans et al. (2011) will be used to estimate your clients' percentage of body fat. Keep in mind that as a clinician, you are not collecting data to determine the minimal detectable change. Rather, you are using other people's data to either calculate the minimal detectable change or using the minimal detectable change they have calculated for you. In this case, we use the data of Lubans et al. to calculate the minimal detectable change. The standard error of the measure calculated before for the adolescent boys was 1.5%. Using the minimal detectable change formula, the minimal detectable change for the boys is 2.1% or:

$$MDC = \sqrt{2} \cdot 1.5 = 2.1$$

Thus, an adolescent in the diet and exercise program would have to have a 2.1% decrease in percentage of body fat for the treatment plan to be deemed real change and not error.

Like the standard error of the measure, the minimal detectable change represents the 68% confidence level for true change. However, some practitioners prefer to be very confident that a real change has taken place. To be more confident, one can calculate the 95% confidence interval for the minimal detectable change (MDC_{95}), which represents a 95% confidence that real change occurred. The minimal detectable change can be converted to the 95% confidence interval for the minimal detectable change by using the following formula:

$$MDC_{95} = 1.96 \cdot MDC$$

Using this formula, the 95% confidence interval for the minimal detectable change would be 4.2. Thus, to be 95% confident that a real change in body fat occurred, an adolescent would have to have a 4.2% change.

Minimal Important Difference

The **minimal important difference** is the amount of change in an outcome that represents an important change to the patient. A variety of methods can be used to determine a measure's minimal important difference, and these methods can be divided into four basic approaches: the anchor-based approach, the sensitivity and specificity-based approach, the distribution-based approach, and the social comparison approach (Copay, Subach, Glassman, Polly, & Schuler, 2007).

Anchor-Based Approach

The first approach is the anchor-based approach. An anchor is an outcome instrument with established reliability and validity against which an alternative outcome can be compared. For example, it may be worth knowing how much change on a region-specific outcome measure (e.g., the Foot and Ankle Ability Measure) is important to the patient. To do that, the Foot and Ankle Ability Measure would be anchored to another outcome such as the global rating of change. In other words, the goal would be to determine how much change on the Foot and Ankle Ability Measure makes the patient feel better. Alternatively, the Foot and Ankle Ability Measure could be anchored to the Short Form 36 to determine how much change is needed to improve health-related quality of life.

One way change is measured is across time in the same group of patients (i.e., the within-subjects method). In this case, each subject in the research study would be measured at regular periodic intervals on both the Foot and Ankle Ability Measure and the global rating of change. The researcher would make some decision about how much change on the global rating of change was important (e.g., "much improved"). At the end of the study, the average score of the Foot and Ankle Ability Measure when the patients reached "much improved" would be used as the minimal important difference. If some patients did not reach "much improved," they would not be included in the calculation. Some patients may have exceeded the score of "much improved," and in these cases only the Foot and Ankle Ability Measure score that occurred at the "much improved" time point would be used.

Figure 4–12 is an example of this method based on four subjects. If the global rating of change rating 4 equals "much improved," then the circled value for Foot and Ankle Ability Measure represents the minimal important difference for each patient. The average Foot and Ankle Ability Measure value at the global rating of change of 4 (i.e., 74) would be the true minimal important difference for this group of patients. Keep in mind that in practice, a

Minimal important difference: The smallest amount of change in an outcome that represents an important change to the patient.

Connections 4-2
Remember that region-specific outcomes are usually less relevant to the patient and more relevant to the clinician. Anchoring a region-specific outcome makes the measure more interpretable (see interpretability, later in this chapter).

The Critical Consumer 4-2
When the researcher decides how much change is important, it is a somewhat arbitrary decision. Thus, as a consumer you need to consider whether this best fits your needs and whether the researcher has made this decision based on a sound rationale. Unfortunately, there are no clear guidelines for a sound rationale.

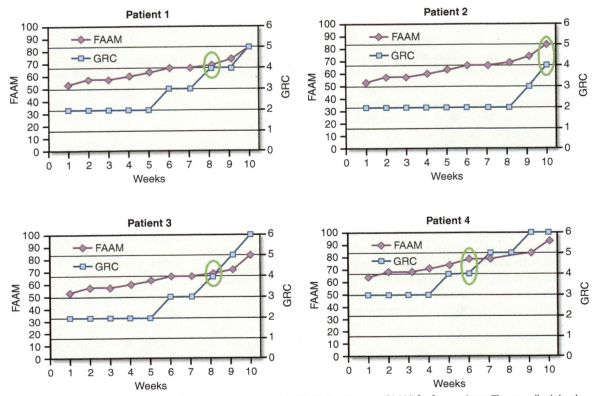

Figure 4–12 The minimal important difference of the Foot and Ankle Ability Measure (FAAM) for four patients. The overall minimal important difference for the Foot and Ankle Ability Measure would be the average of the individual minimal important differences. In this example, the individual minimal important difference is the value associated with a predetermined global rating of change (GRC) equal to 4 (identified by the circle).

much greater patient pool would be used to determine the minimal important difference.

An alternative to the within-subjects method is the between-subjects method. In this case, rather than measuring subjects across time, two different groups of subjects are compared. Specifically, at a specific point in time, subjects are grouped based on the global rating of change. For example, in month six of a cardiac rehabilitation program, patients would be divided into two groups based on the global rating of change ratings of "much improved" and "little improved." After division of the groups, the minimal important difference for quality of life as measured by the Chronic Heart Failure Questionnaire (Guyatt et al., 1989) is determined by comparing the questionnaire scores of the two groups.

It is important to understand that the between-subjects method controls for the dimension of time. In the within-subjects method, time is allowed to vary. In the between-subjects method, time has been fixed. In the previous example, time was fixed at 6 months, and the 6-month minimal important difference was calculated. If the time had been set at 3 months, then the 3-month minimal important difference would have been calculated. It is possible, and likely, that the 3-month and 6-month minimal important difference would be different and thus not interchangeable. As a practitioner, it is important to make that distinction and to be certain to use the correct method for the correct time point.

Issues and Cautions Using Minimal Important Difference

As a property of an outcome, the minimal important difference seems to be gaining popularity. However, it is not perfect, and several limitations have been identified (Copay et al., 2007). First, the different methods described previously often produce different values for the minimal important difference. It is probably not appropriate to suggest that one method is better than another. Rather, it may be best simply to acknowledge the differences and have clinician practitioners decide which best matches their experience or conditions of practice.

Second, the cost of treatment is seldom considered in the size of the minimal important difference. It is possible that even if a patient improved, the patient may deem the monetary or time costs too high for the treatment to be worthwhile. For example, if therapy for neck pain requires daily exercise for an entire lifetime after injury, would a patient be likely to value that treatment? Probably not. If not, the patient would not likely be compliant with the treatment program. Thus, the treatment may reduce neck pain but not be valued by the patient.

Third, the minimal important difference rarely considers the side effects of treatment. Chemotherapy is frequently associated with nausea, a common side effect of treatment. Is tolerating this side effect worthwhile to receive the benefit of treatment? Most patients would say yes, if the chemotherapy is likely to cure the cancer or extend one's lifetime by several years. However, what would the patient decide if the chemotherapy was expected to produce severe nausea and extend life by 2 weeks? How would that decision be affected if the 2 weeks was added to a life expectancy of 1 month versus 6 years? Clearly, these are personal decisions, but they have a direct effect on how the minimal important difference should be interpreted.

A fourth concern with the minimal important difference is that it depends on the baseline value. This is true of many outcomes when made across time. Baseline is the score on an outcome that an individual receives when it is first measured. For example, from a strength training perspective, we know and expect that untrained persons will have a greater response to a strength training program than an elite athlete. This is because untrained persons have more room for improvement. This same principle is true for minimal important differences, and it has two implications. First, minimal important differences for very ill patients may be quite different from those for relatively healthy persons. Second, the amount of change expected by the practitioner or patient must be interpreted in the context of the patient's baseline.

Sensitivity- and Specificity-Based Approach

Another alternative to generating a minimal important difference is to use the sensitivity and specificity approach. Sensitivity is a diagnostic test's ability to detect disease when the disease is truly present (i.e., true positive). Tests with high sensitivity are helpful in ruling out a disease. Specificity is a diagnostic test's ability to detect the absence of disease when the disease is truly absent (i.e., true negative). Tests with high specificity are useful in confirming that a patient has the disease. Both concepts are discussed in detail in Chapter 7. By using this technique, a cutoff score can be created for the outcome of interest (in our examples, the Foot and Ankle Ability Measure or fitness level) that corresponds with improvement on the anchor measure (e.g., the global rating of change). The challenge is finding a cutoff that balances a good sensitivity value with a good specificity value. You will see in Chapter 7 that a test may have good sensitivity but poor specificity or vice versa.

Distribution-Based Approach

The distribution-based approach uses measures such as the standard error of the measure, minimal detectable change, and effect size (standardized mean difference; see Chapter 9) to identify the minimal important difference. This approach differs from the others in that it examines how the target outcome varies from normal values, and it relies less on the patient's perception of improvement on an anchor measure. However, in most cases establishing minimal important difference, this way is based on previous studies using anchor approaches. Research supports that the minimal important difference is typically equal to 0.5 standard deviations of the target measure (Norman, Sloan, & Wyrwich, 2003). In other words, if a patient's score on the target outcome (e.g., the Foot and Ankle Ability Measure) improves by 0.5 standard deviations, the patient will perceive this as an important change in health-related quality of life. This general rule seems to apply across a variety of different outcomes.

Interpreting the minimal important difference is straightforward. Using the Foot and Ankle Ability Measure example of the minimal important difference of 74, any patient who reached this value while undergoing treatment would be judged to have had important improvement. This does not mean that the treatment should be stopped, only that the treatment has had an effect. Conversely, if your treatment does not reach this value within a reasonable amount of time, then a change in treatment may be warranted.

Social Comparison Approach

The social comparison approach is one in which patients are paired (Copay et al., 2007). In this rarely used approach, patients discuss their condition and compare themselves to each other. The minimal important difference is the difference in scores between pairs of patients who identify as a "little better" or a "little worse" versus pairs who identify themselves as "about the same."

Minimal Clinical Important Difference

Minimal clinical important difference (MCID) is the amount of change in a measure that represents an important change to the practitioner and maybe the patient. It is very similar to minimal important difference, and the two are often used interchangeably. This is probably because the methods for deriving the minimal clinical important difference are identical to those for deriving the minimal important difference. The dissimilarity is conceptual rather than methodological. The key is understanding the meaning of the term "clinical." In this context, clinical refers to anchor measures that have meaning to the clinician and maybe the patient (Revicki, Hays, Cella, & Sloan, 2008). Life expectancy is one example. It is known that high blood pressure is a risk factor for stroke, and stroke may cause death, and it is understood that decreasing blood pressure to normal levels reduces the risk of stroke. Thus, it may be important to know the minimal change in blood pressure that causes an increase in life expectancy. Unlike the minimal important difference, the minimal clinically important difference is not developed from anchor measures that the patient can report directly (e.g., global well-being as measured by the global rating of change). Rather, the minimal clinical important difference is anchored to measures such as decreases in the occurrence of strokes, heart attacks, and death or increases in longevity. To emphasize, minimal clinical important differences may be important to the patient, but they cannot be directly reported by the patient (i.e., a patient cannot tell what his or her blood pressure is; it has to be measured).

Minimal clinical important difference (MCID): The smallest amount of change in an outcome that represents an important change to the clinician and maybe the patient.

The outcomes may be of interest only to the practitioner, because the practitioner recognizes a relationship that the patient does not. We know that ankle instability is associated with poor balance. It could be hypothesized that poor strength leads to poor balance. Thus, a clinician may be interested in the minimal clinical important difference of strength needed to improve balance. In this case, having better balance may not be something directly reported by the patient or valued by the patient. Conversely, the clinician understands an important clinical connection between poor strength and poor balance, which relates to ankle stability. Because this set of relationships is important to the clinician but not necessarily to the patient, the preferred usage is minimal clinical important difference rather than minimal important difference.

Because they are calculated the same way, interpreting the minimal clinical important difference is identical to interpreting the minimal important difference. The only dissimilarity between the measures is the conceptual differences of being important to the patient (minimal important difference) or to the practitioner and maybe the patient (minimal clinical important difference).

Responsiveness

Another important property of outcomes is **responsiveness**. Simply stated, responsiveness is an outcome's ability to change when it is expected to change. For example, we would expect a measure of strength to increase across time in a group of people who were strength training. If the measure did not change across time, it would have little value and be considered unresponsive.

Interpretability

Interpretability is defined as its ability to assign qualitative meaning to a quantitative score (Eechaute, Vaes, VanAerschot, Asman, & Duquet, 2007). Back pain is an example. How much reduction in back pain is needed to allow some patients to return to work? A change in pain has little meaning by itself. However, when the quantitative measure can be translated into the context of everyday life, the outcome becomes relevant and interpretable.

Floor and Ceiling Effects

Floor effect and **ceiling effect** are defined as a measure's inability to distinguish among subjects at the extreme ends of the scale. Floor and ceiling effects are conceptually the same, but they occur at either the top (ceiling) or bottom (floor) of a scale.

Pros and Cons 4-1

The minimal important difference is important to the practitioner and the patient because it is a measure that indicates health or injury status in terms of the patient's perspective. However, improvement from the patient's perspective does not necessarily indicate a change in outcome (e.g., balance or strength). The minimal clinical important difference does inform the practitioner about these changes. When working with patients or clients, it is best to use a combination of these measures to obtain the most complete picture.

Responsiveness: An outcome's ability to change when it is expected to change.

Interpretability: The ability to assign qualitative meaning to a quantitative score.

Floor effect: A measurement error indicating that the measurement scale range is too narrow, and very low data points cluster at the bottom end of the scale.

Ceiling effect: A measurement error indicating that the outcome scale range is too narrow, and very high data points cluster at the top end of the scale.

For example, the Foot and Ankle Ability Measure has a ceiling effect. When uninjured subjects complete the Foot and Ankle Ability Measure, they usually have a perfect or nearly perfect score. Thus, the Foot and Ankle Ability Measure poorly distinguishes (or discriminates) among subjects without injury. This means that the Foot and Ankle Ability Measure has limited use in quantifying ankle health in uninjured subjects. Conversely, subjects with injured ankles tend to have scores that spread out along the scale, thus making the scale more useful in injured subjects.

SUMMARY

Different outcomes have different qualities, and not all of them are equal. Thus, it is important to understand several different properties of outcomes. An outcome's reliability simply refers to its repeatability. Reliability comes in different forms, and each form is specific to the outcome's purpose. Validity is a second quality of outcomes, and it refers to an outcome's ability to measure what it purports to measure accurately. Although reliability does not guarantee validity, the lack of reliability compromises an outcome's validity. There are several types of validity, but criterion validity is most often used in exercise science and health care. Reliability and validity are hallmarks for all outcomes. However, some outcomes have additional qualities related to how they are applied in the professional settings. These include properties such as the minimal detectable change, minimal important change, responsiveness, interpretability, and floor and ceiling effects. These properties are important to understand so that the outcomes may be applied to the patient or client.

CRITICAL THINKING QUESTIONS

1. When summarizing data, which measures of central tendency and of variability are best?

2. What is the difference between the standard error and the standard error of the measure?

3. If you had to pick one, which is more foundational to a quality measure reliability or validity?

4. Which are more useful to you as a practitioner, the reliability and validity of an outcome or the clinimetric properties?

5. Why are there different types of reliability and validity

■ **TRUST AND APPLY**

Ditroilo, M., Forte, R., McKeown, D., Boreham, C., & De Vito, G. (2011). Intra- and inter-session reliability of vertical jump performance in healthy middle-aged and older men and women. *Journal of Sports Sciences, 29*(15), 1675-1682.

Locate the foregoing article, and using this article, address the following questions:

1. Which of the outcomes was the most reliable? Was this different for men and women?

2. Were intrasession or intersession measures more reliable? Was this different for men and women?

3. Select one of the outcomes, and interpret the amount of change needed for the change to be considered a real difference.

4. In this article the standard error of the measure was not reported. Using the intraclass correlation coefficient and standard deviation, calculate the standard error of the measure.

5. Compare the formula for the minimal detectable change used in this chapter with the minimal detectable change formula used in the article. How are they the same or different? Is there another formula in this chapter that matches the formula used in this paper?

■ **RESEARCH SCAVENGER HUNT**

1. Using an outcome of interest:
   ● Locate an article that assesses that outcome's reliability and validity.

Then answer the following questions:

   A. What type of reliability was assessed?

   B. Was the reliability high or low?

   C. Was the standard error of the measure calculated for the outcome? If not, calculate the standard error of the measure.

   D. Was the minimal detectable change calculated for the outcome? If not, calculate the minimal detectable change and the 95% confidence interval for the minimal detectable change.

2. Using an outcome of interest:
   ● Locate an article that assesses that outcome's clinimetric properties.

Then answer the following questions:

   A. Using Table 4-4, how many of the clinimetric properties were assessed?

   B. Based on the clinimetric properties that were reported, would you use this outcome in your practice? If so, how?

REFERENCES

Copay, A. G., Subach, B. R., Glassman, S. D., Polly, D. W., & Schuler, T. C. (2007). Understanding the minimum clinically important difference: A review of concepts and methods. *Spine Journal, 7*(5), 541-546.

Eechaute, C., Vaes, P., VanAerschot, L., Asman, S., & Duquet, W. (2007). The clinimetric qualities of patient-assessed instruments for measuring chronic ankle instability: A systematic review. *BMC Musculoskeletal Disorders, 8,* 6-6.

Grotle, M., Garratt, A. M., Jenssen, H. K., & Stuge, B. (2012). Reliability and construct validity of self-report questionnaires for patients with pelvic girdle pain. *Physical Therapy, 92*(1), 111-123.

Guyatt, G. H., Nogradi, S., Halcrow, S., Singer, J., Sullivan, M. J., & Fallen, E. L. (1989). Development and testing of a new measure of health status for clinical trials in heart failure. *Journal of General Internal Medicine, 4*(2), 101-107.

Janz, K. F., Lutuchy, E. M., Wenthe, P., & Levy, S. M. (2008). Measuring activity in children and adolescents using self-report: PAQ-C and PAQ-A. *Medicine and Science in Sports and Exercise, 40*(4), 767-772.

Lubans, D. R., Morgan, P., Callister, R., Plotnikoff, R. C., Eather, N., Riley, N., Smith, C. J. (2014). Test-retest reliability of a battery of field-based health-related fitness measures for adolescents. *Journal of Sports Sciences, 29*(7), 685-693.

Norman, G. R., Sloan, J. A., & Wyrwich, K. W. (2003). Interpretation of changes in health-related quality of life: The remarkable universality of half a standard deviation. *Medical Care, 41*(5), 582-592.

Revicki, D., Hays, R. D., Cella, D., & Sloan, J. (2008). Recommended methods for determining responsiveness and minimally important differences for patient-reported outcomes. *Journal of Clinical Epidemiology, 61*(2), 102-109.

Roth, S. M. (2012). Critical overview of applications of genetic testing in sport talent identification. *Recent Patents on DNA & Gene Sequences 6*(3), 247-255.

Establishing Cause and Effect

The evidence that you will use in your professional practice is created by researchers using tried and true practices; these practices are known as the scientific method. Within the scientific method, true experimental designs have features that allow you to assume that causes and effects are linked; without these features, the relationship between cause and effect cannot be distinguished from chance events (see Chapter 5). These experimental designs can further be refined into clinical trials, which use specific methods of planning and interpretation to maximize their application to professional practice.

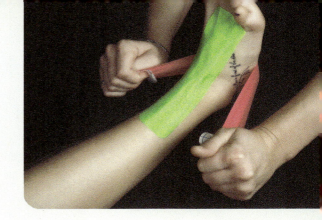

5

Experimental Research

Where Have You Been?

Chapter 4 focused on the properties of outcomes, with a strong emphasis on describing reliability. Reliability can take on many forms, but the most common form encountered in health care and exercise science is test-retest reliability. Relatedly, Chapter 4 discussed ways in which outcomes are used in the clinical setting and the value of knowing the clinimetric properties of outcomes. Finally, that chapter addressed the concepts of accuracy, bias, and validity. Without reliable and valid outcomes, the foundation of research is weak. Thus, the hallmark of any line of research is establishing that the outcomes to be used are reliable and valid and measure qualities that are important.

Where Are You Going?

The concept of validity is not limited to outcomes. As you will see, validity also applies to experiments. This chapter addresses the structures and methods used in experimental research. It discusses different options a researcher has in designing an experiment, as well as the three types of validity associated with experiments: internal, construct, and external. Each of these is important in different ways, and each determines the degree to which research results can be trusted and applied to your own set of circumstances. The content of this chapter lays the groundwork for understanding how to categorize evidence into the levels previously discussed. It addresses the strengths and weaknesses of the typical research designs so you can distinguish good research designs from poor designs.

Learning Outcomes

After reading this chapter, you should be able to answer these questions:

1. What is an experiment?
2. How is cause-and-effect established?
3. Do the research results apply to my situation?
4. What is meant by "experimental validity"?
5. How does the experiment fit into the levels of evidence?

Key Terms

Confounder
Construct
Construct validity
Control group
Dependent variable

Experimental research
Experimental group
External validity
Independent variable
Internal validity

Quasi-experimental research
Random assignment
Random sampling
Threat

Experimental research is one of the most common forms of research encountered in exercise science. It is often considered synonymous with laboratory research. Although much laboratory research *is* experimental, as you will see, it is frequently nonexperimental as well. The classic definition of an *experiment* is research with at least two separate groups. One of the groups must serve as the **control group**, which receives no treatment or a standard treatment. The other serves as the **experimental group** and must receive a treatment that is different from that of the control group. The groups must be formed by **random assignment** of subjects. Research designs that do not meet these criteria are not true experimental designs and are defined as nonexperimental or quasi-experimental, depending on the structure of the design. Examples of these types are given later.

◼ THE BASIC EXPERIMENTAL DESIGN

Let us assume you are interested in conducting one of two different experiments. In the first experiment, you want to know whether a particular strength training program improves strength. People volunteering for the experiment would be randomly assigned to the training group (experimental group) or to the control group. The control group would continue with normal daily activities without strength training, and the experimental group would participate in strength training. In the second experiment, you want to know whether ice, compression, elevation, and electrical stimulation (experimental group) reduce swelling from an ankle sprain better than the standard treatment of ice, compression, and elevation (control group). Ideally, the control group would receive no treatment; however, withholding all treatment would be unethical in this case. Thus, the control group would receive the standard treatment. This type of standard treatment control group is common in clinical trials.

The main purpose of a true experimental design is to establish *cause and effect*. More specifically, you want to know whether an independent variable causes change in a dependent variable. By definition, an **independent variable** is a variable that the researcher controls, and the **dependent variable** is the outcome that is measured. In your first experiment, strength training would be the independent variable, and some measure of strength (e.g., one-repetition maximum) would be the dependent variable. In our second experiment, the treatments would be your independent variable, and a measure of swelling (e.g., ankle volume) would be the dependent measure. Changes in a dependent variable must always follow the independent variable in time, to establish cause and effect. In most experiments, the dependent variable is measured at least twice, once

Experimental research: Method of research in which the researcher manipulates variables. An experiment classically conducts tests on two randomly assigned groups, a control group and an experimental group, and compares the different outcomes of the tests for each group. Also called true experimental design.

Control group: In a true experimental design, this group (arm) receives no treatment or receives standard treatment. This group can be compared with the treatment or experimental group. Also called a control.

Experimental group: In a clinical investigation, a group that receives a treatment that is different from that of the control group.

Random assignment: A method used to place subjects in groups based on a random process, rather than based on some personal characteristics or by personal choice. The intent of random assignment is to create equal groups.

Connections 5-1
As seen later, experimental designs in clinical research are also known as *randomized controlled trials.*

Independent variable: In a research study, the variable that the research controls.

Dependent variable: In a research study, the outcome that is measured.

before the treatment and once after the treatment. For example, you can measure strength before and after the strength training program. Because you are interested in the change in strength from the strength training, this measurement must be taken before (baseline) and after. Change can occur only *after* the treatment.

◼ INTERNAL VALIDITY OF RESEARCH

As previously indicated, the purpose of experimental research is to establish cause and effect. To do that, an experiment must have internal validity. If a study is internally valid, then confounders (i.e., alternative explanations) for the cause and effect have been eliminated as much as possible. The best way to understand internal validity is to understand the *threats* to internal validity and ways in which we can eliminate those threats.

Threats

A threat to validity (internal or otherwise) is anything that potentially confuses or confounds the results of research. To achieve the goal of experimental research of establishing cause and effect, these threats must be identified, understood, and minimized. The threats to internal validity are described next.

Selection Bias

Selection refers to the way in which subjects are assigned to either the treatment group or the control group. In experiments, subjects are randomly assigned, or *randomized.* Random assignment occurs when subjects are placed in groups based on a random process, rather than assigned to groups based on some personal characteristics (e.g., body weight) or by personal choice. Assume for your strength experiment that you allowed subjects to choose groups. One possible result is that highly motivated people who wanted to be stronger would sign up for the strength training group, whereas less motivated people would likely pick the control group. At the end of the experiment, the subjects in the training group would be stronger than those in the control group. However, you would not know whether the difference between groups was the result of the training, the subjects' motivation, or some combination of the two. Thus, the cause-and-effect relationship would be confounded by motivation. By randomly assigning subjects to groups, the presumption is that, on average, motivation (and other factors) will be equal across both groups; therefore, any strength differences found will be caused by the training.

Internal validity: The degree to which a researcher controls or eliminates all extraneous variables, including cofounders, of a study.

Confounder: An extraneous variable that affects the outcomes that are being studied such that the test results do not reflect the actual relationship between the outcomes that are under investigation. A variable that the researcher fails to control or eliminate such that it damages the internal validity of an experiment. Also called confounding variable or third variable.

Threat: Any factor that potentially confuses or confounds the results of research.

A similar situation could exist for the ankle treatment study. If electric stimulation were believed to be especially beneficial for severe ankle sprains, participants with more severe sprains would therefore be assigned to the group receiving the stimulation. As a result, participants with less severe sprains would receive the standard treatment. Now consider that the participants with more severe sprains had more swelling and thus had more room for improvement. At the end of the study, the group receiving stimulation would likely have improved the most, but, as a researcher, you would have to ask yourself whether this result occurred because the participants had more swelling or because the stimulation was beneficial. It is impossible to know which of these is true. If the groups were randomized, the severity of injury would likely be evenly distributed across both groups. In this case, any benefit seen by the stimulation group could be attributed to the treatment.

History

History refers to any event that occurs during a study that may have caused a difference between groups. Similar to selection bias, it is controlled by random assignment. For example, for the ankle sprain study, subjects with more severe sprains may self-medicate with pain relievers that are also anti-inflammatory agents. The result could be a more rapid decline in inflammation and swelling among those participants. If all the participants with severe sprains were purposely assigned to the stimulation group, the use of anti-inflammatory agents could make it appear that the stimulation treatment worked when, in fact, the anti-inflammatory agents would have been responsible for the improvement in condition. Regardless of the specific history effect, random assignment to groups generally helps to equalize these effects across both groups.

Maturation

Maturation occurs when subjects naturally change across time. It is controlled for by the inclusion of a control group. The clearest examples are studies that involve children. If the strength training study involved children, you could reasonably expect that the children would grow stronger with age. Without the control group of students of similar age, you could confuse this natural change with the effects of the strength training. Similarly, in the other experiment, even if you do nothing, ankle sprains are expected to improve with time. Thus, without a control group, you could not possibly know whether the electrical stimulation added any benefit over the standard treatment or whether the improvement was the result of the natural course of time.

Regression

Regression is the tendency of extreme scores to move back toward the average score. It is a natural phenomenon that occurs when subjects are selected based on extreme scores. For example, assume for the strength training study that subjects were selected from a larger pool of subjects and that the subjects selected were those who performed the worst on the one-repetition maximum test (i.e., they were the weakest). With or without strength training, their one-repetition maximum scores would improve the next time they were measured. The reason for this is that measures are imperfect. Every measure contains error, and the size of that error varies randomly. Extreme scores are most likely caused by high error at the time of measurement. This effect tends to make low scores lower than expected and high scores higher than expected. When a measure is taken a second time, the error tends to be smaller, thus resulting in a score change that moves toward the mean. This change can be mistaken for a treatment effect.

In clinical studies, regression can occur when subjects are allowed to self-select to participate in research. For example, patients with arthritis are likely to seek help when their arthritis is at its worst. However, these same people are likely to feel better because symptoms tend to regress back to normal levels.

You should be aware that regression also operates across measures taken simultaneously. For example, if subjects with ankle sprain are selected based on large amounts of swelling, pain scores measured at the same time are unlikely to be equally high. That is not to say that people with extreme swelling will not have a great amount of pain; they may. Rather, the people with the most extreme swelling are not likely to be the people with the most extreme pain. Thus, selecting subjects based on extreme scores on one measure does not mean that subjects will have extreme findings on all measures.

Regression can be combated at least two ways. First, subjects selected for their extreme scores should be randomly assigned to groups. Doing this distributes the effects of regression to both groups. Second, because regression is largely a measurement phenomenon, using outcomes that are very reliable will minimize the effects of regression.

Attrition

Attrition refers to subjects dropping out of a study. One reason attrition is important is that differences between small groups are harder to find than differences between large groups. In addition, if more subjects drop out of one group than the other, the results of the research could be affected. For example, in the strength training study, subjects may drop out of the study if they find the strength training too demanding. If too many subjects drop out, it may appear that the training did not work, even though it did. Similarly, subjects with relatively minor ankle sprains may decide that the treatment regimen is too onerous and drop out of the study. Because of the attrition, minor sprains would be overrepresented in one of the groups, and the results of the study could be affected.

As with most of the other threats, random assignment helps to reduce this effect. However, in the case of attrition, random assignment may not always solve the problem. Even if mild and severe ankle sprains are equally represented in the control and treatment groups, attrition can significantly change the experiment. For example, if all the participants with minor sprains dropped out of the study, leaving only those with severe sprains, the results would no longer be valid for ankle sprains in general; instead, the results would be restricted to severe sprains. Although the results could still reveal an important finding, as a practitioner, you must be mindful of how attrition can change the initial purpose and meaning of a research study and that attrition can be an outcome in itself.

Testing Effects

Testing effects refer to the way in which test scores or performance can change because of a subject's interaction with the test. Testing effects occur when the same test is done repeatedly. For example, with the strength study, having someone perform a one-repetition maximum on the first day means that this person will likely perform better on subsequent days even without strength training because of practicing the procedure.

One way to account for this effect is to have both the control and treatment groups do the exact same testing protocol, including practice. Although this step does not eliminate the testing effect, it does ensure that the testing effect is consistent across both groups. Alternatively, testing effects can be minimized by having long periods between testing. If your training study tested strength only before and after a 12-week training program, the testing effect would be unlikely to have an important impact on the final result.

One thing to keep in mind is that repeated testing does not necessarily expose an experiment to testing effects. For example, if you measure ankle swelling by using water displacement, this method is not a measure that subjects can improve by repeated testing. In this case, the testing effect would be nonexistent.

Most testing effects are expected to *improve* test performance. However, this is not always the case. For example, when testing physical performance, fatigue from repeated testing can have a detrimental effect. There is more than one way to combat fatigue effects, but the most effective way is to use appropriate rest inter- vals. Fatigue is a short-term effect and is not a concern when tests are completed several minutes or hours apart. However, if the one- repetition maximum test used in the strength training study was repeated multiple times with short rest intervals, strength could actually decline during the testing. This effect could result in a lower one-repetition maximum, thus making the strength training appear more potent than it actually is.

Instrumentation

Instrumentation effects refer to changes in the instruments during the course of the study. These effects can take a couple of different forms. For example, different weight scales could have different calibrations or a weight scale's calibration could change over time; thus, a person's recorded weight could change because of the scale's calibration, not the experiment. With measures that require the examiner to be skilled, a change over time could be the result of the examiner's improved skills. For example, one way to meas- ure ankle swelling is with circumference measures. This method requires the examiner to place the tape measure across the correct anatomical landmarks. With practice, the examiner would likely become more proficient at this procedure, thus improving accu- racy. This change in accuracy could mistakenly be interpreted as the result of the treatment.

One way to negate this threat is to use the same equipment throughout a study. Different measurement devices (e.g., weight scales) may have different calibrations, so changing measurement devices during the course of a study can affect the results. For the same reason, the same equipment should be used for all groups. This way the calibration remains the same across groups. Finally, when possible, the calibration of equipment should be checked periodi- cally. The required frequency of this inspection depends on the equipment and the stability of its calibration. Human testers should have adequate training and practice before the start of a study and should be periodically tested to confirm their accuracy and consistency.

Threat Combinations

More than one of the previously discussed threats can exist simul- taneously. Sometimes the effects may partially, or totally, cancel each other out. However, these combined threats may also add together, similar to adding $3 + 4 = 7$. In this case, the result is larger than either single threat alone. However, if the threats interact (i.e., are multiplicative), the result can be much larger than the threats individually, just as $3 \times 4 = 12$.

One possible threat combination is selection-attrition. For example, for the ankle experiment, imagine creating the two groups with all the severe ankle sprains in one group and all the mild ankle sprains in the second group. The severe sprain group would have more tissue damage (i.e., selection) and thus would be more likely to have greater swelling than the mild sprain group. Additionally, assume that the severe sprain group has two unidentified subgroups, very severe and moderate, and assume that moderate sprains heal faster than very severe sprains. Because of this fast healing, subjects may elect to drop out of the study earlier and at a higher rate (i.e., attrition). The likely result of this combination of attrition and selection would be that the participants with the most severe sprains would remain in the study. Consequently, the severe sprain group would become even more extreme. Moreover, because more severe sprains are likely to take more time to heal, this combination could make the treatment appear less effective than it really is.

Expectancy

Another threat to internal validity is expectancy. It can apply to the subject in the study, as well as to the experimenter. For instance, if an investigator was studying the effects of two different vertical jump training programs, bias could be unconsciously induced based on the hypothesis that one training program is better than the other. This bias could occur at the time of the intervention or during testing of the outcome.

To control for expectancy, research designs often use placebos and blinding. A placebo is a "treatment" given to the control group that increases the similarity between the control group and the experimental group, but it still allows the groups to be different on the independent variable. Suppose a supplement manufacturer wants to test a product that is expected to increase 400-m running performance. In this case, the subjects could be randomly assigned to an experimental group or a control group. Both groups would ingest a product, but the control group would be taking a placebo that is similar to the real supplement in all ways (such as taste and appearance). The only difference between these two products would be the presence of the active ingredient.

Even in animal studies, investigators often use "sham" surgical procedures or treatments to make sure the animals are treated the same way except for the independent variable. This may include inert implants, or even just making sure that both groups of animals spend the same amount of time being handled by the investigators or in a certain environment.

Blinding a design occurs when either the investigator or the research participant does not know which group to which the participant is assigned. In the supplement example mentioned previously, the research participants would not know who is in the supplement group or who is in the placebo group. If the investigators were also blinded to the group membership, it would be a double-blind study. In the vertical jump training study, the participants would likely know that they are in a given training group that is different from the other, but the testers can be blinded to the group membership to help control for expectancy.

▣ ELEMENTS OF CONTROL

As previously mentioned, experiments have two key elements of control. The first is the control group and the second is random assignment. To have a true experiment, both must exist.

Control Group

As described in the section on threats to internal validity, a control group is important to serve as a baseline for comparison. In theory, whatever history, maturation, or attrition effects occur in an experiment will be the same for both groups. Thus, the control group provides a standard against which the treatment group can be compared. For example, assume you are interested in the effects of exercise on childhood obesity. You put the children on an exercise program and measure body composition before and after the exercise program. As expected, at the end of the exercise program, the children's body composition changes. However, did this change occur because of the exercise or because the children matured over the course of the study? If no control group is used for comparison, you will not know because you have two competing explanations. A control group eliminates maturation as a competing explanation, or confounder.

Random Assignment

Random assignment is the second element of experimental control. As previously indicated, *random assignment* refers to the way in which the experimental and control groups are selected. Through random assignment, every subject in an experiment has an equal opportunity to be in either group. The intent of random assignment is to equalize the groups. For example, if ankle sprain severity (mild versus severe) results in different attrition rates, randomly assigning participants with ankle sprains to the treatment and control groups should result in equal numbers of severe and mild sprains in each group. Thus, in theory, the two groups would be equal in overall severity.

You should be aware that, just because random assignment is used, equality of the two groups is not guaranteed. For example, a coin has two sides; thus, with each coin toss, the probability of turning up heads is 50%. If you toss a coin 10 times, you would expect to have five heads and five tails. However, if you have ever tried tossing a coin in this way, you know that it is possible to have three heads and seven tails or some combination other than five and five. In any of these other cases, the two groups would not be equal. This result is frequently described as a failure of randomization. On the contrary, however, it is a normal result of randomization. Although beyond the scope of this discussion, this imbalance in randomization can be partially accounted for in the statistical analyses used to test hypotheses.

RESEARCH DESIGNS

Research designs can be placed into basic categories. Not every one of the designs in a given category controls internal validity equally; some do it better than others. A list of designs and examples of their structure are provided in Table 5–1.

Pre-experimental Research Designs

To be an experiment, random assignment and control groups are required. Pre-experimental designs have neither. The basic pre-experimental design is the one group posttest design, or "one-shot" design (Fig. 5–1). In this design, one group is given an experimental treatment and is assessed after the treatment to determine whether a change occurred. For example, you could treat someone with an ankle sprain with ice and compression and determine whether that person improved after the treatment. In this case, the assumption is that the change occurred in close proximity to the treatment, meaning that the treatment must be the cause. Nevertheless, it should be quite obvious that it is impossible to know what really caused the posttreatment change, and this design is never used in the scientific literature.

Another flaw of the one-shot design is that most measures require some type of a baseline to know whether change has occurred. For example, to know whether a person's strength has changed, you really need to know what his or her strength level was before training. One way to improve the design is to add a pretreatment measure (i.e., pretest) before the treatment followed by a posttreatment measure (i.e., posttest) (Fig. 5–2). Now you have a reference to determine change. However, this design also fails to control the threats to internal validity because it has no control group.

Table 5–1 Summary of Pre-experimental, Experimental, and Quasi-experimental Designs											
Name	**Group**			**Design**							
Pre-experimental											
One-shot	Treatment					T	O				
One group pretest-posttest	Treatment				O	T	O				
Static two-group comparison	Treatment					T	O				
	Comparison						O				
Experimental											
Randomized two-group	Treatment	R				T	O				
	Control	R					O				
Randomized three-group	Treatment 1	R				T_a	O				
	Treatment 2	R				T_b	O				
	Control	R					O				
Randomized two-group pretest-posttest	Treatment	R		O		T	O				
	Control	R		O			O				
Randomized two-group crossover	Group 1	R		O		Ta	O	Tb	O		
	Group 2	R		O		Tb	O	Ta	O		
Quasi-experimental											
Nonequivalent control group	Treatment			O		T	O				
	Comparison			O			O				
Time series	O	O	O	O	T	O	O	O	O	O	O

O, observation; R, randomized; T, treatment.

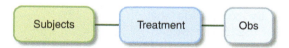

Figure 5–1 The one-shot design. (Obs = Observation)

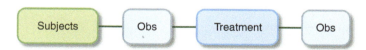

Figure 5–2 The one-shot pre-post design. (Obs = Observation).

Although neither of these designs should be used for an experiment, it is worth noting that this is how people commonly understand their daily experiences. For example, you have a headache (pretest). You take an aspirin (treatment). Your headache goes away (posttest). You conclude that the aspirin worked. Did it?

Maybe you also took a nap and the nap caused you to relax, which made the headache go away. In this simple example, knowing what made the headache go away is clearly impossible. It was probably the aspirin, but without a true experimental design, you cannot be certain. Nevertheless, this is a good example of how people conduct experiments in their normal lives, and these types of designs can give you a starting point for more appropriate designs.

A design that more closely approximates a true experimental design is the ex-post facto, or static two-group design (Fig. 5–3). In this design, groups are formed after some group has received the treatment. For example, patients entering a clinic for ankle rehabilitation may receive electrical stimulation treatment from clinician A, whereas patients seen by clinician B do not receive electrical stimulation. After completion of therapy, the two groups are compared. As you could guess, one of the confounders in this study would be treatment differences related to the different clinicians rather than the use of electrical stimulation.

True Experimental Designs

True experimental designs are the only designs that can unequivocally establish cause and effect. These designs can take on a couple of different forms, but all include random assignment to one or more treatment groups and a control group. The basic design includes two groups with a posttest measure (Fig. 5–4). This measure allows direct comparison of the treatment with the control. A more advanced design is a two-group design that includes a pretest (Fig. 5–5). This is probably the most commonly used design in health-care and exercise science. By comparing the groups' pretests, one can assess whether the two groups differ on subject characteristics or the dependent variable. By comparing the groups' posttests, one can determine whether the treatment had an effect. By comparing the pretest and posttest of the control group, one can determine whether history or maturation affected

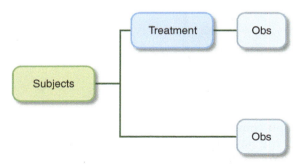

Figure 5–3 The static two-group design. (Obs = Observation).

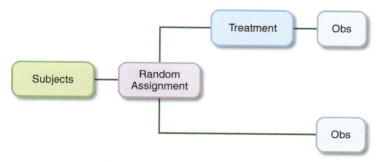

Figure 5–4 The random two-group design. (Obs = Observation).

the result (but not which one). Finally, by comparing the pretest and posttest of the experimental group, one can quantify the magnitude of the change the treatment produced. As you can see, simply adding a pretest increases the information available to the researcher.

One of the shortcomings of the pretest-posttest design is the testing threat to internal validity. Recall that a pretest can sensitize subjects to the testing in a way that makes them perform differently on a posttest. In exercise science, this is not always the case. For example, measuring ankle swelling before treatment is not likely to affect the posttest measure of swelling. Similarly, because of the length of a typical strength training program, a pretest measure of strength is not likely to affect the posttest. However, as a consumer of research, you need to be mindful of these possibilities and assess their effect on a study's results.

For simplicity, the examples previously described involved only one treatment group. However, both the previously discussed designs can be extended to two or more treatment groups. The number of groups used depends on the purpose of the research and the resources available. Using more groups means having more subjects and using more resources, such as supplies, equipment, time,

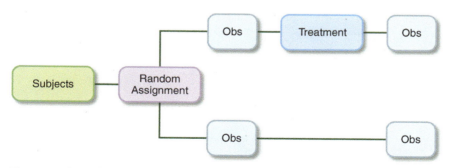

Figure 5–5 The random two-group design with a pretest. (Obs = Observation).

and so on. Therefore, although using more groups is sometimes possible, it is not always pragmatic.

Crossover Designs

Another alternative to the basic experimental design is the crossover design seen in Figure 5–6. In this design, all subjects receive all treatments. For example, in the ankle study, subjects would be divided into two groups. Group one would receive the standard treatment; group two would receive the experimental treatment. After the treatment, both groups would be measured for changes in swelling. Subsequently, each group would receive the opposite treatment and then be measured for swelling again. Thus, both groups would be "crossed over" to the other treatment.

This design works only when treatments do not have permanent effects. For example, if the first treatment in the ankle study produced a permanent change in ankle swelling, then the second treatment would not likely produce additional improvement. When treatments do not produce permanent effects, the crossover design is a very efficient design. It allows both treatments to be tested on more subjects, thus allowing for more confidence in the results.

Quasi-experimental Designs

Another type of research found in exercise science and other clinical professions is that using **quasi-experimental research** designs. These designs have a variety of forms, but the most commonly used designs in health-care and exercise science are described here. These designs can be very important in understanding intact or naturally occurring groups. However, naturally occurring groups often differ in many ways, not just on the characteristic of interest. For example, if you divide participants with

Pros and Cons 5-1

Experimental designs are ideal for establishing cause and effect. They allow for tight control of confounding factors. However, the more control you have, the less likely the experiment will look like the real world.

Pros and Cons 5-2

Crossover designs are very efficient. They allow multiple treatments to be studied with fewer subjects than true experiments. However, these designs risk having one treatment interact with the second if insufficient time is allowed between treatments. They also are not useful when treatments effects are permanent.

Quasi-experimental research: Method of research similar to experimental research except without the random assignment to groups. Also called quasi-experimental design.

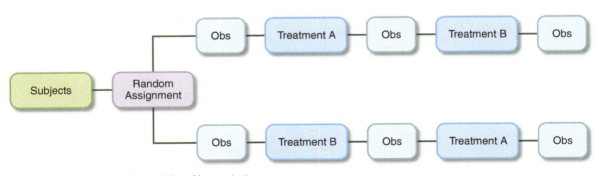

Figure 5–6 The crossover design. (Obs = Observation).

ankle sprains into severe and mild groups, you have to be aware that the mechanism of injury of severe sprains may be different from that of mild sprains. It may also be the case that people with severe sprains may participate in more hazardous sports (e.g., football). Thus, the category of severe sprains is actually very complex and may represent factors other than what you would define as injury severity. Furthermore, these other factors may be more influential than the characteristic of interest. For this reason, determining cause and effect is often difficult or impossible with these designs.

Nonequivalent Control Group Design

A nonequivalent control group design looks like a true experiment, but it lacks random assignment to groups (Fig. 5–7). Thus, instead of having a control group, it has a comparison group. This design is different from the static two-group design in that the groups are formed for a specific reason. Typically, the goal is for the two groups to be as equal as possible. For example, the strength study could be modified so that it takes place in a health club environment. In this case, clients in the morning could use free weights, and clients in the afternoon could use only machine weights. Because the groups are not randomly assigned, they cannot be presumed equal. You should also note that, unlike the static two-group design, these groups are formed before beginning the treatment, and a pretest is used. The pretest allows some assurance that, at the start, the two groups are approximately equal. If the groups are different at pretest, then this difference must be recognized as a possible confounder.

Interrupted Time-Series Design

The quasi-experimental design previously described is a variation on the experimental design. An alternative is the interrupted time-series design (Fig. 5–8). In this design, a control or comparison group

Connections 5-2

Because quasi-experimental designs do not use randomization, they are lower on the evidence pyramid.

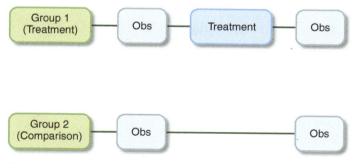

Figure 5–7 The nonequivalent control group design. (Obs = Observation).

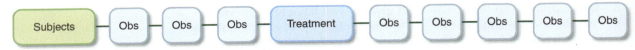

Figure 5–8 The interrupted time-series design. (Obs = Observation).

may or may not be used. The typical time-series design does not use a comparison group. The basic time-series structure is for a group of subjects to be measured on a series of pretests. Once a stable baseline is established, the treatment is administered, and a sequence of posttests follows. For example, if the ankle sprain study were done as a time-series study, the subjects would undergo a period of no treatment (e.g., several days), and ankle swelling would be measured each day. By examining the data, the researcher would determine when a stable baseline was established and then initiate the treatment. Once the treatment was started, posttest swelling measures would be made daily. After a sufficient course of treatment (a concept that can be very subjective), the posttest measures would be compared with the pretest measures. Rather than standard statistical testing, the typical mode of analysis is comparison of pretest and posttest data patterns. In this example, the researcher could look for changes in swelling level or in the rate (or slope) of swelling change.

The interrupted time-series design is best used when experimental and quasi-experimental designs are not feasible. For example, the number of subjects may not be sufficient to form two groups. This design is common when studying limited populations, such as amputees. This design should not be used for mere convenience. In fact, it is commonly more challenging to employ because maintaining rigorous control can be more difficult than with group designs.

Single-Subject Designs

The final type of quasi-experimental design is the single-subject design. This design is a variation on the interrupted time-series design, and its name is somewhat of a misnomer. It follows the same pattern as the interrupted time-series design, except that a smaller number of subjects are used. In theory, this design could be used with a single subject; however, more typically, three to five subjects are used. This design is best used when a disease or pathological process is rare (e.g., high [syndesmosis] ankle sprains), thus making recruitment of a large number of subjects very difficult. These designs are also challenging to implement and maintain control on threats to internal validity. Thus, they should not be viewed as substitutes for other study designs.

Although clinicians may not realize it, single-subject designs are commonly used in clinical practice. For example, a physician notes that a patient has borderline high blood pressure. Because this is the first observation, the physician asks the patient to return in 6 months for a recheck. At the recheck, the patient's blood pressure is still high, so the physician decides to prescribe blood pressure medicine for the patient and asks the patient to follow up again in 6 months. At this recheck, the patient's blood pressure is normal. At subsequent annual physical examinations, the physician rechecks the patient's blood pressure. Without doing so intentionally, the physician has used a single-subject design to make a clinical decision. Although this example is probably common in clinical settings, note that for research purposes, at least three blood pressure observations would be required to establish a baseline before a treatment is begun. For many measures used in single-subject designs, more than three observations are required to establish a stable baseline.

CONSTRUCT VALIDITY

Up to this point, the discussion has focused on internal validity, its threats, and the remedies to those threats. However, a second type of validity, called construct validity, must also be considered. Constructs are difficult to understand conceptually. They are typically described as those entities you seek to understand but are not directly observable. Constructs are important because they connect an experiment to theory and to the language of practice (Shadish, Cook, & Campbell, 2002). For example, one construct that commonly occurs in exercise science is "the athlete." What is the definition of an athlete? If you wanted to measure a person to determine whether he or she is an athlete, how would you do that? Other examples could include the constructs "physically active," "strength," and "ankle sprain." Intuitively, you have a notion of what these constructs are. However, in science, they must be able to be defined. Often, it is necessary to use multiple measures to capture a construct. One complex construct is "quality of life." One measure commonly used for quality of life is the Short Form 36 (SF-36) (Ware & Sherbourne, 1992), a 36-item questionnaire that assesses multiple dimensions of life, including a person's ability to do work, emotional health, and ability to complete roles at home and at work. Thus, quality of life cannot be assessed with a single item, but rather as a combination of multiple items.

In any research, multiple constructs exist simultaneously:

- **Subjects:** The first construct to consider is the subjects used. Who were the subjects, and how were they defined? For example, what is the age group, activity level, ethnic breakdown, or degree of injury?

- **Setting:** The next construct commonly encountered is the setting. For example, what is meant by a clinical setting? Is it a hospital, physical therapy clinic, or athletic training room?
- **Treatment:** The third construct is the treatment (i.e., independent variable). What were the parameters for the treatment, and how was the treatment implemented? How long was the treatment applied, what was the intensity, or what was the volume?
- **Outcomes:** The final construct is the outcomes (i.e., dependent variables). How were the outcomes measured? Are they appropriate for the research question? Are they important to the group of subjects being studied?

When you encounter constructs in research, they are typically defined in one of two ways. The first is in the form of a simple description. This is common for the subjects in the study and the setting. Treatments and outcomes, however, may be described or have an operational definition. For example, the construct "biceps brachii strength" may be operationally defined as "the maximum force produced during a set of three 6-second isometric contractions at ninety degrees of elbow flexion."

As a consumer of research, your focus should be on whether these constructs match your needs. For example, is the subject pool similar to the clients or patients you normally encounter? If not, do the differences mean that research is not applicable to your clients? These same questions apply to the setting and the outcomes. The exception to these questions is the treatment construct. The definition of the treatment (i.e., the treatment construct) may be very different from your version of the treatment, but often that is the point of the research. For example, in the fictitious ankle study, maybe you do not typically use electrical stimulation. However, if the group receiving stimulation has greater improvement than the control group, this result could be a justification for you to change your treatment to the better treatment.

Fourteen threats to construct validity have been identified (Shadish, Cook, & Campbell, 2002). Some of these threats are common to exercise science and health care; others are less common. The typical threats and examples of these threats are provided in Table 5–2.

EXTERNAL VALIDITY OF RESEARCH

The final type of validity encountered in research is external validity. Like internal validity, external validity concerns the cause-and effect relationship. More specifically, it relates to whether that relationship applies across different groups of subjects, settings, treatments, or outcomes. In other words, to what extent are the results generalizable? To emphasize, internal

---

The Critical Consumer 5-2
Construct validity is commonly ignored. However, as a consumer, this concept should be very important to you. If the measures, treatments, subjects, and so forth are not defined correctly, then they will have little applicability to your clinical needs.

External validity: The degree to which the results of a study can be generalized to other groups of subjects, settings, treatments, or outcomes.

Table 5–2 Common Threats to Construct Validity	
Threat	**Example**
Inadequate definition of construct	Defining "ankle sprain" as "an injury to the ankle" may be inadequate because the pathological process may be medial ligament damage or lateral ligament damage.
Construct confounding	Defining strength as the maximum force produced by a muscle would be the result of two related (i.e., confounding) constructs: the ability to produce muscle tension and the cross-sectional area of the muscle.
Mono-operation bias	Assessing the effectiveness of a training program using only strength measurements is limiting. It may be that adding measures of muscle power to strength measures would be a better assessment of the program.
Monomethod bias	Measuring health with only physiological measures, such as blood pressure, blood cholesterol, and body fat, is limiting. Alternatively, paper-and-pencil measures of quality of life could be added.
Reactive self-report	If subjects know they are being assigned to groups, they may purposely alter pretest self-report measures (i.e., questionnaires) to have a better chance of entering their preferred group.
Compensatory rivalry	If subjects know which group they have been assigned to (i.e., treatment or control), the groups may compete for better performance. This can be remedied by blinding the subjects to their group membership, as is typically done by using a placebo as the control condition.
Resentful demoralization	Subjects not receiving the group they desire, usually the subjects assigned to the control group, may be unhappy and thus may not perform as expected. This can be remedied by blinding the subjects to their group membership, as is typically done by using a placebo as the control condition.
Experimenter expectancies	If the experimenter expects one group to perform better than another (e.g., the experimental group versus the control group), the experimenter may apply the treatment more rigorously or be more encouraging to subjects.

validity is specific to whether the proposed cause (treatment or independent variable) produced change in the outcome (dependent variable). External validity relates to whether the treatment produces a change in the outcome if, for example, the subjects are different. Using the strength study as an example, if the subjects used were college students, the results would likely apply to college students but would not directly apply (or be generalizable) to an older population. To make the results more generalizable, you as the practitioner could consider selecting research that uses subjects who are most representative of the population with which you are concerned.

Targets of Generalization

Five "targets of generalization" have been identified (Shadish, Cook, & Campbell, 2002). These targets represent the typical ways research findings are generalized beyond a study's context.

Narrow to Broad

Narrow to broad is the typical generalization consumers of research wish to make. Do the results apply to broader conditions? This commonly means, do the results from the study population apply to the general population? It can also relate to the setting (e.g., do laboratory results apply to a real-world clinical environment?). It may also apply to the treatment (e.g., do the results from one type of strength training apply to all types of strength training?).

Broad to Narrow

Broad to narrow is often overlooked by researchers but has significant application to clinicians. The key issue is whether the research from a relatively large study (i.e., one with a large number of subjects) applies to a single person (i.e., a specific patient)? Individual patients commonly have specific characteristics that do not match the study population. These individual characteristics could mean that the response of an individual patient to a treatment will differ from that of the larger group.

At a Similar Level

This target relates to whether the results actually apply to similar population samples at the same collective level. For example, if a smoking-cessation program is found to be effective at a large western university, will it apply to a large southern university? Initially, you may not expect differences between east and west, but cultural traditions could be one reason differences exist. Many of the southern states have a rich tobacco history because this area has historically been where tobacco is grown and the tobacco companies are located. Thus, the acceptability of tobacco use may be relatively lower in the western states than it is in the southern states, and this difference could change the applicability of research findings.

Similar or Different Kind

Another common target of generalizing is applying the results with similar subjects to different subjects. Typically, researchers worry about whether results will cross over to different types of subjects. In exercise science, the classic concern is whether results found with men will apply to women and vice versa. Concern about whether results in adults will apply to children is also common. For example, can an exercise program designed for controlling adult obesity be applied to obese children? A more subtle question is whether the results apply to similar subjects. For example, does the ankle treatment work the same way for a patient treated in clinic A versus patients treated in clinic B?

Random Sample to Population

The final generalization target is rarely encountered, and it involves a concept called random sampling. In contrast to random assignment, random sampling occurs when subjects are randomly selected (i.e., sampled) from the total population. This type of sampling is rarely done because it is logistically very difficult. However, when it is done, the question arises whether the sample is in fact representative of the whole population. Just as tossing a quarter multiple times does not produce equal numbers of heads and tails, random sampling does not always result in a good representation of the population.

Random sampling: A method of randomly selecting subjects from the population to participate in a study.

Threats to External Validity

Five threats to external validity have been identified. These threats relate to whether the cause and effect apply to the targets of generalization. The five threats are listed in Table 5–3.

◼ TRADEOFFS BETWEEN INTERNAL AND EXTERNAL VALIDITY

One of the challenges of research is that internal and external validity continuums are commonly in opposition to each other. To ensure the integrity of the cause-and-effect relationship, strict controls are usually used in an experiment. For example, experiments are commonly conducted in laboratory settings, to allow the researcher to control the environment. However, as the environment becomes more controlled, it begins to look less like the real world. Unlike the laboratory, the clinical setting has many distractions for a patient that can affect treatment. For example, different clinicians may provide treatment on different days. Patients in the

Table 5–3 Threats to External Validity	
Threat	**Example**
Causal relationship varies with subjects	The results of strength training for men may not apply to women.
Causal relationship differs with treatment variations	Free-weight strength training may not produce the same results as training with machine weights.
Causal relationship differs with outcome measure	An ankle sprain treatment program may be effective in reducing swelling but may not affect range of motion.
Causal relationship differs with setting	A treatment for ankle sprains may work in an athletic training room setting but may not work in a physical therapy setting.
Causal mechanisms differ per context	A strength training program is found to improve quality of life. For athletes, this change may result from true strength increases that enhance performance. In the general population, the improvement in quality of life may result from social interactions in the health club. The same benefit from the same program occurs by different mechanisms.

real world may miss appointments, whereas in a controlled setting this may happen rarely or not at all. Similarly, a strength study done in a laboratory environment may be much more controlled than the same program in a health club setting.

Alternatively, research can be conducted in an environment very similar to the real-world environment or in the real-world environment itself. Although doing so typically improves the external validity of the study, conducting research in a real-world setting often means a loss of control. In other words, the chance that internal validity is lost increases.

There is no single solution to this problem. Often, a multistep approach is used. For example, it is often best to perform a laboratory study first, to determine whether a treatment works under ideal conditions. If it does not work, then there is no point in trying it in the real world. Conversely, if the treatment does work in the laboratory, the same protocol can then be tested in the real world. The first study establishes internal validity; the second study establishes external validity. Several studies on a given topic may be conducted along the internal-external validity continuum.

■ LINKS AMONG INTERNAL, CONSTRUCT, AND EXTERNAL VALIDITY

The concepts of internal validity, construct validity, and external validity are interrelated. Using the strength study as an example

Research Study

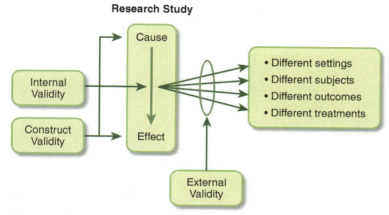

Figure 5–9 The interrelationships among internal, construct, and external validity.

can help to illustrate this point. The first thing to remember is that both internal validity and external validity address the cause-and-effect relationship. Assume that the strength training protocol used in the strength study is a three-set, 10-repetition exercise using the subjects' 10-repetition maximum. Assuming that subjects are randomly assigned to the control and experimental groups, and the integrity of the treatment is maintained across time, the study will have internal validity. In addition, if the subjects used were college students, the study would be externally valid for other college students, but not necessarily for the general population. Now assume that the subject population was selected from the general population; in this case, the study would be externally valid for the general population, including college-age students and older persons. Finally, consider a change in the treatment to a weight training program of five sets of 30 repetitions at 10% of maximum voluntary contraction with the load adjusted weekly. You would probably not view this as a strength training program; to call it strength training would violate the validity of the strength training construct. However, this violation has no effect on the internal validity (assuming you have randomly assigned subjects to the treatment and control groups), and it has no effect on external validity (provided you used subjects to which you want to generalize). The overall structure of these relationships is illustrated in Figure 5–9.

Retention Questions 5-2
1. Which forms of validity are associated with the cause-and-effect relationship?
2. Which form of validity is related to how things are defined?
3. Define the maturation threat, and identify whether it applies to internal or external validity. What is the typical relationship between internal and external validity?

▪ SUMMARY

One of the key elements to all research is validity. As a consumer of research, it is important for you to know whether the results of a study are trustworthy and applicable. Trustworthiness is addressed through internal validity and relates to whether the cause (i.e., treatment) actually produced the effect (i.e., outcome). To achieve internal validity, research must employ specific experimental research designs that include random assignment and control groups. When experimental designs cannot be used, quasi-experimental designs may be appropriate. However, the tradeoff with quasi-experimental designs is a loss of some degree of internal validity. Applicability is addressed through construct and external validity. When you consider applying research findings to your own practice, you must be sure that the construct is defined in a meaningful way and the results of the research apply to the environment or people you treat. When consuming and applying research, you must be aware of all three and the threats to each.

◼ CRITICAL THINKING QUESTIONS

1. If you were going to design an experiment, what would you need to consider for establishing cause and effect?

2. If you were going to define the construct "quality of life," what elements would you consider?

3. What issues would you consider in applying a study's cause-and-effect relationship with your work or practice situation?

4. What level of evidence should be applied to each of the research designs discussed in this chapter?

◼ TRUST AND APPLY

Maenhout, A. G., Mahieu, N. N., De Muynck, M., De Wilde, L. F., & Cools, A. M. (2013). Does adding heavy load eccentric training to rehabilitation of patients with unilateral subacromial impingement result in better outcome? A randomized, clinical trial. *Knee Surgery, Sports Traumatology, Arthroscopy, 21*(5), 1158-1167.

Locate the foregoing article, and using this article, address the following questions.

1. Identify the independent variable.
   a. Was the independent variable defined in a meaningful way?
2. Identify the dependent variables.
   a. Were the dependent variables defined in a meaningful way?
   b. Was improvement in shoulder pain/function defined in more than one way? Was more than one measure used?
3. Identify the type of research design.
   a. Use a flow chart to diagram the design, being sure to identify randomization, treatment, and observations. Be specific in identifying these elements by using information in the article (e.g., variable names).

4. Using the threats to internal validity, assess whether each threat has been controlled and how.

5. Using the targets of generalization and the threats to external validity, assess whether the study is externally valid.

▬ RESEARCH SCAVENGER HUNT

1. Using a research topic of your own:
   - Locate an experimental study and diagram the design.
   - Locate a quasi-experimental design.

Then answer the following questions.

   A. Which design best controlled internal validity?

   B. Which design had better external validity?

   C. Did either study use pretest measures? How did this improve the study design?

2. Using a research topic of your own:
   - Locate a crossover study and diagram the design. Be specific in identifying the elements by using information in the article (e.g., variable names).

Then answer the following questions.

   A. Was enough time allowed between each treatment?

   B. What is the advantage of this design?

▬ REFERENCES

Shadish, W. R., Cook, T. D., & Campbell, D. T. (2002). Construct validity and external validity. In *Experimental and quasi-experimental designs for generalized causal inference* (pp. 65-102). Boston, MA: Houghton Mifflin.

Ware, J. E., Jr., & Sherbourne, C. D. (1992). The MOS 36-item short-form health survey (SF-36). I. conceptual framework and item selection. *Medical Care, 30*(6), 473-483.

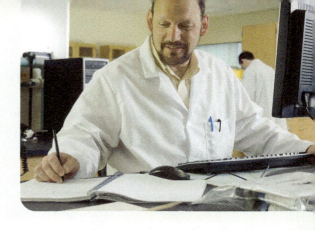

Clinical (Therapeutic) Trials

Where Have You Been?

Up to this point, you have learned how to find research that you could apply
to your clients or patients. That has included finding the evidence using electronic databases and then applying it to your practice situation. You have also
learned to evaluate different aspects of the research you find. Among those
key elements are identifying the type of outcome used in the research and determining whether those outcomes meet your need. This includes identifying the
performance aspect of the outcome or where on the disablement continuum
each of the outcomes belongs; whether the outcome is patient based or clinician
based, and whether it is disease oriented or patient oriented. For an outcome to
be worthwhile, it must also meet technical requirements such as validity, reliability, responsiveness, and interpretability. You have also learned classic research
designs frequently encountered in exercise science and rehabilitation research.
Each of these designs has strengths and weaknesses that make them useful for
particular circumstances. Furthermore, depending on the design and scope of the
study, the study may or may not be internally valid for establishing cause and
effect. You also learned that internal and external validity often oppose each
other, and that research is often a compromise among competing goals.

Where Are You Going?

The previous chapters have focused on the basics of research. In this chapter,
these concepts are extended to apply to true clinical research. You will learn that
clinical research organizes research questions into a hierarchy, and the measures
that were previously discussed fit within this hierarchy. Research designs in clinical research are either similar or identical to the designs you previously learned.
However, they may go by a different name. Clinical trials may be described as
occurring in phases. This is very common in pharmaceutical research, and these

phases are described in the context of exercise science and rehabilitation research. You will also learn the importance of random assignment of research participants and how different methods of randomization work. Finally, you will learn how to calculate two clinical measures: *numbers needed to treat* and *numbers needed to harm*. These measures are useful in interpreting research and can be easily calculated with data presented in the clinical trials results if the authors have not done so.

Learning Outcomes

After completing this chapter, you will be able to answer these questions:

1. What are the differences among primary, secondary, and ancillary research questions?

2. What is the difference between a treatment's efficacy and effectiveness?

3. What are the key features of treatment arms, and what combination of treatment arms is best for establishing cause and effect?

4. Which form of blinding is best, and why should it be used?

5. How many samples are in a population?

6. Which randomization procedure is best?

7. When clinical trials are divided into four phases, exercise and rehabilitation trials are most likely to be in which phase?

8. If a clinical trial cannot be designed as a randomized controlled trial, which design would be the best choice?

Key Terms

Absolute risk reduction (ARR)
Active comparator arm
Adverse effects
Adverse event
Ancillary question
Block randomization
Control event rate (CER)
Double blind
Effectiveness
Efficacy
Equivalency study
Experimental arm
Experimental event rate (EER)
Factorial design
General adverse event

Group allocation designs
Historical control design
Intent-to-treat analysis
Natural history
No intervention arm
Nonrandomized concurrent
  control
Number needed to
  harm (NNH)
Number needed to
  treat (NNT)
Per protocol analysis
Phase I trial
Phase II trial
Phase III trial

Phase IV trial
Placebo arm
Primary question
Randomized controlled
  trial (RCT)
Secondary question
Serious adverse event
Sham arm
Simple randomization
Single blind
Stratified randomization
Study arm
Triple blind
Withdrawal studies

Clinical trials are a form of research that have historically emphasized the development of pharmaceutical agents. However, clinical trials can be the application of research methods to any intervention with the intent of establishing the intervention's usefulness in humans. One of the key features of a clinical trial is a specified population (e.g., patients with cancer or a heart attack) to which the therapy is directed. In other words, the trial has a very specific, intended target population. This is not always the case in experimental research, in which the intent is to establish whether a treatment can produce a change in a group receiving the treatment. In experimental research, control groups are not patients, but rather individual subjects that may provide the best experimental control. For example, if you wanted to know whether a fitness program actually improved cardiovascular function, one strategy would be to select healthy persons who do not exercise regularly. These subjects would then be randomly assigned to either a control group or the group receiving the fitness program. Why would you pick these subjects? The main purpose would be to improve experimental control. First, the treatment is more likely to have an effect in untrained persons. Thus, you have maximized the possibility of finding an effect. Second, by selecting healthy subjects you eliminate confounding factors, such as cardiovascular disease, that could interfere with the treatment. This type of experiment is useful in establishing whether the treatment (i.e., fitness program) works. A more important clinical question would be this: "Does this fitness program improve the cardiovascular function of patients with diagnosed heart disease?" Because this latter question identifies a specific clinical population, the resulting experiment would be more appropriately labeled as a clinical trial.

In reality, no differences exist between clinical trials and the experimental research designs you learned about previously. Many of the designs from Chapter 5 are incorporated into clinical trials. The key differences between the two can be broadly identified as differences in terminology and emphasis. As you will see, some of the designs and research components presented in Chapter 5 are used in clinical trials, but with different names. As suggested earlier, you will also see that clinical trials place emphasis on clinical populations. Because of this emphasis, different components of the research are managed differently. Nevertheless, at the heart of every clinical trial are the same issues as in experimental research.

Clinical trials, by their design, are intended to be more clinically focused. As such, the conditions of clinical trials are more similar to real clinical circumstances. Because of this, clinical trials are viewed as having more external validity or real-world applicability. Put another way, clinical trials better translate to real patient care.

EFFICACY VERSUS EFFECTIVENESS

As suggested earlier, one of the differences between clinical trials and other research methods is what they emphasize. One key shift in emphasis is from testing efficacy to testing effectiveness. Efficacy is defined as a positive result for a treatment under ideal, experimentally controlled conditions. Effectiveness is defined as a positive result for a treatment under normal, real-world conditions. This includes using typical clients or patients and using typical practitioners to provide the treatment. For example, an experiment testing a strength training protocol conducted on healthy, untrained persons (half to the training group and half to a control group), training 3 days per week under the supervision of the research team, would qualify as an efficacy trial. Conversely, if a similar trial was conducted with the clients at a fitness club (i.e., a real-world rather than laboratory condition), this experiment would qualify as an effectiveness trial.

Efficacy: A positive result for a treatment under ideal, experimentally controlled conditions.

Effectiveness: A positive result for a treatment under normal, real-world conditions.

TYPES OF QUESTIONS

Clinical trials are designed to address multiple questions simultaneously. This is in contrast to more traditional experiments in which controlling for internal validity often limits the questions that can be asked. Typically, five types of questions (Table 6–1) can be asked as part of a clinical trial (Friedman, Furberg, & DeMets, 2010e).

Primary Questions

The primary question is the specific question that the study is designed to answer. It represents the question that is of the greatest interest. Identifying this question is critical to the planning of research because the resources used in the research will be directed at this question. Without a primary question, the research can be unfocused and at risk of being unable to answer any question.

The primary question can focus on any part of the disablement continuum, depending on the goal of the study. For example, in orthopedics, a study of anterior cruciate ligament surgery could focus on whether the surgical procedure reestablishes normal knee mechanics (i.e., body function). However, the primary question could instead focus on whether the surgical procedure allows the patient to return to sport activities (i.e., participation). Alternatively, a study on strength training could be interested in whether fitness levels improved (i.e., activity) or, more narrowly, whether strength improved (i.e., body function).

Connections 6-1

Efficacy is the clinical term used synonymously for internal validity. Effectiveness is the clinical term used synonymously for external validity. Internal validity and external validity are opposite ends of a continuum. As one increases, the other typically decreases. The more experimental control that is applied (increasing internal validity), the less the experiment resembles the real world. Conversely, conducting research in the real world often means that experimental control cannot be tightly maintained. For example, in the real world, different clinicians may be responsible for applying the same treatment. However, different clinicians may have different skill levels. Thus, the quality of the treatment may vary depending on which clinician provides the treatment.

Primary question: One of a group of five types of questions that can be asked as part of a clinical trial. The primary question is the specific question that the study is designed to answer.

Table 6–1 Questions Asked in Clinical Trials	
Question Type	**Definition**
Primary questions	The specific question that the study is designed to answer representing the question that is of the greatest interest.
Secondary questions	Questions that are not the main reason for the study and focus on assessing different dependent measures from the primary question.
Ancillary questions	Those questions that are not specifically planned but can be tested with the study data.
Natural history questions	Questions that address the natural history of a disease. These questions are addressed by the no intervention arm of the trial.
Adverse effects questions	Questions that document adverse events encountered during the course of the trial. These types of questions are typically unplanned because adverse advents cannot usually be predicted.

Currently, clinical trials are more typically asking primary questions that focus on the higher end of the disablement continuum, such as functional limitations and disability. This is because of the desire to shift from a disease focus to a patient focus in health-care research. In specific cases, asking primary questions that are focused on the health condition (e.g., what makes osteoporotic bone grow stronger) are appropriate. However, limiting questions to the lower end of the continuum often does not help understand what makes the patient feel better.

Secondary Questions

Secondary questions are those that can be answered by the study but were not the reason the research was conducted. One type of secondary question focuses on assessing different dependent measures from the primary question. For example, assume that your primary question is whether a fitness program improves quality of life and general health. Your secondary question could be whether strength is improved (or maximal oxygen consumption) with the fitness program. Alternatively, a study on balance exercises on a sprained ankle could have the primary question of whether the therapy improves walking and/or allow rapid return to competition. Your secondary question could be whether the balance training improves ankle strength.

Another type of secondary question focuses on subgroups within the study. For example, the fitness study would probably include men and women. However, it is not certain that men and women will respond equally to the fitness program. Thus, a secondary question could be to compare fitness improvement between men and women. For the ankle study, it may be that medial and lateral

Connections 6-2

Primary and secondary questions should include references to the outcome measure of interest. Different researchers have different emphases for the study. However, it is common for primary questions to focus on patient-based, patient-oriented outcomes and for secondary questions to focus on more clinician-based, disease-oriented outcomes. It is also often the case that primary questions focus on the upper levels of disability continuums (e.g., handicap), whereas secondary and ancillary questions are more focused on the lower levels (pathophysiology).

Secondary question: One of a group of five types of questions that can be asked as part of a clinical trial. The secondary questions are questions that are not the main reason for the study and focus on assessing different dependent measures from the primary question.

ankle sprains are included. The secondary question could be whether medial and lateral ankle sprains respond equally well to balance training. Other comparisons in this category could include differences among age groups, rural versus urban patients, and differences in socioeconomic status. Which groups are selected entirely depends on the purpose of the study.

Ancillary Questions

Ancillary questions are those questions that are not specifically planned but can be addressed with the study data. These are often considered substudies within the main study. For example, in the fitness study, you may be interested in understanding who the most frequent participants were. Although the intent at the outset of the study would be to have all participants participate equally, this seldom occurs. Nevertheless, attendance data may reveal that younger participants were likely to participate regularly, whereas older participants did not. This could be further analyzed to understand what *caused* the lack of participation. It could be that older individuals have more family obligations, or they thought the program was too time intensive or too strenuous. For the ankle study, if part of the therapy was a home program, it could be worth knowing how often participants did the home component of the program. The effectiveness of the program could depend on how well the home program was followed. Thus, ancillary questions can be very important in understanding the primary questions.

Ancillary question: One of a group of five types of questions that can be asked as part of a clinical trial. Ancillary questions are not specifically planned but can be addressed with the study data. These are often considered substudies within the main study.

Natural History

Another question that can be addressed is the natural history of a disease or injury. This type of question can be addressed only with a no intervention trial arm. In other words, this group must be receiving no treatment or a placebo (although placebo effects can be present and should be interpreted cautiously). The purpose of natural history questions is to better understand how the disease progresses over time. Questions concerning the naturally occurring complications, symptoms, and signs of the disease are considered. Put another way, "What happens if the disease is allowed to run its course to its natural end?"

For some diseases, these types of studies have ethical issues. For example, the natural end of untreated cancer is death. Is it ethical to deny someone a promising treatment for cancer? Maybe not, if the new treatment is truly unsupported. In this case, review boards are established to monitor the progress of the group receiving the new treatment. If the treatment group overwhelmingly responds favorably to the treatment, the control group is switched to the new treatment. Thus, both groups receive the benefit of the new treatment.

Natural history: Questions that address the origins, evolutions, and interrelationships of a disease. These questions are addressed by the no intervention arm of the trial.

For other conditions such as ankle sprains, ethical concerns are less problematic. For example, a typical ankle sprain improves in 6 weeks regardless of the treatment. Thus, the ethical issue would be considered minor because the treatment would affect the speed of recovery and not the final result. Nevertheless, if the treatment group was showing much faster improvements, then switching the control group to the treatment would be appropriate.

These latter two examples provide other problems to be considered. When moving the control group to the treatment group, this effectively ends the planned experiment because you no longer have a control group. In addition, starting the control group on the treatment later in the progression of the disease may not produce the same effectiveness for the treatment. For example, for an ankle sprain, providing ice, compression, and elevation 2 weeks after the sprain is likely to have minimal effects when compared with applying these measures at the time of the sprain. Thus, any data collected from the control group participants after they start receiving the treatment should be analyzed more carefully.

Adverse Effects

The final question that can be asked during a clinical trial is about the existence of adverse effects (i.e., side effects). The details of these questions are not typically planned because they cannot be predicted. Moreover, if substantial adverse events begin to occur as part of the research, the research is often stopped early to prevent injury to participants. Because of this, the evidence for these side effects is often inconclusive. When the treatment's benefit to the client is limited, it is preferable to stop a trial early than subject participants to harm. In the case of the strength training study, injury resulting from the intervention could be an adverse effect that would stop the trial.

Adverse effects: One of a group of five types of questions that can be asked as part of a clinical trial. Adverse effects (side effects) questions document adverse events encountered during the course of the trial. These types of questions are typically unplanned because adverse advents cannot usually be predicted.

■ STUDY DESIGNS

Like all experimental research, clinical trials may use one of several possible designs. There are potentially eight study designs of clinical trials that may be encountered in exercise science and sports medicine research (Friedman, Furberg, & DeMets, 2010b). Many of these are experimental designs, but by a different name or with an enhancement related to clinical research.

Randomized Controlled Trial

The randomized controlled trial (RCT) is the "true" experimental design. In Chapter 5, you learned that this design consisted of a treatment group and a control group and that participants were randomly assigned to each group. It is also possible that more than one treatment group may be used. In clinical research, these groups are often

Randomized controlled trial (RCT): A study design that consists of a treatment and a control group and in which the participants are randomly assigned to each group. It is considered the "true" experimental design.

called study arms (i.e., treatment arm and control arm). The use of "arm" instead of "group" relates to the nature of clinical trials rather than experiments. Clinical trials tend to be studies conducted over long periods of time, with extensive follow-up with patients. For example, in a clinical trial of a knee operation, patients may be followed for up to 10 years to determine the effectiveness of the surgical procedure. Although traditional experiments may last this long, they typically have a much shorter duration.

Study arm: In a clinical trial, each group or subgroup of participants receiving experimental treatment or no treatment.

Treatment Arm Types

There are five typical treatment arms (Table 6–2) used in clinical trials (clinicaltrials.gov, 2012). Generally, at least two of these types are used in every trial.

Experimental Arm

The experimental arm is the treatment arm of the study. This is the group that receives the new treatment being studied. The primary questions address the effectiveness of this arm in relation to the control groups. In exercise science, this arm could be a strength training protocol. Clinically, this could be a new form of rehabilitation. This arm is present in all clinical trials.

Experimental arm: The clinical trial arm in which the participants receive the experimental treatment. One of five typical treatment arms used in clinical trials.

Active Comparator Arm

The active comparator arm is a type of control group. The experimental arm is compared with this type of control group, but this control group also receives a treatment (Fig. 6–1). This second treatment is considered effective; thus, this comparison is between a new treatment and an existing standard treatment. In rehabilitation, this could be a comparison between the standard treatment for a joint sprain of ice, elevation, and compression

Active comparator arm: The clinical trial arm in which the participants receive the standard, clinically effective treatment (sometimes identified as the comparison group). It is one of the five typical treatment arms used in clinical trials.

Table 6–2	Commonly Encountered Clinical Trial Arms
Arm	**Definition**
Experimental arm	The clinical trial arm in which the participants receive the experimental treatment
Active comparator arm	The clinical trial arm in which the participants receive the standard clinically effective treatment (sometimes identified as the comparison group)
Placebo arm	The clinical trial arm in which the participants receive a fake drug or medication in the form of a similar-appearing inert substance
Sham arm	The clinical trial arm in which the participants receive a fake treatment or therapy that does not include the key components necessary to make the treatment effective
No intervention arm	The clinical trial arm in which the participants receive no treatment (sometimes identified as the control group)

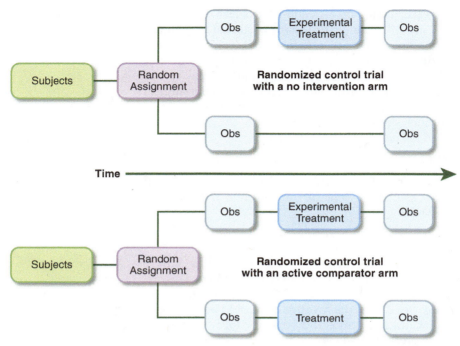

Figure 6–1 No intervention versus active comparator. The upper panel shows a typical randomized controlled trial with a no intervention arm. The lower panel shows the same design with active comparator intervention. (Obs, Observation)

(active comparator) and an experimental arm that receives the same treatment in addition to electrical stimulation. In exercise science, it could be a comparison of aerobic training using a standard treadmill (active comparator) with the same program using an elliptical trainer. In experimental research, this would be known as a comparison group.

Pros and Cons 6-1

Active comparator arms are very useful alternatives to no intervention arms. When a well-established treatment is in common use, including it in the study is the best way to test a new treatment. It allows participants in both the treatment and active comparator arms to receive treatment. Thus, there are no ethical concerns about denial of treatment to some participants. The results are limited to comparison between the treatment and active comparator arms. Comparisons with other treatments are inappropriate. Furthermore, use of active comparators cannot establish how effective a treatment is over no treatment at all.

Placebo and Sham Comparator Arms

Placebo arms and **sham arms** use fake treatments (clinicaltrials.gov, 2012). Placebos are typically inert substances that look and taste like a drug or other substance used in the treatment arm. Similarly, a sham is a procedure or device that appears identical to the treatment but does not include the key components necessary to make the treatment effective. Although placebos are most commonly used in drug trials, they may also be used in a trial of a nutritional supplement. Thus, the experimental arm would receive the actual supplement while the placebo arm would receive something that looked or tasted like the supplement. One way this may be done is by putting both substances into identical-looking capsules that are swallowed whole. Another way may be to include the supplement in another food such as a protein shake.

A sham treatment may be used in rehabilitation research. For example, a study on therapeutic ultrasound could be conducted by removing the quartz crystal from the device. By doing so, the device would look normal and otherwise operate correctly. The clinician would proceed to apply the treatment as normal except that no ultrasound would be produced. Thus, participants in the sham arm would appear to be receiving ultrasound, and the clinician could also be blinded to the groups.

Placebo arm: The clinical trial arm in which the participants receive a fake drug or medicine in the form of a similar-appearing, inert substance. It is one of five typical treatment arms used in clinical trials.

Sham arm: The clinical trial arm in which the participants receive a fake treatment or therapy that does not include the key components necessary to make the treatment effective. It is one of five typical treatment arms used in clinical trials.

No Intervention Arm

The **no intervention arm** is simply an arm that receives no treatment. Inclusion of a no intervention arm is the best way to ensure internal validity of the research. However, in clinical trials this is not often possible because ethical considerations may not permit denial of treatment to a patient. Thus, active comparator arms are more common.

No intervention arm: The clinical trial arm in which the participants receive no treatment (sometimes identified as the control group.) It is one of five typical treatment arms used in clinical trials.

Pros and Cons 6-2

Placebos and shams can perform very important functions in research designs. Often clients have a response to a treatment just because they are receiving treatment, not because the treatment is effective (i.e., the placebo effect). Use of placebos or shams allows you to establish how much of a treatment's effectiveness is caused by simply receiving treatment. Conversely, it is important to remember that placebos and shams are not equal to no treatment and cannot be interpreted as a no treatment or control arm. It may be that a treatment's effect will be smaller when compared with a placebo than when compared with no treatment because of the placebo's effect.

Retention Questions 6-1

1. What is the distinction between an active comparator arm and an active control arm?
2. When would a researcher choose an active comparator versus a no intervention arm?
3. What is the distinction between a sham and a placebo?
4. What is the difference between a no intervention arm and a control group?

Randomization

Randomization is one of the key components of a randomized controlled trial. It is this process, combined with the treatment arm and some type of comparison arm, that makes these studies true experiments. Randomized studies are considered to have good-to-strong internal validity. Randomization is typically done one of three ways: simple, block, or stratified (Fig. 6–2) (Friedman, Furberg, & DeMets, 2010d).

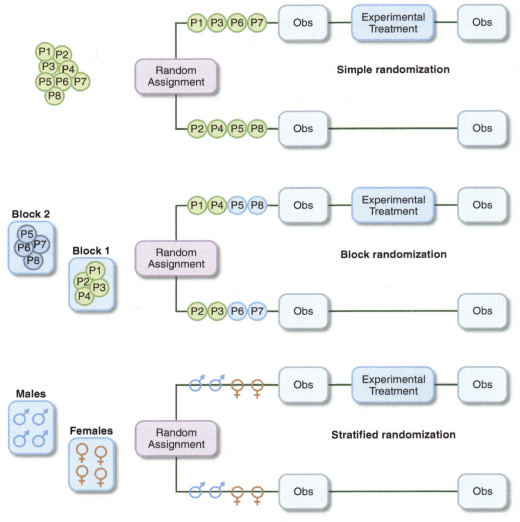

Figure 6–2 Methods of randomization. Upper panel shows the result of simple randomization of 8 participants (P). The middle panel is block randomization. Each block is randomized separately into the trial. The lower panel is stratified randomization. Male and female subjects are randomly assigned to each arm separately. (Obs, Observation)

Simple Randomization

Simple randomization is performed as each subject is enrolled in the study. Some mechanism such as a random numbers table is used to indicate the treatment group to which the participant is assigned. A random numbers table is a table of two-digit numbers that have been randomly generated. The investigator picks a starting point on the table and moves across the rows and columns while looking up each number. If the number of the table is an even number, then the next participant is assigned to the treatment arm. If the number is odd, then the participant is assigned to the study's other arm. If three treatment arms are used, numbers ending in 1 would indicate the first arm, numbers ending in two the second arm, and numbers ending in 3 the third arm. Numbers ending in other digits would be ignored.

One of the shortcomings of this process is that it can produce an imbalance in subject assignment. For example, if you toss a coin 10 times, on average 5 heads and 5 tails should result. However, this is only the average result of many sets of 10 tosses. In actuality, it is possible to have 7 heads and 3 tails. This same thing can happen with subjects initially entering a clinical trial. In other words, early in the trial more subjects may be entered in one arm than the others. Over the course of the trial, this imbalance will disappear because eventually the arm will fill up, thereby forcing subjects to be assigned to the other arms. This type of imbalance may cause bias. It may be that patients with the most severe cases are recruited and assigned first. If this is true, then these participants with severe cases could be assigned to the treatment arm more often than the other arms. Thus, the treatment arm results are a combination of the treatment and the severity of the disease or injury. To avoid this type of imbalance, other randomization procedures are used.

Simple randomization: A process of randomly assigning participants to study groups as they enroll, typically by using a random numbers table.

Block Randomization

An alternative to simple randomization is **block randomization**. Block randomization assigns participants to blocks first and then randomly assigns the participants from each block. For example, assume you are conducting a strength training study with strength training as one arm and no strength training the other arm. Also assume that you want to block randomize in blocks of four. You would enroll the first four subjects and randomly assign them to the two groups. The result would be two subjects in the strength training arm and two in the no intervention arm. You would then enroll the next four subjects and randomly assign them to the two groups and continue repeating this until all subjects were enrolled. The advantage of this process is that the problem of imbalance between the arms is avoided. When blocks are created, they are

Block randomization: A process of assigning individual subjects to study groups. The researcher divides participants into subgroups called blocks and then randomly assigns individuals within each block to treatment conditions.

created in multiples of the arms. For the foregoing example there were two arms; thus, groups of two, four, six, and eight would work. If it had been a three-arm study, then groups of three, six, and nine could be used. Larger blocks can be used, but if the blocks become too large, it is possible to have an imbalance in the assignment similar to simple randomization.

Stratified Randomization

Stratified randomization is randomization from groups created by the researcher for a specific purpose. It is similar to block randomization in that subjects are in groups. In this case, the groups are formed around some preexisting factor such as sex. Assume in the strength training study with a treatment arm and a no intervention arm that you wanted to study differences between men and women. Rather than using simple randomization, which could result in more women in one group or the other, you would randomly assign the women and men to the arms separately. By doing this you ensure that equal numbers of men and women are assigned to each arm.

Stratifying subjects into groups can be done for any purpose. Stratifying subjects into different age groupings is another example. In exercise science, you may also want to stratify based on ability, fitness level, or sport. One of the hidden problems with stratification is that related factors are also stratified. For example, if participants are stratified for age, you are coincidentally stratifying for different diseases, in that some diseases are more likely at different ages. When you stratify for sex, you may also be stratifying for profession because some professions are predominant in one sex or the other. Often these other factors that are coincidentally stratified can be predicted. It is also possible that unrecognized factors may also be stratified and affect the results. Thus, although stratification is frequently used and is useful, its shortcomings must also be considered.

Blinding

Blinding is another important aspect of clinical trials research. Blinding is the process by which participants in research are prevented from knowing who has been assigned to which treatment arms. Blinding may apply to the persons receiving the treatment, the clinicians providing the treatment, or both. In studies that are **single blind,** the subjects receiving the treatments (e.g., patients) or the investigators do not know to which treatment arm they have been assigned. This is important because patients' or investigators' behavior can change if they know the arm assignment. For example, if patients are being rehabilitated following knee operations and they know that they are in the experimental arm

Stratified randomization: A process of assigning individuals to study groups in which the researcher creates groups for a specific purpose, such as some preexisting factor (e.g., sex), and then randomly assigns individuals from the groups to a treatment group.

Single blind: A method of conducting a study in which either the participants receiving treatment or the clinicians providing care know whether the participants are in the control group or the experimental group. Single-blind studies attempt to eliminate observer or subject bias, depending on which group is "blinded."

that potentially produces better results, they may be more enthusiastic and diligent in adhering to the treatment. Conversely, patients who know they have been assigned to the standard treatment may believe they are not receiving the most advanced care. Because of this, they may not be as careful about adhering to their treatment. Similarly, if investigators know the arm assignment, they may be more encouraging to patients in the treatment arm and less so to those in the comparison arm. One or both of these situations are possible, and if they occur, they may affect the results by producing an overly favorable result for the experimental arm.

In studies that are **double blind**, both the participants receiving treatment and the clinicians providing care are blinded to the members of each group. The participants are blinded for the same reasons as in single blinding. The clinicians are blinded for similar reasons. If the investigators are not blinded, the experimental arm's results may be larger than expected because of the investigators' enthusiasm. Double blinding also prevents the clinicians from accidentally violating the blinding of the participants. In a single-blind study, it is possible that the clinicians will mistakenly reveal the group to which a participant is assigned. This could be done verbally by accidentally telling the participant, or sometimes the actions of the clinician (e.g., a lack of enthusiasm) can give the participant a clue. If the clinician does not know the arm assignment of the participants, then every participant is theoretically treated in the same way.

Rarely, a study that is **triple blind** is used. Triple blinding is an extension of double blinding in which a data monitoring board is also blinded to participant assignment (Friedman, Furberg, & DeMets, 2010c). Most large clinical trials have a data monitoring board that periodically reviews the results during the course of the study. This is done to ensure that participants in the experimental arm are not put at excessive risk of injury and to ensure that participants in the other arms are not denied the experiment treatment should it prove effective. With triple blinding, the data monitoring board reviews the data without knowing which groups are the experimental arm and which are not. This process supposedly improves the committee's objectivity, but it can also compromise the committee's safety role. Without knowing the results from each group, it becomes impossible to know whether an improving group is the treatment group, an active comparison group, or a placebo group. If the placebo group is improving, this would suggest allowing the trial to continue as is. However, if either the treatment group or the active comparison group is improving, this would suggest the need to give the other patients that treatment. Thus, knowing group assignment can affect the decision-making process.

Double blind: A method of conducting a study in which neither the participants receiving treatment nor the researchers know whether the participants are in the control group or the experimental group. Double-blind studies attempt to eliminate observer and subject bias.

The Critical Consumer 6-1

Unfortunately, most studies in exercise science are not done with double blinding. When the researchers who are evaluating the outcome know who is receiving the treatment, this can lead to bias in the study. Even unintentionally, researchers can interact with the intervention (e.g., offering encouragement) in a way that that the no treatment arm does not receive. Thus, any study that uses no or single blinding should be viewed as less internally valid than a double-blind study.

Triple blind: A method of conducting a study in which the participants receiving treatment, the clinicians providing care, and a data monitoring board do not know whether the participants are in the control group or the experimental group.

Nonrandomized Concurrent Control

Nonrandomized concurrent control studies are an alternative to randomized controlled trials. They are alternatively known as nonequivalent control group designs (see Chapter 5). In clinical trials, this design can be more convenient than some others. It is often easier to assign subjects to treatments based on a naturally occurring group. For example, rather than randomly assigning a patient who needs a knee replacement to two different treatments, it may be easier to assign clinic A to perform one therapy and clinic B to perform the alternative therapy. Patients entering clinic A would receive only the treatment assigned to that clinic. In other words, patients would freely pick which clinic they wanted to go to, rather than be randomly assigned to the treatment. Ideally, these patients would not know which treatment is being offered by each clinic. Thus, to the extent that patients randomly select clinics, the treatment assignment would be random. However, patients often pick the most convenient clinic or favor a clinic for other reasons. Because of this, the assignment cannot be considered random and may introduce bias into the process. For example, if patients select a clinic because they perceive the clinicians to be more competent or friendly, that may produce a placebo effect that favors that clinic regardless of the treatment.

This type of arrangement may also be applied to health clubs and experimental fitness programs. It is important to recall that nonrandom assignment (in experiments or clinical trials) means that the different groups cannot be considered equal, and differences between groups may result in differences at the time of group assignment. One protection is to detect these differences by pretesting the participants on important variables before starting the treatments. This way you know whether differences exist before the treatment begins, and you can compare the pretest and postintervention differences.

Nonrandomized concurrent control: Studies in which participants are not randomly assigned to a control group or an experimental group. Also called nonequivalent control group designs.

Historical Control Designs

Historical control designs are studies that compare a treatment arm with a set of control participants who are cataloged in a database. Often, these control participants have participated in a previous study or are part of a larger database of medical patients (Fig. 6–3). For example, assume you had conducted a strength training study using a no treatment arm and a high-volume strength training arm, and the strength training program was effective. Now that the study is completed, you want to know whether the training volume can be lower but produce the same effect. One option would be to conduct a randomized controlled trial with a control group and a low-volume training arm. Alternatively, you could conduct a historical

Historical control design: A clinical study that compares a treatment arm against a set of control participants who were observed at some time in the past or for whom data are available through a database.

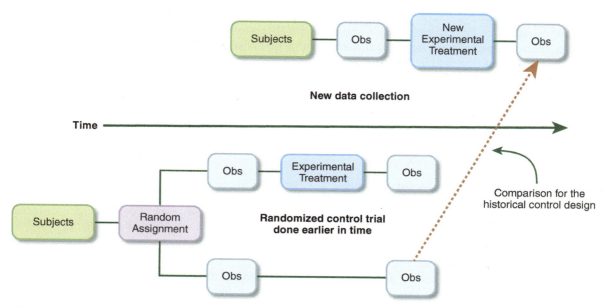

Figure 6–3 Historical control design. Subjects enrolled in the new data collection with the new experimental treatment are compared with the no intervention arm of a previous trial. (Obs, Observation)

control study with a single low-volume training arm and compare it with the previous study's treatment arm. This would allow comparison between arms with high and low work volume.

This type of design is considered weak because the control arm and the treatment arm are not run simultaneously. This means that the control arm conditions are not identical to the treatment arm conditions. For example, assume that the high-volume arm was conducted in the winter months when the participants could not go outdoors and exercise. In this case, these participants may have seen the strength training study as their exercise program for the winter and thus participated regularly. Conversely, if the low-volume arm was conducted in the summer, participants may not have consistently participated because they would rather be outside than in the gym. In this case, the low-volume arm may have not been effective because participants did not follow the program, not because the low-volume protocol was truly ineffective. You may think that a solution to this would be to run the low-volume arm in the winter season, although in a different year. Although that could improve the study, there is no guarantee that the winters would be identical, and thus the same problems would arise.

Environmental factors are not the only threats to historical control designs. Anytime two groups are not run simultaneously, external factors may be different and alter the results. It is also possible that participants recruited at different times of the year are in some way inherently different. For example, study subjects with children may be less likely to participate in the summer because of vacations with the family. It is impossible to predict or identify all the potential differences that may occur when study arms are not implemented simultaneously, but differences are inevitable. Thus, these designs are generally avoided and should be used only when no other options are available.

Crossover Designs

Crossover designs, as discussed in Chapter 5, are also used in clinical trials research. To emphasize, these designs have the advantage that every participant serves as his or her own control. This means that every participant receives all treatments, and the design is very powerful for testing hypotheses. It also means that some participants will receive the treatment before the control, and vice-versa. Because of this, treatments are limited to only those treatments that will wash out. Washout means the elimination of a treatment effect after a known period after the treatment is withdrawn. For example, when a blood pressure medication is stopped, the effect of the medication will wash out, and the patient's blood pressure will return to higher levels. Because of this, a crossover design could be used to study blood pressure medication. However, when the treatment is strength training, the increase in strength is not likely to wash out immediately. In this case, the crossover design would not be efficient because either the strength gains would never wash out, or at least it would take a long time to do so. As with all designs, this design can be very useful, but it must be matched appropriately with treatment.

Withdrawal Designs

Withdrawal studies are defined as studies in which patients receiving treatment are withdrawn from the treatment, or the treatment dose is decreased (Fig. 6–4). For example, patients with ankle instability who are performing balance exercises 5 days per week could have the exercises reduced to 1 day per week to see whether their instability increases with fewer treatments. If the instability does increase, this would suggest that the higher treatment frequency is necessary. Conversely, if the lower frequency produces no change, this would suggest there is no need to use the higher frequency. The same could apply to exercise to control blood pressure. Daily exercise may be reduced to fewer times per week to see whether the reduced blood pressure is maintained.

The shortcoming of this type of study is that participants must be receiving an existing treatment that is believed to be or has been

Connections 6-3

Historical control designs have very weak internal validity. They do not assign participants to groups by random assignment. In addition, because the controls are not studied simultaneously with the treatment group, it is difficult to know whether the two groups are different because of the intervention or as a result of differences in time. Thus, historical control designs cannot establish true cause and effect.

Withdrawal study: A clinical trial in which patients receiving treatment are withdrawn from the treatment or the treatment dose is decreased.

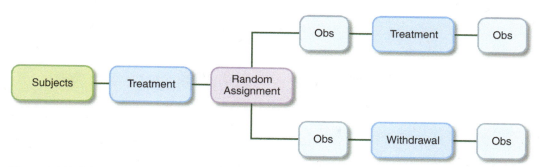

Figure 6–4 Withdrawal design. Randomized controlled trial showing treatment and withdrawal arms. (Obs, Observation)

shown to be effective. In addition, the participants' outcome of interest (e.g., ankle instability, blood pressure) must be known and understood to be stable across time. Because of this, the results of these types of trials are limited to a very specific population. For example, if reduced balance training effectively maintains ankle instability, that finding would apply only to those persons with the type of instability studied. The results would not be generalizable to all people with ankle sprains. Thus, these types of designs can be useful but are limited in their application.

Factorial Designs

The **factorial design** is an extension of the experimental design (Fig. 6–5). The examples previously presented used only two or three treatment arms: the control arm and on or two treatment arms. In the factorial design, four arms are used. These arms are the control arm, treatment arm A, treatment arm B, and treatment arm AB. In the case of the treatment AB arm, participants receive both treatments. For example, a fitness study could include control, strength training, aerobic training, and strength plus aerobic training arms. This design has two advantages. First, it allows multiple treatments to be assessed simultaneously. Second, it allows the effect of each treatment to be assessed separately (as was true in previous designs) and the interaction between the two treatments (i.e., the strength plus the aerobic training arms). As you would expect, the strength plus aerobic training treatment would probably have a combined effect. However, that effect cannot be assumed to be equal to strength effects added to aerobic effects. In other words, if strength produced three units of improvement in fitness and aerobics produced five units of improvement in fitness, combining them is not likely to result in eight units of improvement (i.e., 3 + 5 =8). Rather, in this case the improvements are likely

Factorial design: A clinical study in which four treatment arms are used: the control arm, treatment arm A, treatment arm B, and treatment arm AB. In the case of the last arm, participants receive both treatments.

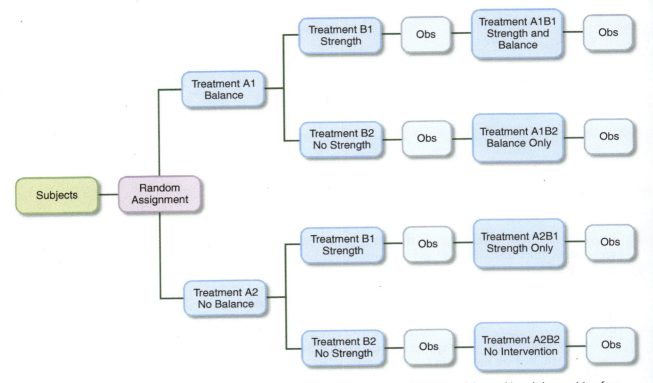

Figure 6–5 Factorial design. Randomized controlled trial with two interventions (Balance and Strength) and the resulting four treatment combinations. (Obs, Observation)

to be reduced in terms of aerobic or strength benefits. The factorial design allows the interaction of treatments to be assessed. Sometimes combining treatments results in improvement over either arm alone, and sometimes there are negative effects. Treatments may interfere with each other and produce a lesser effect than either treatment alone, or they may have no effect on each other. Because of these possibilities, if treatments are possibly combined in clinical practice, it becomes important to study those combinations in clinical trials.

Group Allocation Designs

Group allocation designs randomly assign intact groups to treatments (Fig. 6–6). These groups may be communities, schools, hospitals, clinics, health clubs, or any other grouping that may make sense. What is implied by this design is that there are several existing groups that can be randomly assigned to treatments. For example, 12 middle schools in a large city could be randomly assigned to provide 1 of 2 fitness programs to students as part of

Group allocation design: A process of assigning groups to study arms. The researcher randomly assigns intact groups, such as communities, schools, and so forth, to treatment conditions.

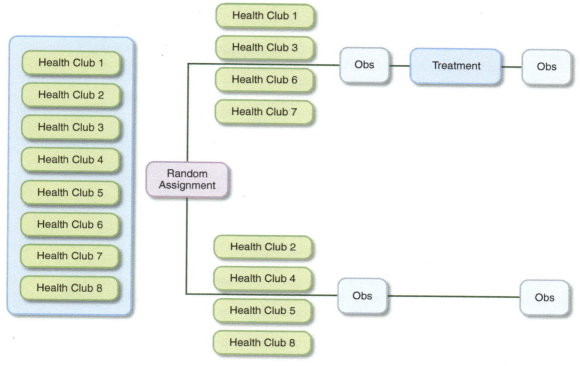

Figure 6–6 Group allocation design. Randomization into treatment and no intervention arms based on the whole group (health club). Individual participants are assigned to treatments based on the health club to which they belong. Statistical analysis is done at the group, not individual, level. (Obs, Observation)

physical education. It might also be that 30 hospitals within a state (or across the nation) are randomly assigned to provide 1 of 2 joint replacement operations for knee arthritis.

This type of design offers convenience in that each site has to administer only one treatment. However, the weakness is that for statistical reasons, only the different sites (i.e., schools or hospitals) can be treated as participants and not the individual subjects themselves. Because of this, for these designs to be effective many sites must be used to gather generalizable results.

The Critical Consumer 6-2

Randomized controlled trials are considered the gold standard in research. However, they generally are expensive and require long periods of time. Thus, they are not always feasible. However, other clinical trial designs are acceptable when randomized controlled trials are not available. Because of this, it becomes important that you understand the strengths and weaknesses of these designs to be certain that they have been appropriately applied, so you can interpret the results accordingly.

Equivalency Designs

Equivalency studies seek to determine whether two treatments are equal. Some effective treatments may be too painful, toxic, unpleasant, or complicated to administer to be desirous. Thus, effort is often made to identify an equally effective treatment that does not have these drawbacks. For example, an existing fitness program may have been shown to be effective for participants exercising 5 days per week. However, in practice many persons may find it too time consuming to exercise this often. Because of this, it may be of interest to determine whether a 2 day per week schedule is just as effective.

There are several challenges to equivalency studies. When equivalency studies are conducted, the goal is to prove that a difference between the treatments does not exist, and this is impossible. If blood pressure was used as the outcome measure for the 5-day and 2-day fitness programs, it could be that decreases in blood pressure for the two programs were the same. Thus, the two programs would appear to be no different. Conversely, measurement error of the blood pressure measures may make the two programs appear equally effective when in fact they are different. Other factors such as random error may also hide the difference. The problem is that whenever there is no difference between the study groups you do not know whether this is really no difference or whether the difference was hidden by other factors.

Because of these complications, equivalency research must be done with very strict rules (Friedman et al., 2010e). First, the standard treatment arm (considered the active control arm) must have the exact same treatment and conditions as in the original research (i.e., the study that proved its effectiveness). Second, the study that established the effectiveness of the active control must be recent enough to ensure that no medical advances or other changes in the standard of care have occurred. Third, the evidence for the active control must be available for comparison. This allows the researchers of the new study to know exactly how much change should be expected. Finally, the variable being measured must be known to be responsive to both the active control and the new treatment.

The final challenge is determining how much difference between the arms will be considered equal. As stated earlier, it is impossible to prove that no difference exists, and in all likelihood some difference between the treatments will exist. Thus, the question becomes how much difference is meaningful. If the active control (i.e., the 5 day/week fitness program) reduces systolic blood pressure by 20 points, how much change does the 2 day per week program need to be considered equal? If the 2-day program reduced systolic blood pressure by 16 points, would that be equal? Would a 12-point change be equal to a 20-point

Equivalency study: A clinical investigation in which two distinct treatments are compared against each other to identify whether one treatment is as effective as another and has fewer drawbacks.

Connections 6-4

Responsiveness is a quality of a measure (see Chapter 4) that indicates that the measure changes when it should change. Thus, it should respond to the intervention if the intervention produces a change.

change? The 12% and 16% differences were given because they represent 20% and 40% changes, respectively. These differences represent typical differences that are accepted as equivalent. As a consumer of research, you should be aware that equivalence between treatments does not mean precisely equal. Rather, it means that the two treatments do not differ by a previously agreed on meaningful amount. Also keep in mind that treatments that are less effective may be preferable to more effective treatments if the less effective treatment is easier to administer, is less painful, less complicated, or generally easier for the patient.

◼ PHASED CLINICAL TRIALS

Clinical trials have been historically defined in phases (Hackshaw, 2009c). Although these phases may not coincide with the type of research you may be using for your evidence-based practice, it is common terminology in health care, and some review is therefore appropriate.

Phase I

Phase I trials have been described as first-in-human studies (Hackshaw, 2009c). This means that before a phase I trial, the treatment has been studied in animals. It also means that animal trials demonstrate enough promise for the treatment that it warrants testing in humans. These trials tend to enroll a small number of participants and focus on biological mechanisms. Thus, the type of outcome measure used is often disease oriented and scientist or clinician based. In exercise science, this could be a strength training study with the goal of determining changes in muscle tissue obtained using a muscle biopsy. In rehabilitation, electromyography could be used to establish a treatment's effect on neuromuscular function. In exercise science or rehabilitation, phase I trials could be used to determine the sequence of exercises for an exercise prescription. They may also be used to determine the most efficient order to administer outcome measures. Finally, they would be used to collect preliminary data to be used for future studies. These types of trials may also be described as "pilot" or "feasibility" studies.

Phase II

Phase II trials are efficacy studies and typically involve hundreds of patients. Phase II studies are small clinical trials (usually randomized controlled trials), that generate data in all the treatment arms. As previously discussed, efficacy studies such as a phase II trial assess the intervention under ideal conditions. The goal is not to determine whether the treatment works in the real world but to determine whether it works at all. Thus, very

Retention Questions 6-2

1. A nonrandomized control trial design would be used when?
2. How are crossover designs and withdrawal studies different from each other?
3. How is a group allocation design different from block randomization?
4. What is the key limitation of equivalency studies?

Phase I trial: A clinical trial in which a treatment is tested on humans for the first time. Before a phase I trial, the treatment has been studied in animals, and the results have demonstrated promise for treatment in humans. Phase I trials tend to enroll a small number of individuals and focus on biological mechanisms. The type of outcome measure is often disease oriented and scientist or clinician based.

Phase II trial: A clinical trial in which an efficacy study is performed to determine whether a given treatment works at all. Phase II trials are typically small (hundreds of patients) and use a randomized control. These types of trials are often thought of as laboratory trials involving humans.

controlled conditions are used to give the intervention the best chance to work. Data are generated to determine whether the treatment works as compared with a control, placebo, or active control, and those data can be used to plan the next trial (Hackshaw, 2009a). This type of trial is often thought of as a laboratory trial involving humans. For example, a phase II strength training trial would be conducted in a laboratory or other strength facility under close supervision of the research team. In a rehabilitation study, balance training such as Tai Chi would be performed in the laboratory or clinical setting under supervision, to ensure that the treatment was performed correctly. Once it is established that the treatment is efficacious, phase III trials begin.

Phase III

Phase III trials are effectiveness trials and typically involve thousands of patients (Hackshaw, 2009b). They are large clinical studies, and like phase II trials, are usually randomized controlled trials. As previously discussed, effectiveness studies assess the intervention under real-world conditions. Thus, a new strength-training program could be administered throughout a chain of health clubs to see whether it produces results in the typical health club client. A Tai Chi program could be administered in nursing homes across the state or country to determine whether it reduces falls. This type of trial is the real test of whether the treatment has value.

Phase III trial: A clinical trial in which an effectiveness study is performed. Phase III trials often involve thousands of patients and use a randomized control.

Phase IV

Phase IV trials are monitoring trials. Once a treatment begins to be used with the general population, these trials are conducted to determine whether the effectiveness and safety of the treatment are maintained. These trials tend to be more observational than intervention driven. They often include large numbers of participants, similar to phase III trials. These studies often are long-term studies and serve the purpose of identifying safety issues and the effectiveness of the intervention. For example, a phase IV trial could be used to determine whether a knee replacement surgical procedure is likely to fail and require another replacement. If so, it could also determine how long the replacement lasts before a new one will be required. Similarly, it could be used to determine whether cardiac rehabilitation decreases the chance of future heart attacks and how that chance changes (increases or decreases) over 5 to 10 years. In other words, these trials focus on the longevity of the treatment as well as long-term complications.

Phase IV trial: A clinical trial in which a monitoring study is performed. These trials are conducted to determine whether the effectiveness and safety of the treatment are maintained. These studies often are long-term studies and serve to identify safety issues and the effectiveness of the intervention.

■ POPULATION SELECTION

As a consumer of research, it is important to know that the sample being studied must be representative of the population of interest. At best, any clinical trial can study only a sample of the population of interest. In addition, even the population of interest may be a subsample of an even larger population (Fig. 6–7). For example, you could start with the population of the United States. From there the research will define the injury or condition of interest. Assume that the injury of interest is an anterior cruciate ligament tear. From this subpopulation, the researchers could further select those patients who have had the ligament reconstructed. From this further restricted subpopulation, researchers enroll subjects into the study. Ultimately, the researchers cannot enroll every possible patient into the clinical trial, and any clinical trial enrolls only a sample of the population of interest. Because of this, the researchers must be very careful to describe their participants' characteristics in detail. As a consumer of research, you must pay close attention to the participants in the clinical trial. You should critically review the participants' characteristics to determine whether they match your client's or patient's profile. If not, then the research likely does not apply to your client. For example, a clinical trial on the success of anterior cruciate ligament replacement

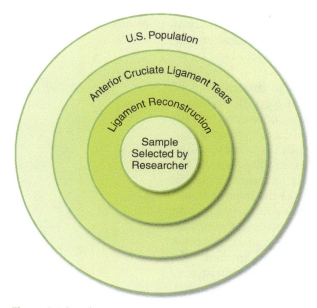

Figure 6–7 Population versus sample. The sample selected by the researcher is a much smaller subset of subpopulations with larger populations.

operations in college athletes may not apply to patients in their 40s and 50s who injured their ligaments skiing. Because of age, both sets of patients may considerably differ in healing ability, motivation, and other important factors. This also applies to trials of fitness and exercise programs. Age and other characteristics of the population may dramatically change the results. To apply the results, the participants should match your client closely.

■ INTENT-TO-TREAT ANALYSIS

It is common to find studies that have excluded participants from the analysis of the interventions because the participants dropped out or did not comply with the study's treatment plan. Analyzing only those participants who completed the study or only those who complied with the treatment protocol is known as per protocol analysis. Alternatively, you may encounter studies that use intent-to-treat analysis (Fig. 6–8). Intent-to-treat is analyzing participants enrolled in a clinical trial as part of the original arm to which they were assigned (Brody, 2012). Although this seems obvious, under some circumstances it is unclear how subjects should be analyzed. For example, if a participant drops out of a study, should he or she be excluded from the analysis? If a participant no longer performs the treatment correctly (e.g., exercises or engages in rehabilitation only 2 days per week instead of 5), should he or she be excluded from the analysis? Finally, if participants do not to meet the studies inclusion criteria after they have been enrolled in the trial, should they be excluded? In intent-to-treat analysis, the answer to these questions is "yes."

The purpose of intent-to-treat analysis is to prevent bias or inaccurate results. Subjects may drop out of a study because a treatment is too cumbersome, painful, or time consuming and for many other reasons. If subjects are not complying or are dropping out of the treatment arm for these reasons, then the treatment may appear to be more effective than it really is. In other words, the remaining participants are those most likely to receive a benefit from the treatment. Very sick patients who see the treatment as a last chance may be more motivated to continue with an unpleasant treatment in the hope of getting better. The opposite may also be true; very sick patients may drop out of the study more often (e.g., they may die). If these types of dropouts are ignored, then only the less sick will remain. In this case, the treatment may appear very effective because the sickest patients are excluded. Either way, the participants who are left in the study likely no longer represent the population of interest.

As a consumer of research, you need to be aware of how dropouts were handled in a given study. If dropouts are ignored,

Connections 6-5

Population selection is critical to the external validity of the study. The participants used determine to whom the study may be applied. If the population selected is unique (e.g., college athletes), then the results will not likely apply to the general population or other subgroups of the general population.

Per protocol analysis: A clinical trial in which data from only those participants who complete the trial and comply with the treatment protocol are included. This is in contrast to the intent-to-treat analysis.

Intent-to-treat analysis: A clinical trial in which data from all participants are included, even if the participants failed to complete the study or comply with the treatment protocol.

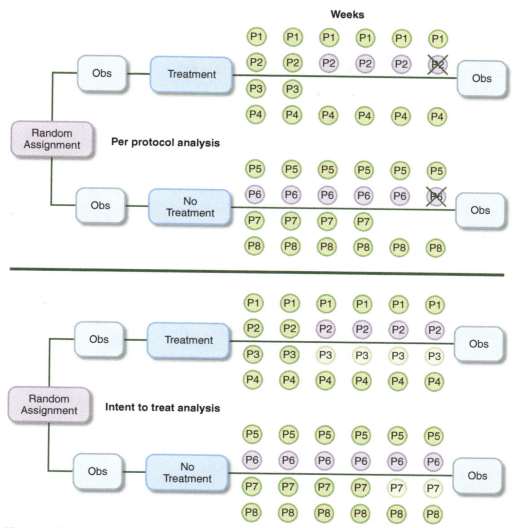

Figure 6–8 Per protocol versus intent-to-treat analysis. The same eight participants (P) are randomly assigned to either a treatment or no intervention arm in a 6-week randomized controlled trial. The upper panel is a per protocol analysis, and the lower panel is an intent-to-treat analysis of the same participants. Participants P2 and P6 stopped following their assigned treatment protocols at week 3 and 1, respectively. Participants P3 and P7 dropped out at weeks 3 and 5, respectively. In the per protocol analysis these participants are ignored, and the analysis is conducted only on participants P1, P4, P5, and P8. In the intent-to-treat analysis, all eight subjects are analyzed as part of their original arm. (Obs, Observation)

then you should expect that the results do not accurately represent the true effectiveness of the treatment. Thus, given the choice between a per protocol analysis and an intent-to-treat analysis, you preference should be for the intent-to-treat analysis because it will most accurately represent the treatment's true effectiveness.

■ NUMBER NEEDED TO TREAT

Most clinical trials used in exercise science and sports medicine focus on outcomes that are measured with units. For example, we can measure strength in units of weight or force. Joint range of motion can be measured in degrees. However, some outcomes are measured as events. The events either happen or they do not and thus are measured dichotomously (i.e., yes/no). For example, a football player who tears his anterior cruciate ligament would be measured as a "yes" event. Heart attacks, falls, stroke, and arthritis are other examples of conditions that may be measured as events.

When events are measured, it becomes possible to compute the **number needed to treat (NNT)**. Number needed to treat is a calculation of how many people would have to be treated to have one positive effect on one person. For example, research has shown that approximately 39 uninjured ankles have to be taped to prevent a single ankle sprain (some of the same data suggest that 143 uninjured ankles would have to be taped) (Olmsted, Vela, Denegar, & Hertel, 2004). Assessing events allows you to assess whether implementation of the treatment will have a real-world impact and to evaluate whether it is financially worthwhile. For example, using the previous numbers needed to treat, taping ankles would cost from $4,100 to $15,300 per season to prevent one ankle sprain. If you are an athletic trainer in a secondary school setting, this is not likely to be an economic option.

Calculating the numbers needed to treat is an easy calculation. Assume you have two study arms. In the treatment arm, you have 100 athletes who have their knees braced. In the no treatment arm you have 100 athletes not being braced. (This means there are 200 knees in each group.) Now assume that in the braced group there were 20 knee injuries. Twenty divided by 200 is 0.10 or 10%. This is known as the **experimental event rate (EER)**. It is simply the percentage of events in the experimental arm. Also assume that there are 50 knee injuries in the control arm. Fifty divided by 200 equals 0.25 or 25%. This is the **control event rate (CER)** or the percentage of events in the no treatment arm. By subtracting the experimental event rate from the control event rate, the **absolute risk reduction (ARR)** results. In this case, CER – EER = 0.15, or a 15% absolute risk reduction. In other words, bracing knees reduces the chance of an injury from 25% to 15%. By taking the reciprocal of the absolute risk reduction you get the number needed to treat.

$$\frac{1}{ARR} = NNT$$

In this example, the number needed to treat equals 1 / 0.15 = 6.7. This means that approximately seven knees need to be braced to prevent one injury.

Number needed to treat (NNT): The number of people needed to be treated so that one person experiences a benefit.

Experimental event rate (EER): The rate at which events occur in the experimental arm, or experimental group, of a study.

Control event rate (CER): The rate at which events occur in the no treatment arm, or control group, of a study.

Absolute risk reduction (ARR): A measure of the change in risk of an experimental treatment in relation to a control treatment. It is calculated by subtracting the experimental event rate from the control event rate.

It is important to realize that the number needed to treat does not add new information. The absolute risk reduction and number needed to treat capture the same information but from different perspectives. The attraction of number needed to treat is that it relays the information very pragmatically. It makes it clear that not every patient will benefit, but it also clearly indicates how much effort (or expense) is required to have a benefit.

■ ASSESSMENT OF TREATMENT HARM

Assessment of harm is most frequently done within the framework of an existing clinical trial, mostly for ethical reasons (Friedman, Furberg, & DeMets, 2010a). It is very difficult to justify conducting a clinical trial for the sole purpose of documenting injuries or other harm. Any injury or other adverse outcome (e.g., heart attack) is defined as an **adverse event**. Three broad categories of adverse events have been defined (Friedman et al., 2010a). The first is a **serious adverse event**. Serious adverse events include events that threaten life or result in a permanent or long-term disability, hospitalization, or a birth defect or congenital abnormality. In rehabilitation and exercise science, most serious adverse events are events that result in hospitalization or disability. The second category of adverse event is that of **general adverse events**. These are defined as those adverse events reported to or observed by clinicians. These events may include muscle soreness from an exercise or rehabilitation program. They may also include pain or swelling that occurs separate from the original injury. The final category comprises special adverse events. These are defined as events in which the investigators have special interest. They can be anything and often are events the researchers have identified because they have a unique impact. For example, although delayed-onset muscle soreness is a normal consequence of exercise, researchers may identify it as a special adverse event because of the impact it may have on implementation of the exercise program.

Occasionally, you may see **number needed to harm (NNH)** reported. This is the number of people who must be treated for one adverse event to occur. This measure is calculated exactly as numbers needed to treat, except adverse events are used rather than positive outcomes. As with number needed to treat, number needed to harm gives you a clear interpretable value for how risky the intervention is. If a study happens to have both numbers needed to treat and numbers needed to harm, then you have an easy way of balancing the risks and benefits of the intervention.

As a consumer of research, you need to evaluate studies that assess or report adverse events the same way as any other study. One of the key considerations is the population. Just because an adverse event is reported does not mean that it will apply to your client.

Pros and Cons 6-3

Number needed to treat is a convenient way of considering how effective a treatment is. It clearly states how many persons would have to be treated to expect one positive result. However, these are only expected results. There is no guarantee that the treatment will be as effective as the number needed to treat suggests (it could actually be better than predicted). In the foregoing example, bracing seven knees does not guarantee that one knee injury will be prevented. It could be higher or lower. Thus, the number needed to treat should be used as an estimate of what to expect on average.

Adverse event: Any injury or otherwise adverse outcome to the health of a participant that happens during a clinical study or within a certain time period after the study is over.

Serious adverse event: An adverse event that threatens life, results in permanent or long-term disability, hospitalization, birth defect, or congenital abnormality.

General adverse event: Any adverse event that is reported to, or observed by, clinicians during a clinical study.

Number needed to harm (NNH): The number of people needed to be treated so that one person experiences an adverse effect, or harm.

You still have to match your client with the studied population and your professional practice circumstances. You should also consider the issues of internal validity. Was the study designed in such a way that you can be certain that the treatment caused the adverse event? Were the investigators blinded to assignment of participants to each treatment arm? Just as internal validity applies to the primary and secondary outcomes, it also applies to harm. Finally, keep in mind that some adverse events may not be known for years. Often the long-term outcome of a new surgical procedure is not known for some time after it is introduced. Similarly, adverse events from a new surgical technique may not be known until later. Thus, just because no adverse events have been reported does not mean they will not occur.

SUMMARY

Clinical trials are research studies specifically focused on establishing the efficacy and effectiveness of clinical interventions. Several different research designs may be used. However, the gold standard is the randomized controlled trial. This type of trial is an experimental design applied to a clinical question and clinical population. Other designs are used when randomizing patients into different treatment arms is not possible. Clinical trials may occur in phases, but these phases are more common with drug intervention studies than with exercise and rehabilitation trials. Finally, although clinical trials are primarily designed to assess efficacy and effectiveness, they may also establish the relative harm of an intervention. Thus, a well-designed clinical trial will provide you with an assessment of the risks and benefits of an intervention.

CRITICAL THINKING QUESTIONS

1. To apply the best treatment program to your patients or clients, what type of clinical trial study design would you prefer to have available and why? What would be your second choice?

2. How would you explain to a client that a double-blind study is better than a single-blind study?

3. How would you define the population from which your clients or patients come? How much younger (or older) would a population have to be before it no longer represented your clients or patients?

4. If randomization was not used, what would be your concerns about the clinical trial?

5. Which would be best to apply to your client or patient, an efficacy study or an effectiveness study?

◼ TRUST AND APPLY

Martinsen, M., Bahr, R., Borresen, R., Holme, I., Pensgaard, A. M., & Sundgot-Borgen, J. (2014). Preventing eating disorders among young elite athletes: A randomized controlled trial. *Medicine and Science in Sports and Exercise, 46*(3), 435-447.

Ridge, S. T., Johnson, A. W., Mitchell, U. H., Hunter, I., Robinson, E., Rich, B. S., & Brown, S. D. (2013). Foot bone marrow edema after a 10-wk transition to minimalist running shoes. *Medicine and Science in Sports and Exercise, 45*(7), 1363-1368.

Locate either of the foregoing articles, and using the article address the following questions.

1. What is the primary question of the research?
   a. Is this a question that applies to your clients?
   b. Is there a secondary question, and does it apply to your client?
2. What is the study design used?
   a. What is the strength or weakness of that design?
   b. Does the design give you more or less confidence in the research?
3. What is the population being studied? Does it match your client group?
4. How was blinding used in the study? Does it give you more or less confidence in the research?

◼ RESEARCH SCAVENGER HUNT

Find a randomized controlled trial that corresponds to your clinical practice. Use that article to answer the following questions:
1. Does the population in the study match the clients or patients you typically see?
2. Was the study double blinded? How does this affect the credibility of the study?
3. Did the study use a no intervention arm? How does this affect the meaning of the study?
4. Was an intent-to-treat analysis conducted? How does this affect your confidence in the results?

◼ REFERENCES

Brody, T. (2012). Intent-to-treat analysis vs. per protocol analysis. In *Clinical trials: Study design, endpoints and biomarkers, drug safety, FDA and ICH guidelines*. London: Elsevier.

clinicaltrials.gov. (2012). Glossary of Common Site Terms. Retrieved from http://clinicaltrials.gov/ct2/about-studies/glossary

Friedman, L. M., Furberg, C. D., & DeMets, D. L. (2010a). Assessing and reporting adverse events. In *Fundamentals of clinical trials* (4th ed., pp. 215-232). New York: Springer.

Friedman, L. M., Furberg, C. D., & DeMets, D. L. (2010b). Basic study design. In *Fundamentals of clinical trials* (4th ed., pp. 67-96). New York: Springer.

Friedman, L. M., Furberg, C. D., & DeMets, D. L. (2010c). Blindness. In *Fundamentals of clinical trials* (4th ed., pp. 119-132). New York: Springer.

Friedman, L. M., Furberg, C. D., & DeMets, D. L. (2010d). The randomization process. In *Fundamentals of clinical trials* (4th ed., pp. 97-119). New York: Springer.

Friedman, L. M., Furberg, C. D., & DeMets, D. L. (2010e). What Is the Question? In *Fundamentals of clinical trials* (4th ed., pp. 37-54). New York: Springer.

Hackshaw, A. K. (2009a). Design and analysis of phase II trials. In *Concise guide to clinical trials* (pp. 39-56). Hoboken, NJ: BMJ Books.

Hackshaw, A. K. (2009b). Design of phase III trials. In *Concise guide to clinical trials* (pp. 57-76). Hoboken, NJ: BMJ Books.

Hackshaw, A. K. (2009c). Fundamental concepts. In *Concise guide to clinical trials* (pp. 1-16). Hoboken, NJ: BMJ Books.

Olmsted, L. C., Vela, L. I., Denegar, C. R., & Hertel, J. (2004). Prophylactic ankle taping and bracing: A numbers-needed-to-treat and cost-benefit analysis. *Journal of Athletic Training, 39*(1), 95-100.

Other Methods in Clinical Research

In addition to knowing research design principles, you must also understand the many other statistical methods that researchers use to generalize their findings (see Chapter 7). Understanding these methods is critical for you to apply those findings to your practice. Beyond this, you also need to understand methods that are used when "traditional" research is not practical or ethical and how these large, "uncontrolled" studies can also contribute to evidence-based practice (see Chapter 8).

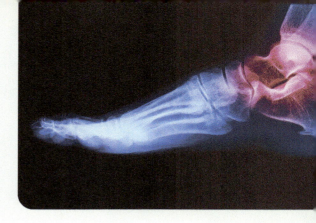

Diagnostic Statistics

Scott E. Ross, PhD, LAT, ATC, FNATA
University of North Carolina, Greensboro, North Carolina

Where Have You Been?

In Chapter 6, you learned that clinical research organizes research questions into a hierarchy. In addition, you learned that clinical trials may be described as occurring in phases, and these phases are applied to exercise science and rehabilitation research. You also were introduced to randomization, which is critical for strengthening the internal validity of a research study. Finally, you learned how to calculate numbers needed to treat and numbers needed to harm, which are two important clinical measures for determining the effectiveness of an intervention.

Where Are You Going?

In this chapter you will learn to apply diagnostic statistics for accuracy of clinical tests. You will learn that sensitivity and specificity indicate the percentage of persons correctly identified as having and not having, respectively, a condition based on a clinical test result. In addition, positive and negative predictive values will be defined and you will learn how these outcomes tell you the percentage of persons with positive outcomes who actually have a condition and the percentage of persons with negative test results, who do not have a condition, respectively. These two predictive statistics are important for "ruling in" or "ruling out" the condition. Related to these accuracy statistics are the positive and negative likelihood ratios, which tell you how many more or fewer times likely a person is to have or not have a condition, respectively. These two statistics are powerful and critical for ruling in (positive likelihood ratio) and ruling out (negative likelihood ratio) a condition. An additional way to examine the accuracy of a clinical test is to plot a receiver operating characteristic curve. This curve plots the sensitivity of a test versus the false-positive rate (test identifies a person as having a condition, but the person really does not have it) to determine the accuracy of a test for identifying those persons with a given condition. Finally, a measure known as area under the curve quantifies the degree of accuracy for a test based on the receiver operating characteristic plot. A high area under the curve value is indicative of an accurate test.

Learning Outcomes

After completing this chapter, you will be able to answer these questions:

1. What are the differences among sensitivity, specificity, positive predictive score, and negative predictive score?

2. What are the differences among scores and rates for true-positive, false-positive, true-negative, and false-negative outcomes?

3. What do positive and negative likelihood ratios tell you about the accuracy of a clinical test?

4. What is a receiver operating characteristic curve, and how is it used to quantify accuracy?

5. How do you determine a clinical meaningful threshold (i.e., cutoff score) on a receiver operating characteristic curve that identifies persons with a given condition?

6. How does an area under the curve value relate to the accuracy of a clinical test?

Key Terms

Area under the curve (AUC)
Cutoff score
False-negative rate
False-negative score
False-positive rate
False-positive score
Likelihood ratio
Negative likelihood ratio

Negative posttest probability
Negative predictive value
Positive likelihood ratio
Positive posttest probability
Positive predictive value
Receiver operating characteristic (ROC) curve
Sensitivity

Specificity
True-negative rate
True-negative score
True-positive rate
True-positive score
Youden index

Applying evidence-based techniques to clinical populations of interest is critical for accurate diagnosis. You should question whether or not a technique can be used on a patient if no evidence exists to support its effectiveness. In a research study, for example, you may want to use a clinical test to identify joint laxity in ankle sprains. Given the opportunity to perform a clinical test for joint laxity on a sprained ankle, you would want to choose a test that is able to detect pathological joint laxity in a person who has an ankle sprain. The chosen test must also allow you to have certainty that your positive result is indicative of an ankle sprain. Although you want this test to identify laxity with an ankle sprain, it must also identify the absence of pathological joint laxity in an uninjured person. You want to have certainty that a negative test result indicates that no injury exists. The clinical test also needs to tell you the degree to which your test results predict whether your client has an ankle sprain. A simple calculation can be performed to derive the probability of having (or not having) an ankle sprain with a specific test result. Although this probability can be computed, you still will need to know whether the probability is even clinically meaningful. With a few easy mathematical formulas, you can determine whether the probability of having an ankle sprain is meaningful enough to diagnose a person as having an ankle sprain. All this information can be summarized with a graph that displays the accuracy of the clinical test as well as an objective score a person needs to reach for correct diagnosis of an ankle. The diagnostic statistics in this chapter are critical for determining both accuracy of a test and clinical applicability. Ultimately, you will learn that diagnostic statistics in the area of evidence-based medicine are crucial in taking the guesswork out of your tests for clinical diagnosis.

DIAGNOSTIC STATISTICS FOR ACCURACY

Sensitivity and Specificity

Researchers investigating the clinical usefulness of a test are examining its ability to differentiate between those with and without a condition (e.g., pathological condition, disease, risk factor). Sensitivity and specificity are key outcome measures in determining the discriminate ability (ability to determine whether the condition is present or not present) of a test. Sensitivity is defined as the percentage of persons with a positive test result in persons who, in fact, have the condition (true-positive test results divided by the sum of positive and negative test results for the condition). For example, in determining whether a person tore the anterior cruciate ligament, a

Sensitivity: The percentage of people who have a positive test result and, in fact, have the condition tested for; true-positive test results divided by the sum of positive and negative test results for a condition.

clinician can employ the Lachman test to assess the degree of joint laxity. The sensitivity of this test has been reported as 0.82, meaning that 82% of persons with an anterior cruciate ligament tear were identified as having a positive Lachman test result (Solomon, Simel, Bates, Katz, & Schaffer, 2001). The definitive test for diagnosing an anterior cruciate ligament tear is magnetic resonance imaging because it has a sensitivity of 99%, thus indicating it is an accurate test for identifying tears in persons who have an anterior cruciate ligament tear (Vaz, Camargo, Santana, & Valezi, 2005).

Specificity is defined as the percentage of persons with a negative test result in persons who, in fact, do not have the condition (true-negative test results divided by the total sum of negative and positive test results for not having the condition). In the previous anterior cruciate ligament examples, the specificity values of 0.94 and 0.95 are associated with the Lachman test and magnetic resonance imaging, respectively (Solomon et al., 2001; Vaz et al., 2005). Thus, 94% and 95% of persons without anterior cruciate ligament tears were not identified as having a tear as determined by negative results on the Lachman test and a magnetic resonance imaging scan, respectively (Solomon et al., 2001; Vaz et al., 2005). Sensitivity and specificity provide targeted information on the performance of a test, and from an evidence-based medicine approach, you will want to employ a test with a high percentage of positive results for clients with the condition (sensitivity) and a high percentage of negative results for those without the condition (specificity).

Figure 7–1 is used throughout this section to help you visualize these diagnostic statistics for accuracy. The set of data presented in Figure 7–1 represent positive and negative test results for a clinical test. The solid circles represent persons with a condition, and the diamond symbols represent persons without a condition. A threshold for a positive test result is the solid line running through the middle of the data. Thus, data points above the threshold line are indicative of positive results, and those below the threshold line are negative results. A greater number of circles above the threshold line compared with the circles below the threshold line indicates that this test has high sensitivity. A greater number of diamonds below the line compared with those above the line indicates that this test has high specificity.

For a given data set, sensitivity and specificity are inversely related in that as one diagnostic statistic increases, the other decreases. To demonstrate this inverse relationship between sensitivity and specificity, we will consider data published by McCrea (2001) on using the Standardized Assessment of Concussion scores for assessing sport-related concussions. The Standardized Assessment of Concussion is an objective and standardized test for assessing an injured athlete's mental status immediately following

Specificity: The percentage of people who have a negative test result and, in fact, do not have the condition tested for; true-negative test results divided by the total sum of negative and positive test results for not having a condition.

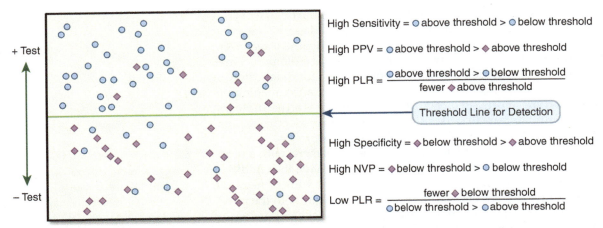

Figure 7–1 Understanding diagnostic statistics. This figure displays positive and negative test results for persons with (solid circles) and persons without (open diamonds) a given condition. The threshold for a positive test result is the solid line in the middle of the figure. Persons above this line have a positive test result, and persons below it have a negative test result. On the right side of the figure are conceptual equations for understanding sensitivity, positive predictive value (PPV), positive likelihood ratio (PLR), specificity, negative predictive value (NPV), and negative likelihood ratio.

a suspected concussion. McCrea (2001) examined difference scores between baseline assessment (mental status without a concussion) and mental status with a concussion. McCrea (2001) recommended a change score of only –1 point (worse performance) to identify decreased mental status in athletes with a concussion. At a change score of –1 in mental status, 60 of 63 athletes with concussions were identified as having this condition (sensitivity = 0.95) and 42 of 55 athletes without concussions were identified as not having a concussion (specificity = 0.76) (McCrea, 2001). At a change score of –3, the sensitivity of the Standardized Assessment of Concussion test dropped to 0.78, whereas the specificity increased to 0.95 (McCrea, 2001). These data indicate that a greater change score misidentified 14 athletes with concussions as not having a concussion, but 52 of 55 athletes without concussions were correctly identified as not having a concussion.

You also can use Figure 7–1 to help visualize this inverse relationship. A clinician may have a more liberal interpretation of the test result that moves three circles and three diamonds above the threshold line. The test now has an increased sensitivity because it identifies positive test results in more patients with the condition. However, the liberal interpretation of the results also decreases the specificity by allowing three more patients to test positive for a condition that they do not have. The clinician essentially increases both the true-positive and false-positive results of this test, and these terms are defined in the next section to help you read and interpret data sets.

True-Positive, True-Negative, False-Positive, and False-Negative Results

In publications, authors typically display a 2 × 2 contingency table for diagnostic statistics, and it is important that you become familiar with these tables so that you can understand the results of the investigations. Table 7–1 displays a 2 × 2 diagnostic contingency table for the computations of sensitivity and specificity values. The columns indicate whether a person has a condition or not, and the rows indicate whether the clinical test result is positive or negative. In the "Positive" row, the true-positive score indicates persons with the condition testing positive on a clinical test, and the false-positive score displays persons without the condition testing positive on the clinical test. In the "Negative" row, the false-negative score indicates persons with the condition testing negative on a clinical test, and the true-negative score demonstrates persons without the condition testing negative on the clinical test. The values in the "Condition Present" column can be used to compute sensitivity, and you are computing the percentage of persons testing positive for "Condition Present" (true-positive test results divided by column total). Thus, you are able to compute a true-positive rate, which is the clinical term for sensitivity. The values in the "Condition Not Present" can be used to calculate specificity, and, again, you are computing the percentage of persons testing negative for the "Condition Not Present" (true-negative test results divided by column total). This computation is the true-negative rate, which is the clinical term for specificity.

True-positive score: The number of persons who actually have the condition and receive positive results on a clinical test.

False-positive score: The number of persons who do not have the condition but receive positive results on a clinical test.

False-negative score: A score that indicates the number of persons who actually have the condition but receive negative results on a clinical test.

True-negative score: The number of persons who do not have the condition and receive negative results on a clinical test.

True-positive rate: The percentage of persons who do have the attribute or disease who receive positive test results. The term used for the true-positive rate is sensitivity.

True-negative rate: The percentage of persons who do not have the attribute or disease who receive negative test results. The term used for the true-negative rate is specificity.

Clinical Diagnostic Usefulness for Sensitivity and Specificity

The clinical application of sensitivity and specificity is somewhat limited for diagnostic purposes, with two exceptions. Take, for

Table 7–1 Calculations for Sensitivity and Specificity Values		
	Condition Present	**Condition Not Present**
Positive test result	tP	fP
Negative test result	fN	tN
	Sensitivity $= \dfrac{tP}{(\text{Column total})}$	Specificity $= \dfrac{tN}{(\text{Column total})}$
	Sensitivity $= \dfrac{tP}{(tP \times fN)}$	Specificity $= \dfrac{tN}{(fN \times tN)}$

fN, false negative; fP, false positive; tN, true negative; tP, true positive.

example, a study published by Michener et al. (2009), who examined the accuracy of the Neer test for diagnosing subacromial impingement syndrome in patients with shoulder pain (Michener, Walsworth, Doukas, & Murphy, 2009). The Neer test had a relatively high sensitivity (0.81) and a low specificity (0.54) (Michener et al., 2009). You may want to jump to the conclusion that this test is good for correctly diagnosing subacromial impingement syndrome. In the case of high sensitivity, however, a patient may test positive, but you still do not know whether the result is a true positive or false positive. Data presented by Michener et al. (2009) indicate that 13 patients had true-positive test results and 18 had false-positive results. All patients had shoulder pain, and you cannot discern whether the shoulder pain is a result of impingement (true positive) or another condition (false positive).

The Neer test can be used, however, to rule out a condition when a patient tests negative. Recall that sensitivity examines only persons with a condition, and high sensitivity indicates that relatively few persons with the condition have negative test results (false-negative test result). A negative test result therefore likely indicates that a person does not have the condition (i.e., it is ruled out). In the paper by Michener et al. (2009), only 3 patients of 16 with subacromial impingement syndrome tested negative (false negative) on the Neer test, whereas 21 patients without impingement tested negative (true negative). Because the true-negative test results outweigh the false-negative test results, a negative test result can be used to rule out subacromial impingement syndrome. The acronym SnNOUT (high sensitivity [Sn], negative test result [N], rules out [OUT]) may help you remember this notion (Sackett, Haynes, Guyatt, & Tugwell, 1991).

Zaslav (2001) published an investigation on the use of the internal rotation resistance strength test for diagnosing intra-articular shoulder impingement syndrome versus subacromial impingement syndrome. The clinical test used in this study had a high specificity (0.96) and sensitivity (0.88) for identifying intra-articular impingement (Zaslav, 2001). As a result of the high specificity, you again may want to conclude that a negative test result can diagnose the absence of intra-articular impingement. A negative result with high specificity for a clinical test does not necessarily rule out a condition because a patient with the condition may test negative (false negative). In the case of high specificity, however, you can rule in the disease when a person tests positive.

Remember that specificity examines only persons without the condition, and high specificity indicates relatively few persons with positive test results (false-positive test results). A positive test result therefore likely indicates that a person has the condition (i.e., rule in). In the paper by Zaslav (2001), only 3 patients without intra-articular impingement tested positive (false positive), and

23 patients with intra-articular impingement tested positive (true positive). Because of the greater true-positive results compared with the fewer false-positive results, a positive test result can be used to rule in intra-articular impingement. The acronym SpPIN (high specificity [Sp], positive test result [P], rules in]) may help you remember this concept (Sackett et al., 1991).

Even with the aforementioned exceptions, these two statistics cannot be used to estimate the probability of having a condition. Sensitivity examines only that proportion of persons with a condition who have positive and negative test results. To compute the probability of having a condition, you need to know whether or not persons without a condition have positive results. Similar to sensitivity, the specificity of a test cannot be used to estimate the probability of not having a condition because you would still need to know whether or not persons with a condition have negative results on these clinical tests. To use sensitivity and specificity effectively to compute the probability of having a condition based on test results, you need to combine them into a single outcome known as a likelihood ratio. This computation is discussed later in this chapter because you first need a sound understanding of predictive values to grasp the likelihood ratio concept fully.

Positive Predictive Value and Negative Predictive Value

The probability that a person with a positive test result will have a condition is known as the positive predictive value or positive posttest probability. Simply put, this measure provides the percentage of true-positive scores in all persons with and without a condition who have a positive test result. The greater number of true-positive scores and fewer false-positive scores will result in a higher positive predictive value. Clinically, you can use this percentage to predict the probability that a person has a condition if he or she tests positive. Take, for example, the use of magnetic resonance imaging in the diagnosis of an anterior cruciate ligament tear that has a positive predictive value of 91.9% (Vaz et al., 2005). The percentage of 91.9% is the probability of having a condition (i.e., anterior cruciate ligament tear) after a positive test result. The negative predictive value examines the probability that a person with a negative test result will not have a given condition. This measure provides the percentage of true-negative scores in all persons with and without a condition who have a negative test result. Magnetic resonance imaging, for example, has a negative predictive value of 99.5%. However, the negative posttest probability is the probability of having the condition given a negative test result, which is computed as 1 minus the value of the negative predictive value. In the case of magnetic resonance imaging, the

Positive predictive value: The probability a person with a positive test result actually has a given condition. It is computed as the percentage of true-positive scores in all persons with and without the condition who have positive test results.

Negative predictive value: The probability that a person with a negative test result does not have a given condition.

Negative posttest probability: The probability of having the condition given a negative test result. It is computed as 1 minus the value of the negative predictive value.

negative posttest probability for an anterior cruciate ligament tear is 0.005 (1 − 0.995) (Vaz et al., 2005).

Let us again use Figure 7–1 to understand positive and negative predictive values conceptually. This time, however, you will pay attention to the data above the threshold line only for positive predictive value and need to worry about data below the threshold line only for negative predictive value. A greater number of circles above the threshold line compared with the diamonds above the threshold line indicates that this test has a high positive predictive value. Thus, most positive test results are associated with persons with a given condition. In contrast, a greater number of diamonds below the line compared with circles below the line indicates that this test has a high negative predictive value. More negative test results are associated with persons without a given condition.

Once again, you need to grasp the concepts in a 2 × 2 contingency table to understand positive and negative predictive values published in literature. Table 7–2 displays a 2 × 2 diagnostic contingency table for the computations of positive and negative predictive values. The columns and rows in this table are identical to those in Table 7–1. In Table 7–2, however, positive and negative predictive value results are computed from the scores in the rows of the contingency table. Again, you can think of positive predictive value as the percentage of true-positive scores from all positive test scores (true-positive result divided by row total). On the contrary, negative predictive value is the percentage of true-negative scores from all negative test results (true-negative results divided by row total).

Relationship Between Prevalence and Predictive Values

For clinical applicability of predictive values, you will need to consider prevalence of the condition, test sensitivity, and test specificity to obtain the correct probability of a person having a condition.

Table 7–2 Positive Predictive Value and Negative Predictive Value Calculations

	Condition Present	Condition Not Present		
Positive test result	tP	fP	$PPV = \dfrac{tP}{(Row\ total)}$	$PPV = \dfrac{tP}{(tP \times fP)}$
Negative test result	fN	tN	$PPV = \dfrac{tP}{(Row\ total)}$	$PPV = \dfrac{tP}{(tP \times fP)}$

fN, false negative; fP, false positive; tN, true negative; tP, true positive.

Prevalence is the proportion of the population with a condition (number of persons with condition divided by the total population). As an example, the prevalence of intra-articular impingement syndrome in a surgical patient population was 24% in the study published by Zaslav (2001) that examined the diagnostic accuracy of the internal rotation resistance strength clinical test in identifying intra-articular impingement syndrome. As indicated previously, the internal rotation resistance strength test had 88% sensitivity and 96% specificity for identifying intra-articular and subacromial impingement, respectively (Zaslav, 2001). These statistics are combined with prevalence to compute the number of patients with a positive test result who, in fact, have intra-articular impingement by multiplying the number of patients by prevalence and then by sensitivity ($110 \cdot 0.24 \cdot 0.88 = 23$). Then, the number of patients who tested positive but do not have intra-articular impingement can be computed by first subtracting specificity from the number 1 and then multiplying the number of patients by the percentage of patients without the condition ($[1 - 0.96] \cdot 110 \cdot 0.76 = 3$). Note that 0.76 is used to indicate that 76% of these patients do not have intra-articular impingement. With this new information, the positive predictive value is 88% (23 / [3 + 23]).

To compute negative predictive value, you first need to calculate the number of patients with a negative test result who, in fact, do not have intra-articular impingement by multiplying the number of patients by the percentage of patients without the condition and then by specificity ($110 \cdot 0.76 \cdot 0.96 = 81$). Next, the number of patients who tested negative but who actually have intra-articular impingements is computed by multiplying the number of patients by prevalence and then subtracting the number of patients testing positive on the clinical test, which was computed earlier ($[110 \cdot 0.24] - 23 = 3$). The negative predictive value is then computed as 96% (81 / [81 + 3]). Thus, after testing these athletes with this clinical test, you can conclude that the positive posttest probability is 88% and the negative posttest probability is 4% ($1 - 0.96$). The problem with these predictive scores is that the values can be applied only to populations with the same prevalence. If the prevalence is greater or lesser than the current, then you will need to perform new computations based on the prevalence of the population under investigation.

So now, let us assume that the prevalence of intra-articular impingement is 5% in 100 swimmers at a high school. You cannot use the positive and negative predictive scores of 88% and 96%, respectively. Using the same clinical test to identify impingement (88% sensitivity, 96% specificity), you now can use prevalence to compute predictive values. The positive predictive value in this population is 50% (4 / [4 + 4]). The numerical values for calculating the positive predictive score were obtained from the number of athletes with a positive test result who, in fact, have intra-articular impingement ($100 \cdot 0.05 \cdot 0.88 = 4$) and the number of athletes who tested positive but who do not have intra-articular impingement ($[1 - 0.96] \cdot 100 \cdot 0.95 = 4$). The negative predictive value in this population is 99% ($91 / [91 + 1]$). The numerical values for calculating the negative predictive score were obtained from the number of athletes with a negative test result who, in fact, do not have intra-articular impingement ($100 \cdot 0.96 \cdot 0.95 = 91$) and the number of athletes who tested negative but who actually have intra-articular impingement ($[100 \cdot 0.05] - 4 = 1$).

Note here in this example compared with the last that the positive predictive score decreased when prevalence decreased, which will be true for any data set you may work with. Furthermore, because of the low prevalence, you still do not have conclusive results given a positive test result. Although both sensitivity and specificity are high for this clinical test, the low prevalence indicates that very few persons have the condition. Thus, very few persons who, in fact, have a condition will test positive. You also know that very few false-positive test results occur because of the high specificity. Given that the prevalence is low, you will not be able to discern whether a positive test result is a true-positive or a false-positive result (recall that four true-positive and four false-positive results were present in the high school swimmer example). To correct this issue, you can explore more powerful diagnostic statistics known as likelihood ratios, which are discussed in the next section.

Connections 7-1

You learned in Chapter 6 about exposed event risk (EER) and control event risk (CER). These terms are used to indicate the risk of developing a given condition after receiving an exposure or intervention (exposed event risk) or not receiving an exposure or intervention (control event risk). These two terms, interestingly, are similar to predictive values and are used to assess the positive outcomes in both exposure and control events. The exposed event risk examines the percentage of subjects developing a condition following an intervention, thus dividing the number of event occurrences by the sum of event and nonevent occurrences in the exposure (intervention) group. Recall that you used this mathematical computation for positive predictive value. The control event risk examines the percentage of subjects developing a given condition without an intervention. The control event risk, therefore emphasizes the percentages of event occurrences divided by the sum of event and nonevent occurrences in the control group (i.e., the percentage of persons who developed the condition in the control group). The computation is identical to the exposed event risk, but the control event risk is computed in the control group.

Positive Likelihood Ratio and Negative Likelihood Ratio

A likelihood ratio defines the percentage of persons with a condition for a certain test result compared with the percentage of persons without a condition for the same test result. The positive likelihood ratio compares the true-positive rate with the false-positive rate of a test to determine the degree to which the probability of having a condition is increased if the test result is positive, thus allowing you to know how much to move the needle in the positive direction for having a condition. With this measure, greater positive likelihood ratio values are indicative of an accurate test because the true-positive rate will outweigh the false-positive rate (percentage of persons with a positive test result for "Condition Not Present"). In the literature, the notation used for false-positive rate is 1 – specificity. The specificity of a test, again, defines the percentage of negative test results in all persons who, in fact, do not have a condition. A quick way to compute the false-positive rate is simply to subtract the specificity value from the number 1 to obtain the percentage of positive test results in all persons who do not have a condition. A test is accurate when it correctly identifies a large number of persons with a condition and misidentifies very few persons without a condition as having it.

Clinically, a positive likelihood ratio is associated with ruling in a condition, and you will know the degree to increase the likeliness that a person has this condition after a positive test result. In the case of magnetic resonance imaging for diagnosing an anterior cruciate ligament tear, the positive likelihood ratio is 21.5 and indicates that a person with an anterior cruciate ligament tear is 21.5 times more likely to have a positive test result than a person who does not have an anterior cruciate ligament tear (Vaz et al., 2005).

The negative likelihood ratio compares the false-negative rate (percentage of persons with a negative test for "Condition Present") with the true negative rate to determine the degree to which the probability of having a given condition is decreased if the test result is negative. The notation used for the false-negative rate is 1 – sensitivity. The sensitivity of a test, again, defines the percentage of positive test results in all persons who, in fact, have a condition. A quick way to compute the false-negative rate is simply to subtract the sensitivity value from the number 1 to obtain the percentage of negative tests in all persons who have a condition. Lower negative likelihood ratio values indicate that a test is accurate because the true-negative rate will be greater than the false-negative rate, thus indicating that the result correctly identifies a large number of persons without a condition and misidentifies very few persons with a condition as not having it.

In the case of magnetic resonance imaging for diagnosing an anterior cruciate ligament tear, the negative likelihood ratio is

Likelihood ratio: The percentage of persons with a condition for a certain test result compared with the percentage of persons without a condition for the same test result.

Positive likelihood ratio: A comparison of the true-positive rate (the probability that a person who has the attribute or disease will test positive) with the false-positive rate (the probability that a person who does not have the attribute or disease will test negative).

False-positive rate: The percentage of persons who do not have the attribute or disease but receive positive test results. The notation used for the false-positive rate is 1 – specificity.

Negative likelihood ratio: A comparison of the false-negative rate (the probability of a person who has the attribute or disease but tests negative) with the true-negative rate (the probability of a person who does not have the attribute or disease but tests negative). The notation used for the false-negative rate is 1 – sensitivity.

False-negative rate: The percentage of persons who do have the attribute or disease but receive negative test results. The notation used for the false-negative rate is 1 – sensitivity.

0.01, and it indicates that the likeliness of having a negative test result for a person with an anterior cruciate ligament tear is 0.01 times of that of a person without an anterior cruciate ligament tear. A negative test result therefore is less likely to occur in a person with an anterior cruciate ligament tear than in a person without a tear. Thus, low negative likelihood values are used in ruling out a condition, such as an anterior cruciate ligament tear. To flip this concept around, you can say that a person without an anterior cruciate ligament tear is 100 times (1 / 0.01 = 100) more likely to have a negative test result than a person with an anterior cruciate ligament tear.

Likelihood ratios transcend patient populations, thereby giving this statistic a distinct advantage over positive and negative predictive values, which have limited clinical applicability to populations with different prevalence rates. Recall that the positive posttest probability is the positive predictive value you have learned, and the negative posttest probability is the 1 − negative predictive value. Likelihood ratios are used to adjust the pretest probability (which is prevalence) to positive and negative posttest probabilities after a test is administered; to give you a sense of whether the change in probability is meaningful.

Ratings scales used in the literature quantify the clinical meaningfulness of likelihood ratios and indicate a considerable change in the posttest probability from pretest probability. As an example, let us compute and examine the likelihood ratios associated with intra-articular impingement in the surgical patient population and high school swimmer examples outlined in the previous sections. The positive likelihood ratio for these groups is 22 (sensitivity / [1 − specificity]; 0.88 / [1 − 0.96]), meaning that posttest probability values (surgical patients = 88%; high school swimmers = 50%) were changed considerably from pretest probability values (surgical patients = 24%; high school swimmers = 5%) after administering the clinical test. Any positive likelihood ratio value greater than 10 indicates that the likelihood of having a condition is greatly increased and that the positive posttest probability has changed considerably from the pretest probability (Grimes & Shulz, 2005).

As an additional reference, low range (2 to 4.99) and midrange (5 to 9.99) likelihood ratio scores indicate small to moderate increases in the likelihood of having a condition, respectively (Grimes & Shulz, 2005). These low to midrange scores can be clinically meaningful and indicate that the posttest probability may be altered sizably from pretest. A score of 1 essentially indicates that no increase or decrease in the likelihood of having a condition exists (Grimes & Shulz, 2005). In the case of the negative likelihood ratio, the value for surgical patients and high school swimmer examples is 0.13 ([1 − sensitivity / specificity; [1 − 0.88] / 0.96]). The negative likelihood ratio value indicates the negative posttest probability (surgical patients = 4%: high school swimmers = 0.65%) is changed considerably from the pretest probabilities. The rating scale for negative likelihood ratio lower than a score of 1 signifies a small (0.2 to 0.99), moderate (0.11 to 0.19), to high (<0.10) decrease in the likeliness of having a condition (Grimes & Shulz, 2005).

In general, likelihood ratio scores higher than 2 and lower than 0.5 should be considered clinically meaningful for positive likelihood ratio and negative likelihood ratio values, respectively (Grimes & Shulz, 2005). The reason that these values can be used to quantify clinical meaningfulness is that the change from pretest to posttest probability is 15% in either the positive or the negative direction, which is considered significant (Grimes & Shulz, 2005). For positive likelihood ratios, you can add 15% to your pretest probability for each increment of small (2), moderate (5), or high (10) likeliness to estimate the posttest probability (Grimes & Shulz, 2005). For example, you add at least 45% to pretest probability to estimate posttest probability if your likelihood ratio is 10 or greater (10 is the third increment; $15\% \cdot 3 = 45\%$). From the surgical patient example we have used, 24% (pretest probability) plus 45% computes a posttest probability of 69%. The computed positive posttest probability is 88%, but the take-home point is that you know, in this case, that the posttest probability is at least 69% without having to compute the true posttest probability.

For negative likelihood ratios, you can subtract 15% from the pretest probability for each decrement of small, moderate, or high to estimate the negative posttest probability (Grimes & Shulz, 2005). In the surgical patient example, 24% (pretest probability) minus 30% provides a negative posttest probability of less than 0% (0.13 is the second decrement; $15\% \cdot 2 = 30\%$), which is slightly less than the 4% negative posttest probability that was computed. The main take-home point is that if you know the likelihood ratios, then you can use these 15% increments or decrements to determine whether your clinical test provides a clinically meaningful probability of having a condition (or not) following the administration of the test.

Figure 7–1 is used one more time to facilitate your understanding of positive and negative likelihood ratios. The process for visualizing these definitions has two steps. First, for positive likelihood ratio, you want to see that a greater number of circles is present above the threshold line than below it, and then, second, you want to see few diamonds above the threshold line. A pattern like the one just described indicates that the test is highly sensitive and has very few false-positive scores; this means that the positive likelihood ratio is a high value. You saw this play out with the surgical patient and high school swimmer examples, which had a positive likelihood ratio of 22 (sensitivity / [1 – specificity]; 0.88 / [1 – 0.96]; 0.88 / 0.04 = 22).

For negative likelihood ratio, you want to see that a greater number of diamonds is present below the threshold line than above it, and then you want to see few circles below the threshold line. A pattern like the one just described indicates that the test is highly specific and has very few false-negative scores; this means that the negative likelihood ratio is a low value. You saw this pattern in the surgical patient and high school swimmer examples, which had a negative likelihood ratio of 0.13 ([1 – sensitivity] / specificity; [1 – 0.88] / 0.96; 0.12 / 0.96 = 0.13).

■ EXAMPLE OF DIAGNOSTIC ACCURACY STATISTICS

The first example illustrates the clinical usefulness of diagnostic statistics for determining balance impairments to identify chronic ankle instability. The purpose of this study was to identify balance impairments in patients with chronic ankle instability. In this study, subjects with and without chronic ankle instability stood on a single leg atop a force plate and remained as motionless as possible for 20 seconds. A force plate collects the forces a person applies to the surface, and balance measures can then be computed. In this study, balance was assessed using a measure known as center-of-pressure velocity (cm/second), which quantifies how quickly a person unintentionally sways back and forth and side to side. The faster a person sways back and forth and side to side, the more it indicates existing balance impairments, which are important to study because these impairments have been linked to ankle sprains.

Table 7–3 outlines diagnostic statistics associated with this study. The sensitivity test value was 0.85, and specificity test value was 0.92. The sensitivity value indicates that 85% of patients with chronic ankle instability were identified as having balance impairments. The specificity value indicates that 92% of subjects without chronic ankle instability were identified as not having balance impairments. These sensitivity and specificity values are indicative of an accurate test. Out of all persons with positive test results for balance impairments, 92% had chronic ankle instability, which is the positive predictive value. Thus, this test is precise and indicates that the positive posttest probability that a person with a positive test result has chronic ankle instability is 92%. In contrast, the negative predictive value demonstrates that out of all persons with negative test results for balance impairments, 86% did not have chronic ankle instability.

Connections 7-2

You will learn about the odds ratio (OR) in Chapter 8. The odds ratio is the probability that an event will occur in a group compared with the probability that an event will not occur in another group. The odds ratio is computed as the positive likelihood ratio divided by the negative likelihood ratio. If you choose to analyze the positive and negative likelihood ratios in a case-control study, you can compute the odds ratio from these data to provide an additional interpretation of the accuracy of your test. Greater odds ratio values (>1.0) indicate that the test is accurate because it has excellent sensitivity and specificity.

Retention Questions 7-1

1. Can you qualitatively define sensitivity and specificity?
2. What additional information do positive and negative predictive scores add to a diagnostic analysis?
3. How do you interpret a clinical test result if the positive likelihood ratio is high (>2) and the negative likelihood ratio is very low (<0.5)?
4. What do likelihood ratio values tell you about the posttest probability?

Table 7–3	Diagnostic Statistics for Balance Impairments with Chronic Ankle Instability	
	Chronic Ankle Instability Present	**Chronic Ankle Instability Not Present**
Positive	11	1
Negative	2	12
Sensitivity	$\dfrac{tP}{(tP + fN)} = \dfrac{11}{(11 + 2)} = 0.85$	
Specificity	$\dfrac{tN}{(fP + tN)} = \dfrac{12}{(1 + 12)} = 0.92$	
PPV	$\dfrac{tP}{(tP + fP)} = \dfrac{11}{(11 + 1)} = 0.92$	
NPV	$\dfrac{tN}{(fN + tN)} = \dfrac{12}{(2 + 12)} = 0.86$	
PLR	$\dfrac{\text{Sensitivity}}{(1 - \text{Specificity})} = \dfrac{0.85}{(1 + 0.92)} = 11$	
NLR	$\dfrac{1 - \text{Sensitivity}}{\text{Specificity}} = \dfrac{(1 - 0.85)}{0.92} = 0.16$	

fN, false negative; fP, false positive; NLR, negative likelihood ratio; NPV, negative predictive value; PLR, positive likelihood ratio; PPV, positive predictive value; tN, true negative; tP, true positive.

The negative posttest probability that a person with a negative test result has chronic ankle instability is 14%. The positive likelihood ratio value of 11 rules in chronic ankle instability and indicates that a person with chronic ankle instability is 11 times more likely to have a positive test result indicative of balance impairments than a person who does not have chronic ankle instability. The negative likelihood value of 0.16 rules out chronic ankle instability and indicates that a person without chronic ankle instability is six times more likely to have a negative test result for balance impairments than a person with chronic ankle instability. Therefore, the likeliness of having a negative test result for a person with chronic ankle instability is 0.16 times of that of a person without chronic ankle instability. Remember for an accurate test, you are looking for tests with high sensitivity and specificity, high positive and negative predictive values, and likelihood ratios greater than 2 for positive ratios and less than 0.5 for negative ratios, as is the case in this example.

Recall the data published by McCrea (2001) on using the Standardized Assessment of Concussion scores for assessing sport-related concussions for this second example. Remember, the Standardized Assessment of Concussion is an objective and standardized test for assessing an injured athlete's mental status immediately following a suspected concussion. McCrea (2001) found that a change score of only –1 point (worse performance) was sensitive to identifying decreased mental status in athletes with a concussion. Table 7–4 outlines the diagnostic statistics associated with a change score of –1. Recall that in the case of high sensitivity, you cannot use a test to rule in a condition, but you can use it to rule out the condition (SnNOUT). With regard to the Standardized Assessment of Concussion, the high sensitivity (0.95) can be used to rule out a concussion, and of the 45 athletes testing negative, only 3 athletes had a concussion and tested negative (false-negative result). Thus, you can be fairly certain that if an athlete tests negative, he or she does not have a concussion. The specificity (0.76) in this example is not considered high, but applying SpPIN even with this moderate value demonstrates that most positive test results (60 of 73) can be used to rule in a concussion.

Table 7–4	Diagnostic Statistics for Standardized Assessment of Concussion Scores for Concussed and Nonconcussed Athletes	
	Concussion Present	**Concussion Not Present**
Positive	60	13
Negative	3	42
Sensitivity	$\dfrac{tP}{(tP + fN)} = \dfrac{60}{(60 + 3)} = 0.95$	
Specificity	$\dfrac{tN}{(fP + tN)} = \dfrac{42}{(13 + 42)} = 0.76$	
PPV	$\dfrac{tP}{(tP + fP)} = \dfrac{60}{(60 + 13)} = 0.82$	
NPV	$\dfrac{tN}{(fN + tN)} = \dfrac{42}{(3 + 42)} = 0.93$	
PLR	$\dfrac{Sensitivity}{(1 - Specificity)} = \dfrac{0.95}{(1 + 0.76)} = 4$	
NLR	$\dfrac{1 - Sensitivity}{Specificity} = \dfrac{(1 - 0.95)}{0.76} = 0.07$	

fN, false negative; fP, false positive; NLR, negative likelihood ratio; NPV, negative predictive value; PLR, positive likelihood ratio; PPV, positive predictive value; tN, true negative; tP, true positive.

The prevalence for the data presented in Table 7–4 is 53%, and after administering this test, you want to know what the posttest probability is for having a concussion. The positive predictive value for the Standardized Assessment of Concussion demonstrates that 82% of athletes with positive test result have a concussion. Your intuition should tell you that this percentage increase over the prevalence (pretest probability) is significant, but you can confirm it by computing the positive likelihood ratio, which is a value of 4. Recall that likelihood ratio values of 2 and greater tend to be clinically meaningful; thus, this test demonstrates that the posttest probability is important. The negative predictive score on the Standardized Assessment of Concussion indicates that 93% of athletes with a negative test result will not have a concussion. The negative posttest probability of having concussion given a negative test result is 7% (1 – negative predictive score). The likelihood ratio of 0.07 indicates that the athlete's chance of having a concussion after a negative test result reduces from 53% to 7%.

RECEIVER OPERATING CHARACTERISTIC CURVES

A receiver operating characteristic (ROC) curve is a graphic way to represent the positive likelihood ratio values for each point in your data set. Recall that the positive likelihood ratio is equal to sensitivity divided by 1 – specificity. Every data point is plotted on a curve based on the sensitivity value and false-positive rate (1 – specificity) value associated with each data point. The values for sensitivity and 1 – specificity can range only between 0 and 1. Sensitivity is plotted on the y-axis, and 1 – specificity is plotted on the x-axis (Fig. 7–2). The value of each data point is called a cutoff score, which is a score used to determine the presence or absence of a condition. The receiver operating characteristic curve therefore has multiple cutoff scores. Scores from a test above a selected cutoff score indicate a positive test result, and scores below it indicate a negative test result. The sensitivity and 1 – specificity values associated with a cutoff score determine the accuracy of a test for that specific cutoff because the probability of having a condition given a positive test result (i.e., positive likelihood ratio) can be computed by dividing sensitivity by 1 – specificity. As a result, a receiver operating characteristic curve demonstrates how sensitivity and specificity vary together, and it is a useful technique for determining appropriate cutoff scores that accurately distinguish between persons with and without a condition.

Figure 7–2 shows how true-positive and false-positive rates vary together, thus taking into account all scores in the contingency table (true positive, false positive, false negative, true negative) for a given data point (i.e., cutoff score). Typically, the true-positive

Receiver operating characteristic (ROC) curve: A graphic way to represent the positive likelihood ratio values for each point in a data set; the sensitivity of a test divided by the false positive rate (1 – specificity).

Cutoff score: The value of each data point on a receiver operating characteristic (ROC) curve that is used to determine the presence or absence of a condition.

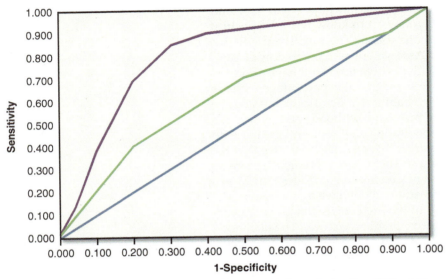

Figure 7–2 Receiver operating characteristic (ROC) curves. This figure displays three ROC curves. The solid black curve running along the vertical axis and across the top of the figure represents a test with perfect accuracy. The dashed black curve represents a test with good accuracy because it is positioned in between perfect accuracy and the solid diagonal line, which represents a 50/50 chance of diagnosing the condition correctly with a given test. The dotted black line represents a test with poor accuracy because it is too close to the solid line. In summary, a test is more accurate the farther away it is from the solid diagonal line and is less accurate the closer it is to the solid diagonal line.

rate will increase to a maximum value with only minimal changes to the false-positive rate. This pattern demonstrates that the test is accurate in identifying those persons with a condition and misidentifies only a few persons without a condition as having it. After this cutoff score, the true-positive rate can increase or plateau, but the false-positive rate begins to increase dramatically; thus, the test begins to lose accuracy because the specificity is decreasing in value. As you move toward the value of 1 on the x-axis, more persons without the condition are identified as having it. A test that has perfect accuracy is displayed in Figure 7–2 as a solid black line that runs along the vertical axis then across the top of the figure. The dashed and dotted lines demonstrate tests with less accuracy. Tests become less accurate the closer the curves are to the solid line running diagonally through the figure.

Optimal Cutoff Score on a Receiver Operating Characteristic Curve

In a research study, you will be interested in knowing the optimal cutoff score, which shows the threshold a person must reach to test positive for a given condition. The first step in identifying this cutoff score is simply to look at the receiver operating characteristic curve and search for the most northwest point on the graph. To do this statistically, you can compute the **Youden index** for each data point by adding the sensitivity and specificity values and then subtract the number 1 (Youden, 1950). The data point associated with a Youden index value closest to 100% is the optimal cutoff score. The most important point to remember is that the optimal cutoff score has the greatest accuracy and corresponds to the score with the greatest true-positive rate and the lowest false-positive rate (i.e., the most northwest data point).

For the balance impairments study previously discussed, the optimal cutoff score in Figure 7–3 is greater than or equal to 6.60 cm/second. The cutoff score of 6.60 cm/second maximized the true-positive rate while at the same time minimizing the false-positive rate. The point 0.23, 1.00 (x, y), however, actually has a Youden index value close to the index value of the optimal cutoff score. The point 0.23, 1.00 (x, y) has a cutoff score greater than or equal to 6.09 cm/second and may be clinically advantageous to select even though it does not have the greatest Youden index value. This thought is elaborated on in Pros and Cons 7-1.

Youden index: A method of summarizing the performance of a clinical test. Computed by adding the sensitivity and specificity values, and then subtracting the number 1, the value ranges from 0 to 1. A value of 1 indicates a perfect test; a value of 0 indicates a useless test.

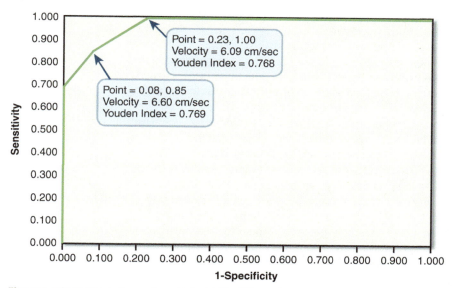

Figure 7–3 Optimal cutoff score for ankle instability. This receiver operating characteristic (ROC) curve represents test results from the balance assessment example. Two northwest points are isolated to demonstrate the use of the Youden index to select a cutoff score. Point 0.08, 0.85 has the greatest Youden index value, indicating that this point captures a high number of persons with chronic ankle instability with balance impairments and few persons without ankle instability with balance impairments. The next best point is 0.23, 1.00 (nearly identical Youden index value), and it identifies balance impairments in all persons with chronic ankle instability. Although this point is more sensitive, it is also less specific and leads to greater false-positive test results.

Pros and Cons 7-1

Clinicians may be willing to use a cutoff score that has a greater false-positive rate than the one identified by the Youden index to achieve a greater true-positive rate. In the balance impairment example, incorrectly identifying persons as having balance impairments will not cause them harm by participating in a balance training program. In fact, the training may have a therapeutic effect on preventing sprains even though these persons should have been identified as not having balance impairments. Clinicians may feel comfortable misclassifying persons to increase the ability of a test to identify persons who actually have balance deficits. In this case, you may not want to use the Youden index (unless your test has perfect to nearly perfect sensitivity and specificity). A cutoff score of 6.09 cm/second from the balance impairment example increases the sensitivity to 1.00 and the false-positive rate to 0.23, which misidentifies three persons without chronic ankle instability as having balance impairments (this cutoff score has the second highest Youden index). The payoff, however, is that the test now identifies all patients with chronic ankle instability as having balance impairments.

In the Standardized Assessment of Concussion example, the Youden index was not used as the cutoff score for identifying decreased mental performance in concussed athletes (McCrea, 2001). The receiver operating characteristic curve for the Standardized Assessment of Concussion is presented in Figure 7–4, and the corresponding 1 – specificity and sensitivity values associated with the Youden index are 0.05, 0.78 (x, y), respectively. Recall that the 1 – specificity and sensitivity values that McCrea (2001) recommended were 0.24, 0.95 (x,y), respectively. If McCrea (2001) had recommended the values associated with the Youden Index, 14 athletes with concussions would have had false-negative test results. Given the high risk for sustaining a second concussion when the first goes undiagnosed, a cutoff score with the second highest Youden index (0.71) was recommended for clinical use because it identifies more athletes as having a concussion at the expense of increasing the false-positive rate (0.05 to 0.24) (McCrea, 2001).

Certainly, using a cutoff score that increases your sensitivity at the expense of increasing your false-positive rate can have clinical advantages. Depending on the medical condition, however, the Youden Index may be better to use in cases of surgical consequences. In the case of an anterior cruciate ligament tear, for example, the Youden index for a Lachman test is important to use in identifying an optimal cutoff score to determine accurately whether a patient has an anterior cruciate ligament tear and to minimize the false-positive rate if the test is being used to recommend a patient for a surgical procedure. Using a cutoff score more sensitive than the one associated with the Youden index will increase the false-positive rate and unnecessarily send patients without anterior cruciate ligament tears to surgical treatment. A clinical test with high sensitivity is very important, but it is as important to maintain a low false-positive rate to minimize sending a person without an anterior cruciate ligament tear to surgical treatment.

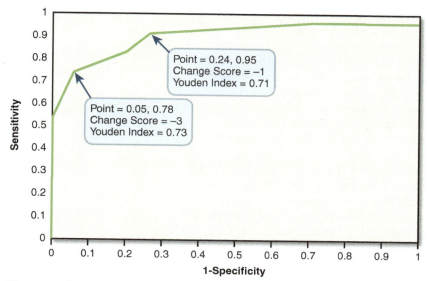

Figure 7–4 Optimal cutoff score for sport-related concussion. This receiver operating characteristic (ROC) curve represents test results from the Standardized Assessment for Concussion example. Two northwest points are isolated to demonstrate the use of the Youden index to select a cutoff score. Point 0.05, 0.78 has the greatest Youden index value, indicating that this point captures a moderate number of persons with concussions who have mental deficits, and few persons without concussions are identified as having mental deficits. The next best point is 0.24, 0.95 (nearly identical Youden index value), and it identifies mental deficits in all but three athletes with concussions. An increased sensitivity associated with this point, however, also decreases the specificity, thus leading to greater false-positive test results.

Area Under the Curve

Up to this point, you have focused on a single data point on a receiver operating characteristic curve, and now you will begin to analyze the curve across its full array of data to examine the accuracy of a test. A measure known as the **area under the curve (AUC)** is an accuracy measure of a clinical test that takes into account all cutoff scores in your investigation and provides the probability that the test result will positively identify a condition. Perfect accuracy is indicated by an area under the curve of 1.0, indicating that the sensitivity is 100% and the false-positive rate is 0%. No apparent accuracy of a test is indicated by an area under the curve less than or equal to 0.50, meaning that the sensitivity and false-positive rate are at or lower than 50%. On a receiver operating characteristic plot, a diagonal line that divides the graph in half indicates an area under the curve of 0.50.

You can use statistical software (e.g., SPSS, IBM, Armonk, New York) to compute the area under the curve for your array of data. The area under the curve is calculated by first computing the

Area under the curve (AUC): An accuracy measure of a clinical test that takes into account all cutoff scores in your investigation and provides the probability that the test result will positively identify a condition.

area of a rectangle (length times width) for each data point, where the width of the rectangle is determined by the difference between two consecutive false-positive rates on the receiver operating characteristic curve and the length of the rectangle is determined by the true-positive rate associated with the greater value of the two consecutive false-positive rates. These area values for each data point then are summed to provide the area under the receiver operating characteristic curve. An example is provided in Table 7–5 on calculating the area under the curve for the data published by McCrea (2001).

The area under the curve value for both the balance impairment and Standardized Assessment of Concussion examples, coincidently, is 0.97. The value indicates that a 97% probability exists that a randomly selected person with a condition (chronic ankle instability or concussion) will have greater deficits on a clinical test than a randomly selected person without the condition. In other words, a high probability exists to identify deficits in a person with either

Table 7–5 Area Under the Curve Value Computation			
Sensitivity	*1 – Specificity*	*Rectangular Area Computation*	*AUC*
1.00	1.00	(1.00–0.98) · 1.00	0.02
1.00	0.98	(0.98–0.96) · 1.00	0.02
1.00	0.96	(0.96–0.91) · 1.00	0.05
1.00	0.91	(0.91–0.78) · 1.00	0.13
1.00	0.78	(0.78–0.65) · 1.00	0.13
1.00	0.65	(0.65–0.24) · 1.00	0.41
0.95	0.24	(0.24–0.18) · 0.95	0.06
0.87	0.18	(0.18–0.05) · 0.87	0.11
0.78	0.05	(0.05–0.00) · 0.78	0.04
0.59	0.00	(0.00–0.00) · 0.59	0.00
0.41	0.00	(0.00–0.00) · 0.41	0.00
0.30	0.00	(0.00–0.00) · 0.30	0.00
0.22	0.00	(0.00–0.00) · 0.22	0.00
0.13	0.00	(0.00–0.00) · 0.13	0.00
0.10	0.00	(0.00–0.00) · 0.10	0.00
		AUC sum	0.97

AUC, area under the curve.

The Critical Consumer 7-1

Area under the curve values range between 0 and 1.0 (i.e., between 0% and 100%) and are classified by the following point scale: 0.90 to 1.00, excellent; 0.80 to 0.89, good; 0.70 to 0.79, fair; 0.60 to 0.69, poor; 0.50 to 0.59, failed (Ross, Guskiewicz, Gross, & Yu, 2009). Statistically significant and meaningful area under the curve values will be good to excellent, unless the study is severely underpowered (i.e., low number of subjects). Michener et al. (2009) presented data on five clinical tests for identifying subacromial impingement syndrome and then plotted a receiver operating characteristic curve that represented the number of positive test results needed to assess impingement. These investigators reported a statistically significant area under the curve value of 0.79 and an optimal cutoff score of three out of five positive test results needed to diagnose subacromial impingement (Michener et al., 2009). The curve rating for these five clinical tests is only considered fair, but the positive likelihood ratio of 2.93 (0.75 / [1 − 0.74]) for the cutoff score of three positive test results can be clinically meaningful (Michener et al., 2009). Recall that positive likelihood ratios greater than 2 can be considered clinically meaningful, and this example demonstrates that the area under the curve values can be fair yet important to a clinician when considering all diagnostic statistics. To take an additional step, the prevalence for impingement was 29%, and the positive likelihood ratio indicates that 15% can be added to the pretest probability to compute, roughly, the posttest probability of 44%. Michener et al. (2009) actually reported a positive posttest probability of 54% for any three positive test results. Thus, three positive test results moved the needle in a positive direction for a clinician to have greater certainty that a patient has impingement. Viewing this result with a critical eye, however, the posttest probability is slightly higher than 50%, and a clinician would want additional testing to diagnose impingement with more accuracy. For other investigations in the literature, statistically significant results also can be found in the lower fair and upper poor ranges. You will need to view these results critically because the area under the curve values are approaching the diagonal line of 0.50, which indicates that the positive likelihood ratios also will approach values that do not have clinical meaningfulness. In other words, you almost have as good of a chance at guessing whether a person has a condition or not.

Retention Questions 7-2

1. How does a receiver operating characteristic curve relate to the positive likelihood ratio?
2. You have a choice of two cut-off scores to determine the threshold of having a condition. The first sits at the far northeast corner of the receiver operating characteristic curve, and the other sits at the far northwest corner of the receiver operating characteristic curve. Which score are you selecting for your cutoff, and why are you not selecting the other?
3. Why is the area under the curve statistic important in determining the accuracy of a clinical test?

condition discussed throughout this chapter (chronic ankle instability or concussion).

Decision-Making With Diagnostic Statistics

You may need a recipe to follow when making clinical decisions because you are now just learning about these statistics. Guidelines are provided in this section for your reference on how to use diagnostic statistics for making clinical decisions. To diagnose a condition, your first step is to know the cutoff score computed from a receiver operating characteristic curve analysis for determining a threshold for a positive test result. Your second step in making a decision is to know the sensitivity and specificity of a clinical test associated with this cutoff score. You may be able to rule out (SnNOUT) or rule in (SpPIN) a condition based on the value of these diagnostic statistics and test results. However, analyzing each of these statistics alone is not as powerful as combining them into a likelihood ratio for correctly diagnosing a condition. Thus, your third step is to apply positive and negative likelihood ratios to your test result.

Positive likelihood ratio values greater than 2 may be meaningful in diagnosing a condition, but you can feel confident that a clinical test result will rule in a condition as the value approaches and rises to more than 10. The negative likelihood ratio is critical to understand how likely a negative test result will rule out a condition. Negative likelihood values lower than 0.50 can be important in ruling out a condition, but you can gain greater confidence that a clinical test result will rule out a condition as the value dips to less than 0.10. Predictive values are not as powerful as likelihood ratios at diagnosing a condition, but analyzing these values is your last step if you can apply them to your patient population.

The major limitation to predictive values is that you cannot transfer published predictive values between populations with different prevalence rates; you can apply likelihood ratios and sensitivity or specificity values to populations that do not have the same prevalence rates. Given that the prevalence rate is the same between your clinical population and those published in literature, predictive scores can indicate the probability of ruling in a condition after a positive test result or the probability of ruling out a condition after a negative test result. When combined with likelihood ratio values, you are able to discern the degree to which your posttest probability changed from your pretest probability and conclude whether the test result is clinically meaningful.

■ SUMMARY

Diagnostic statistics are essential for determining the accuracy, and therefore the clinical meaningfulness, of a clinical test. You first learned that sensitivity and specificity indicate the percentage of persons correctly identified as having and not having a condition based on a clinical test result. The higher the sensitivity and specificity, the better a clinical test is at identifying a person with a condition and the lower the chance is of misidentifying a person without the condition as having the condition. In addition, you learned that positive and negative predictive values tell you the percentage of persons with positive outcomes who actually have a condition and the percentage of persons with negative test results who do not have a condition, respectively. High positive predictive values rule in a condition, whereas low negative predictive values rule out a condition. Recall that positive and negative likelihood ratios tell you how many more or fewer times likely a person is for having or not having a condition, respectively. Greater values of positive likelihood ratios indicate that a person is more likely to have a condition (rule in), and low negative likelihood ratios indicate that the person is less likely to have a condition (rule out). An ROC curve can be plotted to provide a graphic representation of the positive likelihood ratio values across the array of data. From this graph, a cutoff score can be identified as the most northwest point on the plot to serve as a threshold for detecting a condition. Finally, the area under the curve quantifies the degree of accuracy for a test based on the receiver operating characteristic curve, and this statistic summarizes the effectiveness of a clinical test for identifying a condition.

CRITICAL THINKING QUESTIONS

Please refer to Figure 7–5 for the following five questions.

1. The threshold for a positive clinical test in Figure 7–5 is 0.50. The black circles represent test results for patients with a condition, and the diamonds represent test results for persons without a condition. Can you qualitatively determine the degree of sensitivity, specificity, positive predictive value, and negative predictive value?

2. You obtain the clinical test results from a technician but realize that the only diagnostic statistics included is the positive predictive value of 0.54. What information can you relay to your patient to tell him or her about the possibility of having a given condition?

3. You then learn that this clinical test has a sensitivity of 0.83 and specificity of 0.30. Why would you or would you not use this test to determine whether a person has or does not have a condition given a positive test result?

4. You still let the patient know that you do not have all diagnostic accuracy results. The patient asks you to obtain the results, so you call the technician on the phone, but the only additional result that the technician can add to the report is a positive likelihood ratio of 1.17 on the clinical test. Now, what can you tell your patient about having a given condition?

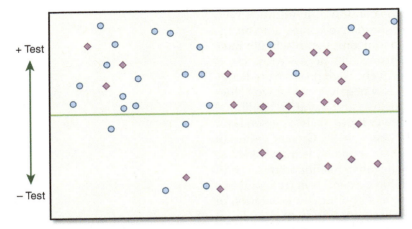

Figure 7–5 Conceptually defined diagnostic statistics. This figure displays positive and negative test results for persons with (solid circles) and persons without (open diamonds) a given condition. The threshold for a positive test result is the solid line in the middle of the figure. Persons above this line have a positive test result, and persons below it have a negative test result.

5. You later learn that the area under the curve statistic on this clinical test is 0.56. You see the patient for a follow-up examination. How will you explain the meaningfulness of this area under the curve value as it relates to his or her test result?

■ TRUST AND APPLY

Croy, T., Koppenhaver, S., Saliba, S., Hertel, J. (2013). Anterior talocrural joint laxity: Diagnostic accuracy of the anterior drawer test of the ankle. *Journal of Orthopaedic and Sports Physical Therapy, 43*(12), 911-919.

Locate the foregoing article, and use the article to address the following questions:
1. What was the sensitivity of the anterior drawer test?
    a. If your patient has a positive test result, how will you explain the accuracy of this test for diagnosing the injury?
    b. What was the specificity for the anterior drawer test, and how does this information contribute to determining the accuracy of this test?
2. What are the values of positive and negative likelihood ratios for the anterior drawer test?
    a. What does the positive likelihood ratio tell you about the accuracy of this test?
    b. What does the negative likelihood ratio tell you about the accuracy of this test?

3. Why do you think that the authors left out positive and negative predictive scores?
   a. Would these predictive scores add meaningful information to the test accuracy results?
   b. Can the other diagnostic statistics provide meaningful information in place of the predictive scores?
4. Based on the accuracy of the anterior drawer test for the ankle, why will you use this test or not use this test for assessing joint laxity in ankle sprains?

RESEARCH SCAVENGER HUNT

Find a published investigation using diagnostic statistics or a receiver operating characteristic curve. Use that article to answer the following questions:

1. How do you quantify the accuracy of the clinical test based on the diagnostic statistics or receiver operating characteristic curve results?
2. What diagnostic statistics information is missing? Would the missing statistics add more meaningfulness to the results? Do the other diagnostic statistics reported in the article substitute for the missing diagnostic statistics?
3. Would you recommend using this clinical test? Why or why not?

REFERENCES

Grimes, D. A., & Shulz, K. F. (2005). Refining clinical diagnosis with likelihood ratios. *Lancet, 365,* 1500-1505.

McCrea, M. (2001). Standardized mental status testing on the sideline after sport-related concussion. *Journal of Athletic Training, 36*(3), 274-279.

Michener, L. A., Walsworth, M. K., Doukas, W. C., & Murphy, K. P. (2009). Reliability and diagnostic accuracy of 5 physical examination tests and combination of tests for subacromial impingement. *Archives of Physical Medicine and Rehabilitation, 90*(11), 1898-1903.

Ross, S. E., Guskiewicz, K. M., Gross, M. T., & Yu, B. (2009). Balance measures for discriminating between functionally unstable and stable ankles. *Medicine and Science in Sports and Exercise, 41*(2), 399-407.

Sackett, D. L., Haynes, R. B., Guyatt, G. H., & Tugwell, P. (1991). *Clinical epidemiology: A basic science for clinical medicine* (2nd ed.). Boston: Little, Brown.

Solomon, D. H., Simel, D. L., Bates, D. W., Katz, J. N., & Schaffer, J. L. (2001). The rational clinical examination: Does this patient have a torn meniscus or ligament of the knee? Value of the physical examination. *JAMA, 286*(13), 1610-1620.

Vaz, C. E., Camargo, O. P., Santana, P. J., & Valezi, A. C. (2005). Accuracy of magnetic resonance in identifying traumatic intraarticular knee lesions. *Clinics (Sao Paulo), 60*(6), 445-450.

Youden, W. J. (1950). An index for rating diagnostic tests. *Cancer, 3,* 32-35.

Zaslav, K. R. (2001). Internal rotation resistance strength test: A new diagnostic test to differentiate intra-articular pathology from outlet (Neer) impingement syndrome in the shoulder. *Journal of Shoulder and Elbow Surgery, 10*(1), 23-27.

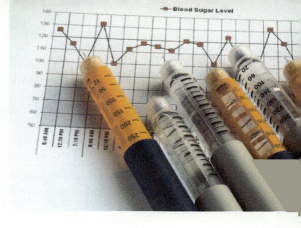

8

Epidemiological Methods in Sport and Exercise Science

Gregory W. Heath
University of Tennessee, Chattanooga, Tennessee

Where Have You Been?

In earlier chapters, our focus has largely been on issues related to measurement and experimental types of research. Particular emphasis has been given to the validity of research and the methods put in place to ensure validity. This has largely meant that studies had to be controlled in various ways. Although this control is very helpful in maintaining internal validity, it sometimes creates an artificial environment. In doing so, internal validity can jeopardize the real-world or external validity of the research. You have also learned that not all research questions can be answered through traditional experimental research. For example, diagnostic trials do not conform to the traditional experimental model. This is an example of how research is modified to meet the needs of the research question. Because of the strict controls and manipulations needed for experimental trials, it may be more appropriate for some research to be done in a more natural environment. Ethical issues may also prohibit the use of experimental methods. For example, to study the cause and effect of a disease implies inducing the disease in individual persons. Clearly, this is unethical. For these reasons, other observational methods can be used to address important questions.

Where Are You Going?

One way of studying disease and health outcomes in a population is in the context of a free-living or natural environment. It is in this context that the observation and collection of population-specific data of epidemiological research methods can be used to generate hypotheses suggestive of causal associations. An understanding of epidemiological methods is important to you as a practitioner to assess and understand the complex relationships among physical activity, inactivity, sport, health, and disease. An understanding of such concepts as the web of causation and the complex interactions among agent, host, and environment in relation to disease or injury and clinical outcomes is essential to the practice of sports medicine, exercise science, and preventive and rehabilitative care. Application of epidemiological measures of disease or injury occurrence, variation in occurrence, and the statistical measures of relative risk, odds ratio, and attributable fraction or population attributable risk contributes to a practitioner's skill level in assessing the potential cause-and-effect relationships reported in the sports medicine and exercise science literature. Becoming familiar with the study methods used in epidemiology, the sport and exercise science professional is better positioned to assess the criteria for cause and effect, as well as critically evaluate the assessment efforts used in meta-analyses and findings of expert review panels (e.g., consensus conference findings).

Learning Outcomes

After reading this chapter, you should be able to answer these questions:

1. What are the different types of epidemiological measures used to study human populations?
2. How is epidemiology different from experimental research?
3. How is causality assessed in epidemiological research?

Key Terms

Agent
Attributable risk
Biological gradient
Case-control study
Coherence
Consistency of association
Cross-sectional design
Cumulative incidence
Direct causal association
Effect modification
Environment

Epidemiological triad
Epidemiology
Host
Incidence
Indirect casual association
Information bias
Odds ratio (OR)
Persistence
Plausibility
Population attributable
  fraction (PAF)

Prevalence
Prospective cohort design
Relative risk (RR)
Secondary association
Selection bias
Specificity of association
Statistically meaningful
  association
Temporality
Web of causation

In the fields of sport and exercise science, epidemiological studies are important for understanding the complex relationships that exist among physical activity, health, and disease. Epidemiology is the study of the occurrence of health-related events and their determinants in human populations (Porta, 2008). The goal of epidemiology is to discover facts essential or contributory to the occurrence of disease or a state of health in a population. The objective of this discipline is to develop effective methods of disease prevention that act directly on causal agents, factors, or determinants. Epidemiology includes the study of where a disease or injury occurs, who has the disease or injury, and who is at risk for developing the disease or sustaining the injury. The importance of epidemiological research is highlighted by the great impact that disease and injury have on society, an impact that is measured in loss of life, disability, emotional anguish, social dysfunction, and economic loss. Because health-care expenditures in the United States now exceed 17.9% of the gross national product, it is imperative that epidemiological research be used to advance knowledge of the causes of disease and injury to reduce their consequences on the individual person and society (National Center for Health Statistics, 2014). The domain of epidemiological research is groups of people, not individual persons, with an emphasis on identifying specific subgroups, explained by age, sex, race or ethnicity, socioeconomic status, educational level, and so forth, and a focus on factors of time, place, and person.

Epidemiology: The study of the occurrence of health-related events and their determinants in human populations.

● EPIDEMIOLOGICAL METHODS

Epidemiologists apply the scientific method practically to problems of the health sciences. The discipline borrows from many specialties and combines them into a viable science. The application of epidemiology requires knowledge of causal factors relative to the occurrence of specific health events. This knowledge is often revealed through measures of association that declare suspected causal factors and specific health events either statistically significantly associated or not statistically significantly associated (i.e., either independent or not independent of one another).

Connections 8-1

Often epidemiological studies are observational and cross sectional, in which cause and effect cannot be directly determined. Instead, associations between possible causes and outcomes such as death or disease are established, resulting in potential hypotheses of cause and effect that, in turn, need to be confirmed by carefully designed experimental or controlled studies.

For those primary associations that are statistically significant, several interpretations are possible. Such a relationship may be direct or indirect. In the case of a **direct causal association**, one event is the cause of a second event. Conversely, an **indirect causal association** is characterized by an event that may be associated with a third event that is really the causal event. A noncausal or **secondary association** is another possibility if the two events are very common and thus are associated but not in a causal fashion.

This can further be explained by the concept of the **web of causation**, an important principle in epidemiology (Porta, 2008). This web (Fig. 8–1) can be defined such that the effect may be the result of a complex interaction of causes, with the understanding that not every effect is the result of a single cause (Caspersen, 1989). An important tenet of epidemiology is that for effective public health interventions to be carried out, they do not require complete knowledge of the web of causation. It is also understood that the web may be sufficiently altered by an attack at one link that may render prevention efforts less effective. For example, when an athlete's host resistance is compromised by a preexisting condition such as asthma, the influenza vaccine may not be as effective as in athletes who do not have asthma. Finally, it is possible that additional unexpected side effects may occur, thus obscuring the relationships within the web of causation.

Direct causal association: A cause-and-effect relationship in which one event is the direct cause of a second event.

Indirect casual association: A cause-and-effect relationship in which one event may be associated with a third event, which is really the causal event.

Secondary association: A cause-and-effect relationship in which two events are very common and therefore associated, but not in a causal fashion. Also called a noncausal association.

Web of causation: An interrelationship of multiple factors that contribute to the occurrence of a disease or injury.

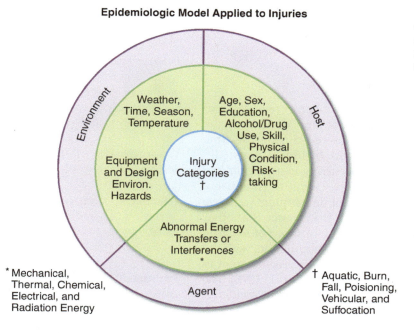

Epidemiologic Model Applied to Injuries

Figure 8–1 Web of causation and the epidemiological triad applied to injuries. *(From National Center for Injury Prevention and Control, Centers for Disease Control and Prevention, Atlanta, GA.)*

Fundamental to understanding the complex nature of a web of causation is the assessment of the critical classes of causal factors, which include the classic paradigm of agent, host, and environment, the so-called epidemiological triad (see Fig. 8–1). The agent in the context of a causation web or multifactorial outcome can be one of any number of factors including, but not limited to, factors that are genetic, physical (e.g., sunlight, fire, radiation, seat belts), nutritive (excess, deficiency), exogenous chemical (e.g., inhalation, ingestion, skin contact), physiological, or psychological, as well as those that are invasive organisms. The host manifests any number of personal attributes that may be linked to increased or decreased susceptibility to any agent or occurrence of disease or injury. These personal attributes include age, sex, immune status, behavioral attributes (e.g., smoking status, physical activity), race or ethnicity, social class, and genetic predisposition. The environment is critical to both the host and agent. Characteristics of the external environment that may influence a host-agent interaction can include physical (e.g., climate, altitude, urban, rural), biological (e.g., food supply, other living things), and social (e.g., population distribution, culture, access to recreation, access to health care). Clearly, the internal environment of both the host and the agent also is important and relevant to the interactions of the host and agent with their external environment.

Epidemiological triad: The traditional model of disease causation, which includes three components: agent, host, and environment.

Agent: A factor whose presence, excessive presence, or relative absence, is essential for the occurrence of a disease.

Host: A person or other living organism that is infected by an infectious agent.

Environment: All the external conditions and influences affecting the life and development of an individual entity.

◼ EPIDEMIOLOGICAL MEASURES

Several measures are used to quantify disease occurrence in the population. Table 8–1 provides an overview of the most common epidemiological measures appropriate to sport and exercise science applications.

Disease or Injury Occurrence

The incidence, or incidence rate, is the number of new cases of disease or injury during a defined period of time, divided by the product of the number of persons monitored during the time period (Savitz, Harris, & Brownson, 1998). Incidence is usually expressed as the number of new cases occurring in a year among a specified population (Kelsey, Whittemore, Evans, & Thompson, 1994). Cumulative incidence is the risk of developing a disease over a defined time period, such as 1 year. Prevalence is another proportional measure; it is expressed as the number of existing cases of disease or injury divided by the total population, with the occurrence of the disease or injury measured at a specific point in time rather than over a certain time period (Savitz et al., 1998). The prevalence of a disease or injury is influenced by both its incidence and its persistence (Kelsey et al., 1994). Persistence is the length

Incidence: A measure of the number of new cases of disease or injury during a defined period of time, divided by the product of the number of persons monitored during the same time period. Also called incidence rate.

Cumulative incidence: The risk of developing a disease over a defined period.

Prevalence: A proportional measure of the number of cases of a disease or injury, present in a specified population, at a specified time period.

Persistence: The length of time the disease or injury remains exposed to risk or mitigating factors.

Table 8–1 Selected Epidemiological Measures	
Measure	**Definition**
Prevalence rate	$$\frac{\text{Number of persons who have attribute/disease at particular time}}{\text{Population at risk of having attribute/disease at this point in time}}$$
Incidence rate	$$\frac{\text{Number of new events in a specified time period}}{\text{Number of person ecposed to risk during this period}}$$
Relative risk	$$\frac{\text{Risk of disease/injury or death in the exposed population}}{\text{Risk of disease/injury or death in the unexposed population}}$$
Odds ratio	$$\frac{\text{Number of exposed cases/Number of unexposed cases}}{\text{Number of exposed controls/Number of unexposed controls}}$$
Population attributable risk	$$\frac{\text{Pe(relative risk} - 1)}{1 + \text{Pe(relative risk} - 1)}$$

Pe, proportion of population exposed.

of time the disease or injury remains exposed to risk or mitigating factors. For example, the prevalence of ankle sprains depends on the number of sprains occurring in the population (incidence) and whether the joint remains inflamed as a result of continued use (persistence). See Table 8–1 for a list of selected measures and their definitions.

Variation in Occurrence of Disease or Injury

A comparison between two groups to reveal the relative frequency of a health-related event is expressed as the ratio of the two rates and is referred to as a rate ratio. A specific type of rate ratio is the **relative risk (RR)**, which is a comparison of the rate in a population subgroup exposed to an agent that is believed to cause a disease, injury, or death with the rate in a population subgroup not exposed (Savitz et al., 1998). A similar measure specific to case-control studies (see the section on epidemiological study methods), often considered synonymous with the relative risk, is the **odds ratio (OR)** or cross-product ratio, which provides an approximation of the relative risk (Savitz et al., 1998). In the instance of both the relative risk and the odds ratio, ratios exceeding 1 are interpreted as conveying greater risk or a greater likelihood of an outcome. A measure used in association with rate ratios to declare their likelihood of not being caused by chance alone is the confidence interval (CI). This represents a range of values for a rate ratio or other variable constructed so that this range has a specified probability of including the true value of the rate ratio. The endpoints of the confidence interval are called the confidence limits

The Critical Consumer 8-1
Be cautious to not confuse incidence and prevalence. Both terms are used to convey the number of injuries or disease cases. However, incidence is a measure of new cases during a set period of time (days, weeks, months, year), whereas prevalence is the number of existing cases at any one time period.

Relative risk (RR): The ratio of the rate in a population subgroup exposed to an agent that is believed to cause a disease, injury, or death to the rate in a population subgroup not exposed.

Odds ratio (OR): The probability that an event will occur in a group compared with the probability that an event will not occur in another group; a close approximation of the relative risk. Also called cross-product ratio.

and, when applied to the relative risk and odds ratio, determine statistical significance when 1.0 is not inclusive of the lower 95% or upper 95% range (Porta, 2008).

Epidemiological Measures of Prevention

Another statistic used to judge the strength of association between a risk factor and disease, injury, or death is the **attributable risk** or attributable fraction (Rothman, 2012). The most common form of attributable fraction is the **population attributable fraction (PAF)**, which indicates the proportion of cases in a population that occurred in a subgroup having the risk factor of interest (Savitz et al., 1998; Kelsey et al., 1994; Rothman, 2012). Epidemiologists assume that the proportion of disease found in that subgroup is the result of, or attributable to, that factor. The population attributable fraction is a function of the both the relative risk of a factor and the frequency or prevalence of that factor in the population. Attributable risk is computed by the following formula where Pe is the proportion of the population exposed to the risk factor:

$$\text{Population attributable fraction} = \frac{\text{Pe (Relative risk} - 1)}{1 + \text{Pe (Relative risk} - 1)}$$

An estimate of the potential percentage reduction in the risk of disease, injury, or death for people who were to change from the exposed group to the unexposed group is the clinical attributable risk. This risk is the proportion of all cases in the exposed group attributable to the factor that defines the exposed group and is computed as $1 - (1\ /\ \text{relative risk})$, where the denominator includes the relative risk of the exposure factor.

The relationship between the relative risk and the population attributable fraction is illustrated in Tables 8–2 and Table 8–3. Table 8–2 lists the measured relative risks from the literature for each of the selected risk factors of smoking, elevated serum cholesterol, hypertension, and physical inactivity for coronary heart disease (Powell, Thompson, Caspersen, & Kendrick, 1987). Note the similarity of relative risk for coronary heart disease for each risk factor. Table 8–3 illustrates coronary heart disease as an outcome in relation to the prevalence of physical inactivity, the relative risk of physical inactivity, and the population attributable fraction in the world's population (Lee et al., 2012). Hence the public health implication of the burden of physical inactivity on coronary heart disease worldwide can be more fully appreciated. Expanding on this example taken from the work of Lee et al. (2012) illustrates the use of population attributable fraction to calculate the disease burden of the population exposed to a specific risk factor in calculating

Attributable risk: The percentage of instances of an illness that can be accounted for by a particular risk factor. Also called attributable fraction.

Population attributable fraction (PAF): The proportion of cases in a population that occurred in a subgroup having the risk factor of interest.

Table 8–2	Relative Risk Estimates for Selected Risk Factors for Coronary Heart Disease	
Risk Factor		**Relative Risk**
Smoking (1 pack/day)		2.5
Serum cholesterol (6.93 mmol/L, ~265 mg/dL)		2.4
Hypertension (systolic blood pressure ≥150 mm Hg)		2.1
Physical inactivity		1.9

Adapted from Powell, K. E., Thompson, P. D., Caspersen, C. J., & Kendrick, J. S. (1987). Physical activity and the incidence of coronary heart disease. *Annual Review of Public Health, 8,* 253-287.

the global burden of selected noncommunicable diseases including coronary heart disease resulting from physical inactivity. Referring to Table 8–4, the population attributable fraction resulting from physical inactivity for the selected noncommunicable diseases of coronary heart disease, type 2 diabetes mellitus, colon cancer, breast cancer, and total mortality are displayed for both population attributable fractions, where the relative risk is unadjusted (use of the foregoing formula), and population attributable fraction, where an adjusted relative risk is made for the confounding of other coexisting risk factors such as sex, age, smoking status, obesity, hypertension, and type 2 diabetes mellitus, where confounding refers to the possible influence of these risk factors on the health outcome of interest, in this case noncommunicable diseases.

Table 8–3	Summary of Worldwide Estimates of Prevalence of Physical Inactivity, Relative Risk, and Population Attributable Fraction for Coronary Heart Disease Deaths	
Parameter		**Estimate**
Prevalence of physical inactivity in population (95% CI)		35.2% (22.3–40.5)
Relative risk (95% CI)		1.16 (1.04–1.30)
Population attributable fraction (95% CI)		5.8% (3.2–7.8)

CI, confidence interval.
Adapted from Lee, I. M., Shiroma, E. J., Lobelo, F., Puska, P., Blair, S. N., Katzmarzyk, P. T., for the Lancet Physical Activity Series Working Group. (2012). Effect of physical inactivity on major non-communicable diseases worldwide: An analysis of burden of disease and life expectancy. *Lancet, 380,* 219-229.

Table 8–4	Summary of the Worldwide Population Attributable Fraction of Physical Inactivity for Coronary Heart Disease, Type 2 Diabetes Mellitus, Colon Cancer, and Breast Cancer				
	CHD	**T2DM**	**CCa**	**BCa**	**Total Mortality**
PAF RR$_{unadj}$ (%)	10.4 (7.2–13.4)	18.1 (10.8–22.8)	11.6 (6.8–15.5)	11.8 (6.8–15.1)	14.2 (8.3–18.0)
PAF RR$_{adj}$ (%)	5.8 (3.2–7.8)	7.2 (3.9–9.6)	10.1 (5.6–14·1)	10.4 (5.7–13.8)	9.4 (5.1–12.5)

BCa, breast cancer; CCa, colon cancer; CHD, coronary heart disease; T2DM, type 2 diabetes mellitus; PAF, population attributable fraction; RR$_{adj}$, adjusted relative risk; RR$_{unadj}$, unadjusted relative risk.
Adapted from Lee, I. M., Shiroma, E. J., Lobelo, F., Puska, P., Blair, S. N., Katzmarzyk, P. T., for the Lancet Physical Activity Series Working Group. (2012). Effect of physical inactivity on major non-communicable diseases worldwide: An analysis of burden of disease and life expectancy. *Lancet, 380,* 219-229.

This latter population attributable fraction is expressed as:

$$PAF = P_d \frac{(RRadj - 1)}{RRadj} \times 100\%$$

where P_d is the percent physically inactive among persons developing the respective disease outcome. Hence the independent contribution of physical inactivity to these noncommunicable diseases deaths can be assessed across the globe, and their impact can be expressed in the number of premature deaths per year (Table 8–5) compared with global premature deaths resulting from the risk factors of tobacco smoking and obesity.

Often, to comprehend the origin of a condition fully, the relationship between or among two or more exposures associated with the disease or injury needs to be understood. This type of relationship is referred to as **effect modification**, and it occurs when the effect of one exposure on disease risk is modified by the presence of another exposure (Rothman, 2012). An example from the literature on smoking is the interaction of cigarette smoking and asbestos exposure in relation to lung cancer, in which exposure to smoking alone carries a relative risk of 10.8, whereas exposure to smoking plus exposure to asbestos carries a relative risk of 53.2, thus increasing the risk of lung cancer by almost 50-fold (Saracci, 1987).

In addition to the impact of interaction on epidemiological studies, bias plays a role. Bias occurs if the observed estimate of a measure tends to deviate from its true value; this deviation then obscures the true relationship between an exposure variable and an outcome. Various types of bias that can be introduced in epidemiological studies are listed in Table 8–5. Examples of bias include **selection bias**, in which only certain subjects from a community are enrolled in a

Effect modification: A cause-and-effect relationship in which the effect of one exposure on disease risk is modified by the presence of another exposure.

Connection 8-2

Bias as defined here is conceptually the same as defined previously. Thus, bias transcends all types of research.

Selection bias: Bias caused by choosing the individual subjects or groups to take part in a study, such as when only certain subjects from a community are enrolled in a study when broader representation is desired.

Table 8–5 Types of Bias in Epidemiological Studies

Selection	Information	Measurement
Ascertainment	Interviewer	Validity
Detection	Recall	Reliability
Response	Reporting	

study when broader representation is desired. An example of **information bias** is when errors in classification of risk status or disease status have been made. Misclassifying physical activity exposure by use of either an incomplete assessment measure that lacks validity or an unreliable instrument would produce significant errors in any study examining the role of physical activity and health outcomes.

Relevant to the issue of validity among exposure or outcome measures used in epidemiological studies is the use of the kappa statistic. This is a measure of the degree of nonrandom agreement between measurements of the same categorical variable (e.g., activity counters versus physical activity questions). If the measures agree more often than expected by chance, kappa is positive; if agreement is complete, kappa = 1; if there is no more or less than chance agreement, kappa = 0; if the measures disagree more than expected by chance, then kappa is negative (Porta, 2008). In developing measures to be used in studies and where a "gold standard" is lacking, the comparison of valid and reliable measures using the kappa statistic is advantageous.

◼ STUDY DESIGNS IN EPIDEMIOLOGICAL RESEARCH

Cross-Sectional Study

A study with a **cross-sectional design** is one in which the relationship between health outcomes and other factors of interest is examined within a defined population at one particular time period. This is the least convincing study design in epidemiology. For example, physical activity or fitness can be measured simultaneously along with a measure of the frequency of disease, injury, or death. Other risk factors may also be measured at the same time. Because this approach is analogous to the "snapshot" in photography (Paffenbarger, 1988), proper temporal sequence is not provided. An example of a physical activity study that uses a cross-sectional approach is the Iowa Farmers Study, which examined the association of physical activity with mortality (Pomrehn, Wallace, & Burneister, 1982).

Information bias: Bias resulting from errors in classification of risk status or disease status.

Connections 8-3
You will recall that to establish a measure as valid it must be in agreement with some form of gold standard measure.

Retention Questions 8-1
1. What is the difference between direct and indirect causal association?
2. What is the difference between prevalence and incidence?
3. What role does the agent, host, and environment play in the epidemiological model?
4. What is the difference between the relative risk ratio and the odds ratio?

Cross-sectional design: A study design in which the relationship between health outcomes and other factors of interest is examined, within a defined population, at one particular time period.

Sixty-two thousand all-cause deaths occurring from 1962 to 1978 in male residents of Iowa 20 to 64 years old were examined. A randomly selected group of 95 farmers was compared with a group of 158 nonfarmers who lived in a city. Farmers had a 10% lower rate of death caused by coronary heart disease, and they were twice as likely to participate in strenuous physical activity compared with the nonfarmers. The farmers were also more fit, as determined by lower exercise heart rate and longer endurance time on a treadmill test. Because the farmers had higher cholesterol levels and a higher body mass index, the apparently protective effect attributed to their high activity and fitness could not be explained by lower cholesterol and body mass. In other words, when these known risk factors for coronary heart disease were controlled for, the farmers still appeared to benefit directly from their higher fitness levels (i.e., some evidence for independence of the effects of physical activity and fitness was present). However, the farmers had lower estimated body fat, as estimated by skinfold thickness, and their rates of smoking and alcohol consumption were half that of the city dwellers. Therefore, the apparently protective effect of physical activity was not fully independent; it could just as likely be explained by the marked reduction among the farmers in the known risks of smoking and drinking alcohol. Thus, a conclusion that the active lifestyle of the farmers protected against coronary heart disease–related deaths must be accepted with an element of caution.

Another application of the cross-sectional study is in determining the prevalence of selected conditions and health behaviors for the purpose of public health planning and surveillance. For example, through the National High School Sports-Related Injury Surveillance System, investigators used the High School Reporting Information Online (RIO), an Internet-based sports injury surveillance system, to examine sports injury data from the 2005 to 2006 through the 2010 to 2011 academic years to determine ankle sprain rates and patterns that were sustained as a function of type of sport and by sex (Swenson, Collins, Fields, & Comstock, 2013). This information is useful in establishing the current prevalence of sports-related injuries among high school athletes and determining patterns among demographic groups (e.g., male versus female), by specific sport, and geographic regions. The High School Reporting Information Online database showed that girls were more likely to have an ankle sprain than boys for sex-comparable sports, whereas rates of ankle injuries were more likely to occur during competition than in practice sessions in both boys and girls (Swenson et al., 2013).

Case-Control Study

When there are no clear-suspected causes of a disease, an epidemiologist operates very much like a detective, attempting to piece together causes after the fact. In this situation, the most common design is the retrospective case-control study. A case-control study compares subjects with the disease (cases) with those absent of the disease (control) and tests for differences between the two groups. This approach can be likened to a flashback in cinematography (Saracci, 1987). An example of a retrospective case-control study is the Seattle Heart Watch Study (Siscovick, Weiss, Hallstrom, Inui, & Peterson, 1982), which examined 1,250 cases of sudden cardiac death among men and women, 25 to 75 years of age, living in the Seattle area to determine the association of physical activity habits with risk of sudden cardiac death. Of these cases, 163 were chosen in which subjects had appeared risk-free before the time of their fatal heart attack. Spouses were interviewed about the decedent's physical activity at work and during leisure time during the year preceding death. Each case was paired with a randomly selected control of similar age, smoking habits, and blood pressure. Low activity on the job and low or moderate activity during leisure were unrelated to death rate. However, people in the top 50% of participants in vigorous leisure physical activities judged by metabolic unit (MET) categories as equivalent to 60% of aerobic capacity or higher (jogging, climbing stairs, chopping wood, swimming, playing singles tennis) had just 40% of the risk for sudden cardiac death when compared with cases who spent no leisure time in those vigorous physical activities (Siscovick et al., 1982).

Another example of a case-control study was the Zuni Diabetes Project (Heath, Leonard, Wilson, Kendrick, & Powell, 1987). This study demonstrated that participation in a community-based exercise program for a mean period of 37 weeks successfully facilitated weight loss in a group of patients with type 2 diabetes mellitus; the mean weight loss for cases was 4 kg (8.8 lb), which was significantly greater than the mean weight loss of 0.9 kg (2.0 lb) for controls (Heath et al., 1987). Furthermore, participation decreased fasting blood glucose values and reduced the need for insulin or oral hypoglycemic agents, or both (Fig. 8–2).

Prospective Cohort Study

A prospective cohort study permits observation of the characteristics and behaviors of a group or cohort of people across time. It permits a natural history of physical activity, fitness, and health-related events to be chronicled as they occur, much like a motion picture. Because it is longitudinal, a prospective cohort design enables an investigator to measure physical activity and health-related events at multiple points in time and consequently to test whether an association between physical activity and a low rate of disease is persistent.

Case-control study: A study that compares subjects with the disease (cases) with those absent of the disease (control) and tests for differences between those two groups.

The Critical Consumer 8-2

Case-control and cross-sectional studies are often confused. Case-control studies collect data in the present, but those data must have existed before the disease or injury (i.e., it is historical data). Cross-sectional studies also collect data in the present but those data are new data (i.e., collected after the disease or injury). The particular challenge with cross-sectional data is that you do not know whether they existed before to the injury or disease, are a consequence of the disease, or have no relationship with the disease.

Prospective cohort design: A longitudinal study that follows a group of similar persons (cohorts), who differ with respect to certain factors under study, to determine how these factors affect rates of a particular outcome. Also called a prospective cohort study (PCS).

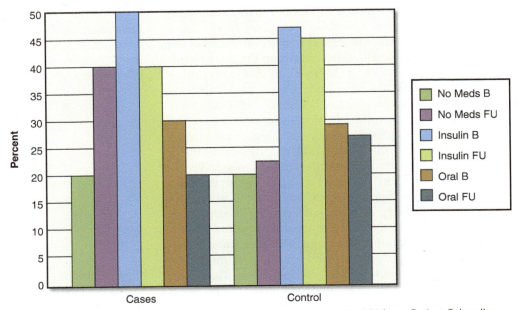

Figure 8–2 Change in hypoglycemic agent status, by percentage, in the Zuni Diabetes Project. B, baseline measure; FU, follow-up; Meds, medications. *(Adapted from Heath, G. W., Leonard, B. E., Wilson, R. H., Kendrick, J. S., & Powell, K. E. [1987]. Community-based exercise intervention: The Zuni Diabetes Project.* Diabetes Care, 10, *579-583.)*

The Aerobics Center Longitudinal Study (ACLS) measured physical fitness defined as endurance time on a treadmill test in more than 10,000 men and 3,000 women at the time they participated in a preventive medical examination (Blair et al., 1989). The men and women were reexamined approximately 8 years later. During the period of observation, 240 deaths among men and 43 deaths among women occurred after approximately 110,000 person-years of exposure. Age-adjusted death rates (per 10,000 person-years of exposure) from all causes were lower with each successive level of fitness in men from the least fit (64 deaths) to the most fit (19 deaths) and similarly in women from the least fit (40 deaths) to the most fit (9 deaths) (Blair et al., 1989). The effects of higher fitness were independent of age, smoking, cholesterol concentration, systolic blood pressure, blood glucose levels, and parental history of coronary heart disease. Much of the decreased death rate was explainable by reduced rates of cardiovascular disease and all-site cancers (Blair et al., 1989).

Another prospective cohort study example addressed the incidence of injuries in a cohort of runners in South Carolina (Macera et al., 1989). Macera et al. (1989) followed 583 runners prospectively for 12 consecutive months to examine the relationship of potential risk factors with the occurrence of running-related injuries of the lower extremities. Running-related injuries were classified as severe if they (1) affected running habits, (2) resulted in a visit to a health professional, and/or (3) required use of prescribed or over-the-counter medication. Runners were asked to keep weekly logs of their running mileage, type of workouts, and competitions, along with injury and illness information. During the 12-month follow-up period, 52% of the men (252) and 49% of the women (48) reported at least one injury. The results identified that running 64.0 km (40 miles) or more per week was the most important predictor of injury for men during the follow-up period (odds ratio = 2.9). Risk also was associated with having had a previous injury in the past year (odds ratio = 2.7) and with having been a runner for less than 3 years (odds ratio = 2.2). These results suggested that the incidence of lower extremity injuries is high for habitual runners and that for persons new to running or those who have been previously injured, reducing weekly distance is a reasonable preventive behavior.

Randomized Clinical Trial or Randomized Controlled Trial

This study design is used to determine whether associations uncovered in epidemiological observations represent cause-and-effect relationships. The validity of the trial depends on having a representative population sample and matching treatment and control groups with respect to characteristics thought to affect outcome. The random assignment of subjects to the treatment or control group is essential to distribute known and unknown confounding variables equally between or among groups.

Examples of a randomized study design in exercise science are the secondary prevention trials among heart attack survivors to determine whether exercise training reduces recurrence rates of myocardial infarction and cardiac arrest.

In a study from Finland, 375 men and women who had survived a myocardial infarction at the time of hospitalization were randomized into a multiple risk factor intervention group, which included exercise, or a control group (Hamalainen et al., 1989). The intervention group had a significant reduction in total cardiovascular mortality and cardiac sudden death rates but not in reinfarction rates. However, because there was no evidence of improved physical fitness on bicycle ergometer testing in the intervention group, the independent effect of exercise was not clearly shown (Hamalainen et al., 1989).

In the United States, the National Exercise and Heart Disease Project was carried out in the mid-1970s (Diabetes Prevention Program Research Group, 2002). Approximately 651 men 30 to 64 years old and from 5 medical centers who had had a heart attack from

1976 to 1979 were randomly assigned to a control group or to a supervised exercise program. The program consisted of 15 minutes of jogging, cycling, or swimming followed by 25 minutes of aerobic games at an intensity of 85% of maximal exercise heart rate. The men were retested after 9 weeks, after 6 months, and at the end of each year. The relative risk of dying in the exercise group versus the control group was 0.63 for all causes and 0.44 for cardiovascular disease during the 4 years following study initiation. These reduced risks were independent of smoking, blood lipid levels, hypertension, and parental history of coronary heart disease (Diabetes Prevention Program Research Group, 2002).

A more recent example of a randomized clinical trial in which physical activity was included as a key component of a lifestyle intervention designed to prevent type 2 diabetes mellitus among persons at high risk for the disease was the Diabetes Prevention Program (LaRosa, Cleary, Muesing, Gorman, & Hellerstein, 1982). In this trial, which sought to compare lifestyle intervention with hypoglycemic agents in preventing type 2 diabetes mellitus, investigators randomly assigned 3,234 persons without type 2 diabetes mellitus but who had elevated fasting and postload plasma glucose concentrations to one of three groups, placebo, metformin (850 mg twice daily), or a lifestyle program with the goals of a weight loss of at least 7% of initial body weight and participation in at least 150 minutes of moderate to vigorous physical activity per week. The mean age of the participants was 51 years, and the mean body mass index was 34.0. Sixty-eight percent of the participants were women, and 45% were members of racial or ethnic minority groups. With an average follow-up period of 2.8 years, the incidence of diabetes was 11.0, 7.8, and 4.8 cases per 100 person-years in the placebo, metformin, and lifestyle groups, respectively. The lifestyle intervention reduced the incidence of diabetes by 58% and metformin reduced the incidence by 31%, as compared with placebo. This trial demonstrated that the lifestyle intervention was significantly more effective than the drug metformin in preventing new cases (incidence) of type 2 diabetes mellitus (LaRosa et al., 1982).

ASSESSMENT OF CAUSALITY

Community-based or clinic-based interventions are based on the presumption that the associations found in epidemiological studies are causal rather than occurring by chance or through some bias. However, in most instances in which epidemiological methods are used to observe health events in the population, the circumstances do not permit the investigator to prove absolutely that

---

Pros and Cons 8-1

Epidemiological research cannot establish the direct cause-and-effect relationship that can be established with experimental research (i.e., randomized controlled trial). However, implementing a "treatment" is often not ethical. For example, to study causes of cancer experimentally, a carcinogen would have to be intentionally given to people assigned to the treatment group. Clearly, this is inappropriate. Because of this, epidemiological studies are the only practical way to study the association between a suspected carcinogen and cancer.

an association is causal. Conversely, several cardinal principles or criteria have been used in epidemiological research for judging the strength of inference drawn from studies about the cause-and-effect relationship between a factor such as physical inactivity and a disease or injury. These criteria were initially coined by Sir Bradford Hill (Hill, 1965). They are often cited as a checklist for causality in epidemiological studies and include the following: strength of association, consistency of association, specificity of association, temporality, biological gradient, plausibility, coherence, and experimental evidence (Hill, 1965).

Strength of Association

The first criterion is that studies show a statistically meaningful association, in this case between physical activity and a lowered prevalence or incidence of disease. A statistically meaningful association is the requirement that the association is not likely to be explainable by random or chance observation. The stronger these associations are, the less likely it is that they are the result of confounding or bias.

Statistically meaningful association: The requirement that an association is not likely to be explainable by random or chance observation.

Consistency of Association

The consistency of association is the requirement that a proposed cause produces similar effects across different conditions. For example, this is achieved when the association of increased physical activity or fitness with lower rates of disease is similar for different types of people, in different geographic regions, and when different measures or components of physical activity or fitness are used. Consistency of association makes a particular bias an unlikely explanation for such a series of observations.

Consistency of association: The requirement that a proposed cause produces similar effects across different conditions.

Specificity of Association

Specificity of association is the requirement that the pattern of reduced risk seen with increasing levels of an agent (e.g., physical activity) must remain in the presence and in the absence of other potential causes of the disease. Even though a study may show a dose-response pattern between increasing levels of physical activity and decreased risk for disease, the pattern of reduced risk seen with increasing levels of physical activity must remain in the presence and in the absence of other potential causes of the disease. An illustration of this criterion, taken from the literature on physical activity and coronary heart disease, is the Harvard Alumni Study carried out by Paffenbarger (Paffenbarger, Hyde, & Wing, 1978).

Specificity of association: The requirement that the pattern of reduced risk seen with increasing levels of an agent must remain in the presence and the absence of other potential casuses.

Temporality

Temporality is defined as the timing between the proposed cause and a lower rate of disease or injury. For a lower rate of disease or death associated with higher levels of physical activity or fitness to be interpreted as being possibly caused by activity or fitness, sedentary or unfit subjects must be just as healthy at the onset of the study as are subjects judged to be more active or fit. In addition, the measurement of activity or fitness must precede the measurement of subsequent events of disease or death.

Temporality: The timing between the proposed cause and a lower rate of disease or injury.

Biological Gradient or Dose Response

Biological gradient is the systematic relationship between a proposed cause and altered rates of disease, injury, or death. If physical activity exerts a protective effect for reducing disease, injury, or death (or conversely, causing some kinds of injury), it should be possible to determine some systematic pattern of relationship between increasing levels of physical activity and altered rates of disease, injury, or death. If rate ratios vary randomly across levels of activity or across differing changes in physical activity, an argument that physical activity was causally responsible for that variation would be uncompelling. The most convincing pattern would be a linear gradient of decreased rate ratios that was proportional to each increment of increased physical activity or physical fitness. It is also possible that the dose-response relationship could be nonlinear, such that each successive increment in physical activity or fitness corresponds to an accelerating change in the rate ratio of disease, injury, or death. A negatively accelerating dose-response relationship would indicate an attenuation of benefit, meaning that the proportionately largest reduction in the rate ratio would be seen at relatively low levels, or across small increases, of activity or fitness, with reductions becoming progressively smaller at the higher levels, or at larger increases, in activity of fitness. A positively accelerating relationship would indicate the converse; in other words, larger benefits would occur at higher levels, or greater changes, in activity or fitness. Finally, it is possible that some threshold of response could occur rather, than a traditional graded pattern. In other words, some minimal level of physical activity or physical fitness may explain all or nearly all of the altered rate ratios. Once the minimal threshold was exceeded, no further change in disease, injury, or death would be observed.

Biological gradient: The systematic relationship between a proposed cause and altered rates of disease, injury, or death.

Plausibility

Plausibility is the ability to explain the association between death and disease and a proposed cause. Even when the preceding

Plausibility: The ability to explain the association between death and disease and a proposed cause.

criteria have been met, the overall case established for cause and effect will remain weak if the association between increased physical activity and decreased disease or death cannot be explained. A convincing explanation requires evidence that physical activity or physical fitness induces biological changes that are coherent with the current etiology (i.e., understanding of the causes and course of development) and the pathophysiology (i.e., the process by which the function of cells and systems deteriorate) of a disease.

Coherence

Coherence is the association between a proposed cause and the known biology and natural history of a disease. Once the proper temporal sequence has been established, it is still important to determine whether an association seen between physical activity or fitness and disease rates holds as time passes and that the evidence is not contradictory to the known biology and natural history of the disease.

Coherence: The association between a proposed cause and the known biology and natural history of a disease.

Experimental Evidence

The most compelling evidence that increased physical activity reduces rates of disease or death would come from an experiment conducted in a large group of initially healthy people drawn randomly from a total population in which participants would be randomly assigned to at least three levels of physical activity of differing intensity or amount or to a control group that remained sedentary for several years.

In the absence of a population-based experiment, confirmation must come from studies of nonhuman animals. Studies using rats, dogs, and nonhuman primates have shown favorable changes in the cardiovascular system after exercise training. In addition, many clinical studies with small groups of human subjects have shown that physical activity can: reduce mild hypertension and alter blood lipid levels, blood glucose concentrations, clotting factors, and white blood cells in positive ways; stimulate bone mineral density; and reduce depression, to name a few benefits. Such clinical experiments are important for demonstrating the efficacy of physical activity for health-related outcomes and for building a stronger case for biologically plausible mechanisms. Nonetheless, they cannot demonstrate that the benefits observed for small, select groups of people are generalizable to the population as a whole.

When all other criteria for judging the scientific strength of cause-and-effect evidence are satisfied, the number of studies finding results that agree determines the confidence with which it can be concluded that physical activity or fitness improves health or

Pros and Cons 8-2

Animal experiments are very useful because they allow for tight control and thus can confirm mechanisms in the absence of human studies. However, animal physiology only resembles human physiology. As such, it cannot be considered to represent the human response. This type of research ranks lower on the evidence pyramid.

longevity. As is the case for the other criteria, the number of studies that agree differs widely according to the disease or health outcome studied. An example of the application of the Hill criterion is the review by Powell et al. (1987) examining the relationship between physical activity and the incidence of coronary heart disease. These investigators set forth a compelling case for the cause-and-effect relationship between increasing levels of physical activity and the prevention of coronary heart disease in their review (Powell et al., 1987).

■ EPIDEMIOLOGICAL DECISION-MAKING

Several useful tools are available within epidemiology for determining when public health action should be taken. These tools are necessary because often relationships between exposure and disease or injury show weak associations in which the relative risk estimate is not too far from the null value of 1.0 (Savitz et al., 1998). These tools include meta-analysis, the use of expert reviewers, and the process of consensus conferences (Savitz et al., 1998).

Meta-analysis

This is a quantitative approach to examining the findings of individual studies systematically and integrating them in an overall evaluation. Petitti described an approach to meta-analysis: identify relevant studies, adhere to explicit inclusion and exclusion criteria for each of the studies selected, assess the quality of the study design and outcome measures used, ensure valid and reliable data abstraction for each of the studies included, assess the appropriateness of the statistical analyses, and be certain that the heterogeneity of the studies has been adequately explored (Petitti, 1994). Meta-analysis is most useful for combining results of multiple small, randomized controlled trials whose results are generally consistent. The method is less useful when trials have found extensive variability through different methods or because the relationship of interest varies across populations. Examples of the appropriate use of meta-analysis from the literature on physical activity and health are the paper by Lee at al. (2012) that addresses the global burden of selected noncommunicable diseases resulting from physical inactivity and the meta-analytic review by Berlin and Colditz (1990) of the relationship of physical activity with coronary heart disease.

Expert Reviewers

An example of using expert peer reviewers to examine epidemiological studies and their relevance to health policies and interventions

Connections 8-4

As you will see when the findings of many studies exist, they can also be statistically combined by a systematic review into a meta-analysis to generate an overall effect of all studies.

Retention Questions 8-2
1. What factors must be present to establish causality in epidemiological research?
2. Of the factors used to establish cause, which relates to the timing of events?
3. Of the factors used to establish cause, which depends on the explanation of the cause-and-effect relationship?
4. How is a prospective cohort study different from a cross-sectional study?

is the 1996 Surgeon General's report on physical activity and health (U.S. Department of Health and Human Services, 1996). This report drew on the expertise of numerous scientists and practitioners from a multitude of disciplines to provide a comprehensive and current assessment of the relationship between physical activity and health. A useful product of this process was a specific set of recommendations about the quality and quantity of physical activity necessary for health that gave rise to particular policy and intervention guidelines for the public's health.

Consensus Conferences

Consensus conferences are similar to the expert review process in which epidemiological evidence is reviewed relative to a specific outcome. The National Institutes of Health (NIH) have used consensus conferences since 1977 to address important issues in public health and medicine. Although the process is similar to the use of expert reviewers, the timeframe is considerably shorter, with the consensus development panel issuing its recommendations within a 2½-day conference (National Institutes of Health, 1996). The National Institutes of Health Consensus Development Panel on Physical Activity and Cardiovascular Health is an example of such a consensus development process (National Institutes of Health, 1996). Specific recommendations were issued from this conference on the importance of regular moderate-intensity physical activity for the health of U.S. children and adults (National Institutes of Health, 1996). This process provided further impetus for enhanced public health policies and community-based physical activity interventions, thereby extending the influence of the Surgeon General's report (U.S. Department of Health and Human Services, 1996).

■ SUMMARY

We have observed that epidemiological research can be an important scientific adjunct for sports medicine and exercise science professionals. Because epidemiology is an eclectic scientific enterprise, it is based on the scientific method and an understanding of potentially causal factors relative to the occurrence of specific health events. The epidemiological measures of rates and proportions, the variation in occurrence of disease or injury, and the application of attributable fraction all provide the sport and exercise scientist with useful tools in understanding the relationships among physical activity, sports participation, health outcomes, and other correlates. The methods of study employed by epidemiologists include cross-sectional study designs, case-control studies, prospective cohort designs, and randomized controlled trials, all of which provide the clinician an array of sources of evidence linking physical activity and exercise to specific health outcomes, all with their inherent strengths and weaknesses. The clinical exercise physiologist thus has the task of assessing the array of evidence from such studies based on a specific set of criteria to determine the causal links among physical activity, exercise, fitness, and health. Finally, the role of expert reviewer processes in assessing the epidemiological evidence for a link between physical activity-related variables and health status can assist the clinical exercise physiologist in establishing appropriate and meaningful health policies on the role of exercise, fitness, physical activity, and health.

CRITICAL THINKING QUESTIONS

1. Of the different measures used in epidemiological research, which measures are most likely to apply to your patients or clients?

2. If you were going to search for an epidemiological study related to your patients or clients, what type of design would you prefer?

3. Given the choice between epidemiological research and experimental research, which would better address your patients' or clients' needs?

4. To feel comfortable that a risk factor for injury (e.g., restricted range of motion) or disease (e.g., high blood pressure) caused the injury or disease, what criteria would need to be met?

TRUST AND APPLY

Lee, D. C., Pate, R. R., Lavie, C. J., Sui, X., Church, T. S., & Blair, S. N. (2014). Leisure-time running reduces all-cause and cardiovascular mortality risk. *Journal of the American College of Cardiology, 64*(5), 472-481.

Locate the foregoing article, and using this article, address the following.

1. What did the authors propose as the cause-and-effect association?

2. What dependent measures were used in the study?

3. Using the criteria of assessment of causality, how many of the criterial were met? Can you give examples of each?

RESEARCH SCAVENGER HUNT

Using your area of interest:
- Locate a cross-sectional study.
- Locate a case-control study.
- Locate a prospective cohort study.

Then answer the following questions.

1. How are the research questions different among the three types of studies?
2. What kinds of measures are used in each study type?
3. How are the conclusions different for each type of study?

REFERENCES

Berlin, J. A., & Colditz, G. A. (1990). A meta-analysis of physical activity in the prevention of coronary heart disease. *American Journal of Epidemiology, 132,* 612-628.

Blair, S. N., Kohl, H. W., Paffenbarger, R. S., Jr., Clark, D. G., Cooper, K. H., & Gibbons, L. W. (1989). Physical fitness and all-cause mortality: A prospective study of health men and women. *JAMA, 262,* 2395-2401.

Caspersen, C. J. (1989). Physical activity epidemiology: Concepts, methods, and applications to exercise science. *Exercise and Sport Sciences Reviews, 17,* 423-474.

Diabetes Prevention Program Research Group. (2002). Reduction in the incidence of type 2 diabetes with lifestyle or metformin. *New England Journal of Medicine, 346,* 393-403.

Hamalainen, H., Luurila, O. J., Kallio, V., Knuts, L. F., Arstila, M., & Hakkila, J. (1989). Long-term reduction in sudden deaths after a multifactorial intervention programme in patients with myocardial infarction: 10-year results of a controlled investigation. *European Heart Journal, 10,* 55-62.

Heath, G. W., Leonard, B. E., Wilson, R. H., Kendrick, J. S., & Powell, K. E. (1987). Community-based exercise intervention: The Zuni Diabetes Project. *Diabetes Care, 10,* 579-583.

Hill, A. B. (1965). The environment and disease: association or causation? *Proceedings of the Royal Society of Medicine, 58,* 295-300.

Kelsey, J. L., Whittemore, A S., Evans, A. S., & Thompson, W. D. (1994). *Methods in observational epidemiology* (2nd ed.). New York: Oxford University Press.

LaRosa, J. C., Cleary, P., Muesing, R. A., Gorman, P., & Hellerstein, H. K. (1982). Effect of long-term moderate physical exercise on plasma lipoproteins: The National Exercise and Heart Disease Project. *Archives of Internal Medicine, 142,* 2269-2274.

Lee, I. M., Shiroma, E. J., Lobelo, F., Puska, P., Blair, S. N., Katzmarzyk, P. T., for the Lancet Physical Activity Series Working Group. (2012). Effect of physical inactivity on major non-communicable diseases worldwide: An analysis of burden of disease and life expectancy. *Lancet, 380,* 219-229.

Macera, C. A., Pate, R. R., Powell, K. E., Jackson, K. L., Kendrick, J. S., & Craven, T. E. (1989). Predicting lower-extremity injuries among habitual runners. *Archives of Internal Medicine, 149,* 2565-2568.

National Center for Health Statistics. (2014). *Health, United States, 2013: with special feature on prescription drugs.* Hyattsville, MD: National Center for Health Statistics

National Institutes of Health. (1996). Physical activity and cardiovascular health: NIH Consensus Development Panel on Physical Activity and Cardiovascular Health. *JAMA, 276,* 241-246.

Paffenbarger, R. S., Jr. (1988) Contributions of epidemiology to exercise science and cardiovascular health. *Medicine and Science in Sports and Exercise, 20,* 426-438.

Paffenbarger, R. S., Hyde, R. T., & Wing, A. L. (1978). Physical activity as an index of heart attack risk in college alumni. *American Journal of Epidemiology, 108,* 161-175.

Petitti, D. B. (1994). *Meta-analysis, decision analysis, and cost-effectiveness analysis: Methods for quantitative synthesis in medicine.* New York: Oxford University Press.

Pomrehn, P. R., Wallace, R. B., & Burneister, L. F. (1982). Ischemic heart disease mortality in Iowa farmers: The influence of lifestyle. *JAMA, 248:*1073-1076.

Porta, M. (2008). *A dictionary of epidemiology* (5th ed.). New York: Oxford University Press.

Powell, K. E., Thompson, P. D., Caspersen, C. J., & Kendrick, J. S. (1987). Physical activity and the incidence of coronary heart disease. *Annual Review of Public Health, 8,* 253-287.

Rothman, K. J. (2012). *Epidemiology: an introduction* (2nd ed.). New York: Oxford University Press.

Saracci, R. (1987). The interactions of tobacco smoking and other agents in cancer etiology. *Epidemiologic Reviews, 9,* 175-193.

Savitz, D. A., Harris, R. P., & Brownson, R. C. (1998). Methods in chronic disease epidemiology. In: R.C. Brownson, P. L., & Remington,,& J. R. Davis, eds. *Chronic disease epidemiology and control* (pp. 27-54). Washington, DC: American Public Health Association.

Siscovick, D. S., Weiss, N. S., Hallstrom, A. P., Inui, T. S., & Peterson, D. R. (1982). Physical activity and primary cardiac arrest. *JAMA, 248,* 3113-3117.

Swenson, D. M., Collins, C. L., Fields, S. K., & Comstock, R. D. (2013). Epidemiology of US high school sports-related ligamentous ankle injuries, 2005/06-2010/11. *Clinical Journal of Sports Medicine, 23,* 190-196.

U.S. Department of Health and Human Services. (1996). *Physical activity and health: A report of the surgeon general.* Atlanta, GA: U.S. Department of Health and Human Services, Centers for Disease Control and Prevention, National Center for Chronic Disease Prevention and Health Promotion.

Synthesizing and Evaluating Research

Because some research syntheses form the top of the evidence pyramid, they can greatly improve your professional practice. However, given that these studies have methods of their own, you must understand those methods before you can apply the studies to your questions. Most importantly, research must be synthesized in a way that minimizes bias and maximizes practical application to your practice. Additionally, Chapter 10 will show you that not all research is created equal. Because the scientific method is not "rigid," researchers make educated decisions on the planning and interpretation of their studies. These decisions affect the quality of the research, and you must be able to discern where the studies you read fall on the continuum of research quality.

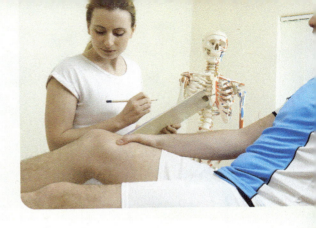

9

Research Synthesis

Where Have You Been?

In Chapter 8, you learned about measures and the properties of measures. This included how these measures may inform your practice and to which measures you may give more attention. You also learned about several different types of research designs. You have learned about how experimental research is conducted and how a cause-and-effect relationship is implied. By extension, you have learned how clinical trials are types of experimental research extended to patient populations, and these trials include establishing both the efficacy and effectiveness of a treatment. You also learned about observational, epidemiological, and diagnostic trials. All these form the basis of how we understand the health and exercise sciences. The problem is that all these different types of research generate tremendous amounts of new information. Because of this, some mechanism of sorting all this information is needed.

Where Are You Going?

One way to sort through the large amount of new research being generated is for you as the practitioner to rely on reviews of the research. Reviews come in two basic forms: traditional narrative reviews and systematic reviews. Both can serve useful purposes. Narrative reviews are more prone to bias and may generate less accurate conclusions. Only the systematic review can establish whether a set of studies consistently supports the research hypothesis. The systematic review can also be extended to include a statistical analysis of the multiple study results. This is known as meta-analysis and is a very powerful tool for making sense of the existing literature.

Learning Outcomes

After reading this chapter, you should be able to answer these questions:

1. What is the difference between a historical review and an expert review?
2. How does bias affect the review process?
3. What are the different types of bias?
4. What are the solutions to bias?
5. What is the difference between a systematic review and a meta-analysis?
6. What is the advantage of a meta-analysis?

Key Terms

Bias
Citation bias
Duplication bias
Effect size
Expert review
Fail-safe N
Fixed effect model
Forest plot
Funnel plot

Historical review
Included study population
Language bias
Meta-analysis
Methodological quality
Narrative review
Overall effect size
Primary study
Publication bias

Random effects model
Raw mean difference
Secondary study
Sensitivity analysis
Standardized mean difference
Systematic review
Trim and fill
Vote counting

Research synthesis is the process of combining preexisting research studies into a single research study for understanding the larger meaning of the research. Research synthesis occurs in three basic forms: narrative reviews, systematic reviews, and an extension of systematic reviews called meta-analysis. To understand the synthesis process, narrative reviews are discussed first, followed by systematic reviews and meta-analysis. However, to understand these three, a distinction must first be made between two basic types of research literature.

PRIMARY STUDY VERSUS SECONDARY STUDY

Up to this point, you have been presented with types of research that generate their own data. Any form of research that generates its own data to answer a research question is known as a primary study. For example, a randomized controlled trial compares a treatment with some type of control. Before this study research, no data exist specific to the research question in the study, and all the data are collected as part of the trial. In epidemiological or nonexperimental research, the same principle applies. Data are collected specifically to study a research problem. In all three cases, the collected data are then analyzed using some type of statistical technique, and conclusions are drawn from them. Although in some cases data may already exist in patients' files, the use of preexisting data to answer a research question still qualifies as primary research. In such cases, the generation of the primary study includes the act of retrieving these data from the patients' files, performing a statistical analysis, and drawing conclusions from the aggregate data.

Primary study: Research study in which researchers directly recruit and collect data on subjects.

A secondary study, is a publication that combines and reviews (or synthesizes) primary studies. Secondary studies use the published results and data analyses of primary studies to make new connections among studies, generate or examine theories, summarize the overall state of the body of literature, identify gaps in the body of literature, or draw new conclusions altogether. To accomplish these goals, two types of research synthesis have been used: the narrative review and the systematic review (with or without meta-analysis).

Secondary study: A publication that combines and reviews primary studies.

NARRATIVE REVIEW

The narrative review is any review that collects, organizes, and synthesizes primary studies without using inclusion or selection criteria. With the narrative review, it is entirely the authors' judgment in determining which studies should be included. The process

Narrative review: Any review that collects, organizes, and synthesizes primary references without using inclusion or selection criteria.

is not systematic, and the method for gathering studies is not reported. Thus, there is no way to determine how studies were included. In effect, the authors are telling the story they want the reader to hear, and this story may or may not be objective. As discussed later, this issue makes narrative reviews prone to bias.

Historical Review

The **historical review** is a narrative review that has the implied purpose of reviewing all the existing literature on a topic. Historical reviews have been the most prevalent in the literature, but you have no way to know how thoroughly the literature has been reviewed. That is entirely dependent on the authors' skills. Even if the review is thorough and includes all the existing literature on a topic, the authors may have misinterpreted the primary studies. It may also be that because of their particular research interest, the authors have focused the review on their particular expertise. For example, maybe the authors have written a narrative review with the goal of presenting the causes of fatigue. Fatigue may be broadly associated with metabolic factors and neuromuscular factors. To accomplish this, the literature would have to be searched for both causes of fatigue. As a reader of the review, your question should be, "Do the authors have the expertise to address both causes of fatigue?" Ideally, the author team would be set up with experts in both areas. However, how would you be assured whether that has been done? Unless you know the authors and their expertise, you may not know. If it is recognized that the authors do not have the correct expertise, you should consider the review with some caution. For example, a group of orthopedists may write a review focusing on the treatment of anterior cruciate ligament injuries. Although the orthopedists would have appropriate expertise to review medical and surgical treatments, they may not have the expertise to address rehabilitation. The part of the review concerning rehabilitation may therefore not be comprehensive, or the interpretation of the studies may be weak. As the reader, you are placed in the position of having to judge the value of the article based on the thoroughness of the review. This requires you either to have some knowledge of the literature or to accept the information at face value. As shown later in the chapter, systematic reviews have methods that are more objective and are therefore easier to judge.

Narrative reviews do not use a systematic process for searching or selecting articles to include. Furthermore, narrative reviews may attempt to draw conclusions from the literature, but these reviews are not typically hypothesis driven, thus making them prone to errors. Searching without a planned process means that articles can

Historical review: A narrative review with the implied purpose of reviewing all the existing literature on a topic.

be missed, and it becomes possible to include articles that do not belong. Mixing randomized controlled trials with other observational studies, for example, may lead to a varied conclusion regarding the value of ankle rehabilitation. This varied conclusion may have nothing to do with the effectiveness of the rehabilitation and may be strictly related to how subjects were selected differently for the randomized controlled trials and the observational studies. In a systematic review, this type of mixing of studies, although rarely done, is clearly delineated in the analysis.

Expert Review

Another type of narrative review is the expert review. Expert reviews are simply narrative reviews written by an expert in the field. These types of reviews can have the same purpose as the more general narrative review and be a survey of the literature by an established expert in the field. This type of review clearly has more face validity than a review written by an unknown or new author. An expert review may also be written solely from the expert perspective. A review of the mechanisms of fatigue, for example, may be written by an expert on peripheral neuromuscular fatigue. This type of review has a limited focus. That focus and the expert perspective, however, increase its value. The limited focus means that it far more likely that the review is comprehensive, and because it is written by an expert, it is more likely to be accurate.

Your challenge as the reader of an expert review is the same as with any narrative review, but you also must determine whether the authors are truly experts. For some fields this is easy. Other fields may have multiple experts, and each one is likely to have his or her own unique perspective on the problem. For example, is ankle instability the result of poor balance, poor reflexes, or poor strength? For each of these causes, there may be a different expert, and within each of these areas, there may be more than one expert with different views. Therefore, there may be no single expert on ankle instability. Because of all the possible variations, even expert reviews challenge you to determine the true value of the review.

Bias in Narrative Reviews

The foregoing descriptions of narrative reviews allude to the key weakness of these types of reviews, in that they are prone to bias. Bias in a narrative review is the presentation of research in a manner that is unrepresentative of all the studies published on a topic (Rothstein, 2005b). The previous example of a fatigue review with the authors focusing only on peripheral neuromuscular fatigue is an example of bias that is intentional. The review is intended to

Expert review: A narrative review written by an expert in the field.

Pros and Cons 9-1

Historical narrative reviews are very useful in quickly conveying an overview of a particular clinical topic. Expert reviews can enhance the historical review by providing more specific coverage on a related topic or on a subtopic of a narrative review. However, these types of reviews are prone to bias. You should recognize them as being very low on the evidence pyramid, falling in the category of expert review.

Bias: A measure of inaccuracy or any effect or interference that produces results that systematically depart from the true value.

Connections 9-1

Bias was introduced previously as the constant error associated with a measure. It is the amount of difference between the real score and the measured score as a result of some fixed amount. Conceptually, bias in narrative reviews is the same. It is the amount that the authors' synthesis of primary studies deviates from a true aggregate of the primary studies.

represent only a portion of the literature on fatigue. This is acceptable provided the authors represent it as a limited review and that you understand it to be such.

Other forms of bias also exist. **Publication bias** is the overrepresentation of articles with statistically significant findings in the scientific literature (Hopewell, Clarke, & Mallett, 2005). Statistical significance is the probability that the study results reflect the treatment or are simply caused by chance. Most research that uses traditional statistical tests determines whether the measured treatment effect is likely the result of chance 95% of time. If the measured result occurs less than 95% of the time by chance, then the result is deemed statistically significant. Publication bias is not the fault of the authors of the review, but rather this is a systemic problem in publication. Journals tend not to publish research unless it has a significant statistical finding. For example, studies on the effectiveness of exercise for reducing blood pressure are far more likely to be published if the exercise program is shown effective (or countereffective). If the exercise program had no effect on blood pressure, then the study would be less likely to be published. Lack of statistical significance can also be a byproduct of poor research design and planning. In any case, publication bias is an unfortunate but well-established limitation in the publication process. In this case, the potential results of publication bias are overrepresentation of studies showing a positive effect of exercise and underrepresentation of studies showing no effect.

Closely related to publication bias is **duplication bias**. Duplication bias is the duplicate publication of results. The most common form of duplication of results is the initial publication in conference proceedings or abstracts followed by publication as a full journal manuscript. Because the results were published twice, they are easier to find and thus are more likely to be included in a review. You should know that this type of duplicate publication is acceptable because the initial publication is brief and preliminary. Duplicate publication of a full paper, however, is considered academic fraud. This type of duplicate publication is defined as "publication of a paper that overlaps substantially with one already published, without clear, visible reference to the previous publication" (International Committee of Medical Journal Editors, 2014).

Publication bias: The tendency of professional journals to publish studies that report statistically significant results more often than studies that report statistically nonsignificant results.

Duplication bias: The tendency to duplicate publication of study results, such as the initial publication in conference proceedings or abstracts followed by publication as a full journal manuscript.

Another form of bias is language bias. This is simply the exclusion of studies that are not in the review authors' native language. Translating foreign language studies is often beyond the resources of authors. These studies, with or without significant results, are often excluded from narrative reviews. You should not consider this exclusion an intentional deception on the part of the authors. Rather, this is a shortcoming of the review for pragmatic reasons.

Citation bias is also possible in narrative reviews. Citation bias is the more frequent citation of studies that have statistically significant results (Hopewell et al., 2005). These studies tend to be overrepresented in the literature, whereas studies with statistically nonsignificant results tend to be underrepresented. This is partially because authors of all research tend to focus on statistically significant results, and less frequently cited studies tend to be more difficult to find.

More subtle errors of the narrative review process can introduce bias. One is the accidental omission of studies, which may result from a poor search strategy by the authors. Without a carefully thought-out search strategy, articles are easily missed. Authors of narrative reviews rarely reveal their search strategy, thereby making it impossible to judge whether the strategy was thorough. This lack of reporting of the search strategy is one of the fundamental weaknesses of narrative reviews.

Another common error in narrative reviews is the inappropriate inclusion of studies. Narrative reviews seldom have explicit criteria for including studies. The inclusion or exclusion of studies is entirely at the authors' discretion. Sometimes authors include every article that can be found. Although this is not necessarily wrong, it can mean that the authors have compared apples with oranges. Narrative reviews, for example, often include both randomized controlled trials and case-control studies. These types of studies have very different methods, as well as different strengths and weaknesses. Whereas randomized controlled trials can determine cause and effect, case-control studies cannot. Narrative reviews include both types of trials as if they both could determine cause and effect, and this leads to a bias in favor of treatments in the authors' conclusions.

Narrative reviews often do not identify subpopulations. For example, the results of an anterior cruciate ligament repair may be very effective for competitive athletes but much less effective for recreational athletes. If this issue is not addressed in the narrative review, the overall summary of results may be biased in favor of the treatment because it works very well in competitive athletes.

One of the typical goals of any review is to combine studies to come to some consensus on what the literature means. The method by which this is done can affect the result. In narrative reviews, the

Language bias: The tendency for authors to exclude studies that are not published in their native language.

Citation bias: The tendency to exclude studies with nonsignificant statistical findings.

Connections 9-2

You will recall that randomized controlled trials are specifically designed to establish cause and effect. However, case-control trials establish only an association between two variables (e.g., artificial turf and knee injuries). Because these designs address different questions with different methods, they should not be combined into one review.

common method is called **vote counting** (Borenstein, Hedges, Higgins, & Rothstein, 2009f). Vote counting is synthesizing studies by simply counting the number of studies with statistically significant results in favor of a new treatment against the number of studies with statistically significant results in favor of the alternative treatment or control group. (Remember that studies with nonsignificant findings are less likely to be published.) The group (new treatment versus alternative treatment) with the greatest number of statistically significant results is preferred. For example, assume you are interested in a review that compares the effectiveness of a drug versus the effectiveness of exercise in controlling blood pressure. Now assume that 10 studies show the effectiveness of drugs, and three studies show the effectiveness of exercise. From this set of studies, it is tempting to conclude that drugs are more effective than exercise. It could also be the case that you are interested only in the effects of medication on blood cholesterol levels, and a review reports three studies showing a positive effect and six studies showing no effect. In this example, using vote counting it is tempting to conclude that the evidence does not support the use of medication.

Although both of the previous conclusions seem logical and are tempting to make, there are at least three flaws in the logic of vote counting. First, you must have all the existing studies on a given topic. In the comparison between medication and exercise, it is possible that the only reason medication seems more effective is that four exercise studies were not found as part of the search strategy. In this case, missing studies can affect the vote count. Second, a study that shows no effect (i.e., no statistically significant difference) does not mean that the treatment was not effective. It could mean that the study was not designed well enough to detect a difference (i.e., poor research design or too few subjects). Third, vote counting does not address the size of the effect or **effect size**. Effect size in this case is the magnitude of the difference between two groups on the dependent variable (see the later section on effect sizes for a more complete definition). For example, the difference (in terms of the standard deviation) in bench press performance between male and female subjects is an effect size. Alternatively, bench press performance between groups with high and low training volume can be expressed as an effect size. This can easily be extended to comparisons among groups undergoing different knee operations for anterior cruciate ligament tears or different rehabilitation protocols for an ankle sprain. (The difference among groups on the dependent variable is only one type of effect size, but it is the most common type.)

The advantage of effect size is that it allows you to understand the magnitude of the effect and not simply rely on whether the

Vote counting: A method of narrative review that simply counts the number of studies with statistically significant results in favor of a new treatment and compares that number with the number of studies with statistically significant results in favor of the alternative treatment or control group.

Effect size: The magnitude of the difference between the control group and the treatment group on the dependent variable or outcome of interest.

result is statistically significant. Just because a research study reports a statistically significant finding, it does not mean that the
finding is meaningful or important. In the blood pressure example,
assume that the seven studies that found that drugs improved
blood pressure produced only a very small improvement in blood
pressure. In addition, assume that the three exercise studies reduced blood pressure by three times as much as the drugs. Seven
studies indicated that drugs work, but three studies indicated that
exercise is three times more effective. This finding suggests that
exercise is the better option because the magnitude of the effect
was greater. Using the second example of studying the effect of
medication on blood cholesterol levels, three studies showed a positive benefit and six showed no benefit. Using vote counting you
may conclude that medication is not very effective, or the effect
may be equivocal. However, given that the three studies showing
benefit had clinically meaningful effect sizes and the other six studies had effect sizes favoring a benefit (although not statistically significant), the overall evidence suggests that medication is effective.
As you can see from these two examples, assessment of the effect
size can greatly alter the interpretation of results.

SYSTEMATIC REVIEWS

Because of the problems associated with narrative reviews, a second type of review has been devised, called the **systematic review**. A systematic review is a review that follows a preplanned
methodology for searching the literature and for determining
which primary studies to include. The purpose of the systematic
review is either to avoid the shortcoming of the narrative review
by applying the systematic process or, when that is not possible,
to identify clearly where potential bias exists.

Methods of Searching for and Assessing Data

As suggested, systematic reviews have a methodology. As in typical research articles, this is explained in a methodology section of
the review. The methodology section usually contains several subsections that address required components. If it is not divided into
subsections, there should at least be a paragraph dedicated to
describing each of the steps.

Hypothesis

One of the key differences between narrative reviews and systematic reviews is that systematic reviews are hypothesis driven.

Connections 9-3

Statistically significant results do
not indicate importance. They indicate only whether a result is by
chance. Understanding whether a
result is important requires different measures such as the effect
size, minimal detectible change,
and minimal clinical important
change.

Retention Questions 9-1

1. What is the difference between an expert review and a
historical review?
2. What is the difference between a primary study and a
secondary study?
3. What is the process of vote
counting?
4. What are the different types
of bias?

Systematic review: A review that follows a
preplanned methodology for searching the
literature and determining which primary
studies to include.

Connections 9-4

Based on the evidence pyramid,
the narrative review sits at the
bottom, in the category of expert
opinion. The systematic reviews,
including those with meta-analysis,
sit at the top of the evidence-
based pyramid.

Figure 9–1 is an example of a hypothesis for a systematic review (Arnold, de la Motte, Linens, & Ross, 2009). The hypotheses are essential because they are what drive the search strategy, the inclusion and exclusion criteria, and other components of the systematic review. Narrative reviews may have a stated or implied purpose, but they do not have hypotheses.

Included Study Populations and Reporting of Subject Characteristics

Another component of a systematic review that is often ignored in narrative reviews is the included study population. In this case, study populations are defined as the participants included in the primary studies. Every systematic review should include a description of the population of participants being included in the review. For example, a systematic review of anterior cruciate ligament repairs may restrict the included population to competitive and recreational athletes. The population may be broadened to include all patients with anterior cruciate ligament reconstructions. In a systematic review of high blood pressure treatments, the included study population may be restricted to patients with high blood pressure only, or it may include those who are prehypertensive. Which populations are included depends on the hypothesis of the systematic review. At times it is possible that the way this is defined depends on the availability of studies. Although this possibility is not ideal, sometimes that is the only way to compile enough studies to complete a meaningful review.

Just as in a primary study in which the characteristics of participants are reported, in systematic reviews these characteristics are reported across all the primary studies. An example of this reporting

Included study population: The participants included in the primary studies.

Hypothesis

On the basis of the above, we identified five hypotheses:
1) Balance is impaired in subjects with ankle instability;
2) Dynamic balance tests will be associated with greater balance impairments than static tests of balance;
3) Within the categories of dynamic and static balance, different measures will produce different effect sizes;
4) Studies clearly stated inclusion criteria will report greater balance deficits than those without stated inclusion criteria;
5) Studies with clearly stated exclusion criteria will report greater balance deficits than those without exclusion.

Figure 9–1 Systematic review hypothesis: an example of a set of hypotheses reported in a systematic review. *(From Arnold, B. L., de la Motte, S., Linens, S., & Ross, S. E. [2009]. Ankle instability is associated with balance impairments: A meta-analysis.* Medicine and Science in Sports and Exercise, 41[5], 1048-1062.)

is shown in Figure 9–2. This type of reporting may be included in narrative reviews, but it is required as part of systematic reviews. It provides a concise means for you to assess whether the subjects are similar to your patients or clients and whether the finding of the systematic review can be applied to them.

Identified Outcomes and Study Designs

The third component of a systematic review comprises identified outcomes and study designs. The outcomes are the dependent variables measured in the primary studies. The study designs are the actual research designs (e.g., randomized controlled trial) of the primary studies that are included in the systematic review. Clear statements of which outcomes and designs were included in the systematic review should be included in the methods section. The outcomes and designs selected depend on the hypothesis. You must determine whether these outcomes have meaning to your practice or to your patients or clients.

Detailed Search Strategy

A detailed search strategy is an important part of the systematic review methodology. Figure 9–3 illustrates a typical search strategy (Arnold, Linens, de la Motte, & Ross, 2009). You can see that the search process included 27 separate steps. You can also see that the

Connections 9-5

Patient-oriented evidence that matters (POEM) is one way to assess a measure's meaning. If the systematic review does not contain POEM measures, you may want to give it less weight. However, you should be aware that finding systematic reviews that focus on POEM measures may be difficult.

Table 3. Characteristics of Participants in the Included Studies

Author(s)	Injured Group			Uninjured Group		
	Age, y	Height, cm	Mass, kg	Age, y	Height, cm	Mass, kg
Bernier et al[13]	22.89	181	80.25	26.22	170	65.08
Hubbard et al[29]	20.3	172.5	72.9	23.3	172.6	71.9
Kaminski et al[14]	19.3	181.5	84	19.5	179.5	82.5
Lentell et al[15]	22 (overall)	Not specified	Not specified	22 (overall)	Not specified	Not specified
Lentell et al[16]	Males: 26.9	Not specified	Not specified	Males: 26.9	Not specified	Not specified
	Females: 25.3			Females: 25.3		
McKnight and Armstrong[27]	FAI: 19.6 R: 18.47	FAI: 171.7 R: 172.9	FAI: 68.55 R: 71.16	21.13	170.84	67.68
Pontaga[25]	21 (overall)	186 (overall)	84 (overall)	21 (overall)	186 (overall)	84 (overall)
Porter et al[26]	22.1	170.3	73.6	21.7	169.5	72.4
Ryan[17]	23 (overall)	Not specified	Not specified	23 (overall)	Not specified	Not specified
Schrader[35]	Not specified	Not specified	Not specified	Not specified	Not specified	Not specified
Sekir et al[19]	21	Not specified	Not specified	21	Not specified	Not specified

Abbreviations: FAI, functional ankle instability group, R, rehabilitation group (prerehabilitation date used for analysis).

Figure 9–2 Participant characteristics: an example of participant characteristics reported in a systematic review. (From Arnold, B. L., Linens, S. W., de la Motte, S. J., & Ross, S. E. [2009]. Concentric evertor strength differences and functional ankle instability: A meta-analysis. Journal of Athletic Training, 44[6], 653-662.)

Table 1. Stepped PubMed/EBSCO Host Search Strategy With the Number of Studies Returned at Each Step[a]

Step	Strategy[a]	PubMed	EBSCO
#27	Search (#18) AND (#26)	189	255
#26	Search (((((#19) OR (#20)) OR (#21)) OR (#22)) OR (#23)) OR (#24)) OR (#25)	428715	108211
#25	Search power*[TIAB]	158385	43558
#24	Search force*[TIAB]	164599	35297
#23	Search isomet*[TIAB]	20238	6081
#22	Search isoton*[TIAB]	10625	850
#21	Search isokin*[TIAB]	3429	4950
#20	Search torque*[TIAB]	8208	4821
#19	Search strength[TIAB]	99872	34248
#18	Search ((#4) AND (#10)) and (#17)	1133	1108
#17	Search (((((#11) OR (#12)) OR (#13)) OR (#14)) OR (#15)) OR (#16)	1770820	136088
#16	Search multiple [TIAB]	457447	39268
#15	Search repetitive [TIAB]	33616	3012
#14	Search functional* [TIAB]	545870	6451
#13	Search recurren* [TIAB]	239173	12473
#12	Search chronic* [TIAB]	566587	51564
#11	Search "Recurrence" [MeSH]	117396	7873
#10	Search ((((#5) OR (#6)) OR (#7)) OR(#8)) OR (#9)	104954	12248
#9	Search inversion [TIAB]	17721	1193
#8	Search instability [TIAB]	44779	5369
#7	Search sprain* [TIAB]	2516	2708
#6	Search unstable [TIAB]	39169	2905
#5	Search "Sprains and Strains"[MeSH:NoExp] OR "Joint Instability" [MeSH]	11935	2395
#4	Search ((#1) OR (#2)) OR (#3)	24851	11741
#3	Search ankle* [TIAB]	22721	11613
#2	Search "Lateral Ligament, Ankle" [MeSH]	191	21
#1	Search "Ankle Joint" [MeSH]	6854	748

(Overlay callout labels: Strength assessment; Ankle instability; Ankle injury; Ankle anatomy)

Abbreviations: TIAB, title and abstract; MeSH, medical subject heading.
[a] *Indicates wild card.

Figure 9–3 Search strategy for a systematic review: an example of a search strategy reported in a systematic review. You can see that the search is divided into four subsections that are then combined in steps 4, 10, 17, 18, 26, and 27. *(From Arnold, B. L., Linens, S. W., de la Motte, S. J., & Ross, S. E. [2009]. Concentric evertor strength differences and functional ankle instability: A meta-analysis. Journal of Athletic Training, 44[6], 653-662.)*

search was divided into four separate subsearches: ankle anatomy, ankle injury, ankle instability, and strength assessment. There are three basic types of steps in the search. The first type (e.g., step 6) accumulates articles. The second type uses the "OR" command to combine subsequent steps (e.g., step 17). In step 17, the six previous steps (steps 11 to 16 inclusive) are combined, and 1.77 million and 136,088 articles were retrieved on PubMed and EBSCO, respectively. The third type interconnects the search terms using the "AND" command. Step 27 is an example that combines search steps 18 and 26. Using these three different steps, an overall search strategy was developed. The first part of the strategy was to search for terms that related to ankle injuries and muscle performance (i.e., the subsearches). The second part accumulated these terms in each group (i.e., steps 4, 10, 17, and 26). The third part, step 17, connected all the ankle terms. The result of step 17 is a collection of primary studies that include ankle injuries that cause instability. The final part of the strategy, step 27, combines primary studies with a strength assessment term (step 26) and primary studies related to ankle instability (step 18) to produce the final result. Thus, you can see that the search strategy was not a random inclusion of terms, but rather a structured search with the goal of optimizing the inclusion of relevant primary studies.

You should also note a couple of other important pieces of the search. First, two search engines were used. PubMed produced 189 studies, and EBSCO produced 255 studies. It may appear at first that this means that a total of 444 (255 +189 = 444) studies were found. Many, if not all, of the PubMed articles were also in the EBSCO search as duplicates. You can see this in Figure 9–4. In the top box, you can see that after duplicates were removed, 291 studies remained. Second, not all of the 291 studies were appropriate, and therefore they were not included in the final systematic review.

After articles were identified in the electronic database search, the authors performed the second phase of the search strategy (Fig. 9–4). This second phase included performing a forward search (stage 2) on studies included from stage 1, a hand search (stage 3) of articles from stage 1 and stage 2, and correspondence (stage 4) with the authors of studies from the first two stages. This process was repeated until no further studies were located. For stages 2 to 4, only one additional study was included.

Inclusion and Exclusion Criteria

Other key components of the systematic review are inclusion and exclusion criteria. Unlike the narrative review, systematic reviews use explicit criteria for including and excluding studies that are explicitly stated in the methods section. For example, in Arnold, de la Motte, et al. (2009), the inclusion criteria were as follows:

1. Primary studies must have "reported means and [standard deviations] for an injured group (or ankles) and an uninjured comparison group (or ankles) or have statistics reported in enough detail that we could calculate effect sizes."
2. Primary studies must have used "an inclusion criterion (or FAI [functional ankle instability] definition) of giving way or frequent sprains or to have described the target condition as FAI."

The application of these criteria to the search and review process can be seen in Figure 9–4.

The purpose of using these criteria was to ensure that studies within the systematic review could be compared with each other. In other words, the goal was to eliminate studies that were insufficiently reported (e.g., no means and standard deviations) or used study populations that were not suitable for the purpose of

Connections 9-6

As you learned previously, the "OR" command requires only that one of multiple search terms be present for the item to be included in the search. In contrast, "AND" requires all search terms to be present.

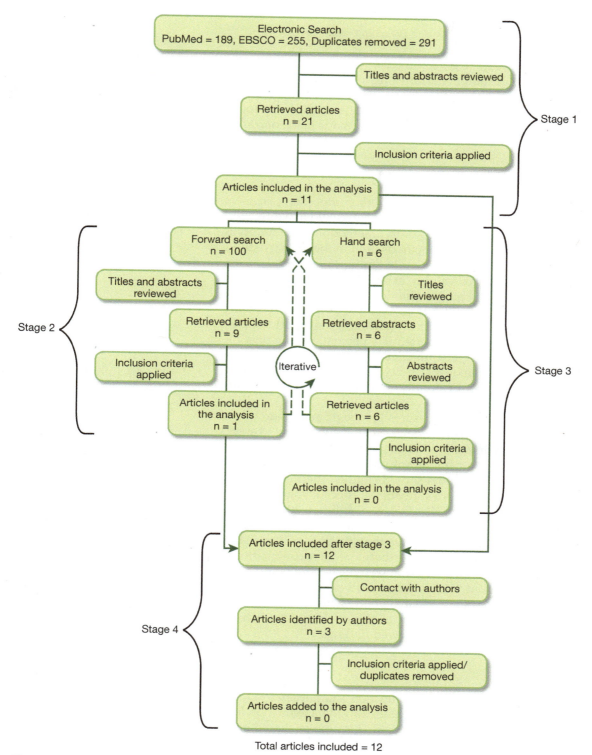

Figure 9–4 Systematic review search flow chart. In this flow of the search process, the authors started with 291 unique articles from two databases. After completing the decision-making process, 12 articles were included in the review. *(From Arnold, B. L., Linens, S. W., de la Motte, S. J., & Ross, S. E. [2009]. Concentric evertor strength differences and functional ankle instability: A meta-analysis. Journal of Athletic Training, 44[6], 653-662.)*

the systematic review (e.g., acute ankle sprains versus chronic ankle instability). Although narrative reviews may be selective in including primary studies, they rarely report specific criteria for including studies. Because of this, it is difficult for you to assess whether appropriate comparisons are being made in the narrative review.

Assessment of Primary Study Quality

Primary study quality assessment is another important feature of systematic reviews. Every systematic review should make an effort to assess the methodological quality. Methodological quality is an assessment of the research methods used in the primary study. In other words, it is an assessment of appropriate controls to ensure validity (i.e., internal validity, external validity, and construct validity). Assessment of quality should be directly reported in the systematic review. Figure 9–5 is an example of quality reporting (Arnold, Linens, et al., 2009). The quality score is reported in the second column. The score reported is a percentage of a possible 20 points. In this case, the instrument used (Fig. 9–6) was a custom-developed survey for ankle instability (Arnold, de la Motte, et al., 2009). Other examples of quality assessment instruments are described in Chapter 10.

    The inclusion of quality measures for the primary studies is a key advantage of systematic reviews. First, it allows you to assess the quality of the primary studies in the systematic review. From that, you can assess how important you think the systematic review is. Similarly, the authors should conduct their own quality assessment. For example, in a study of the effect of yoga on hypertension (Posadzki, Cramer, Kuzdzal, Lee, & Ernst, 2014), the authors used the Cochrane Collaboration's Risk of Bias tool (Higgins, Altman, & Sterne, 2011) and reported their findings on the quality of the included primary studies. Furthermore, they commented in the discussion that the primary studies (which were randomized controlled trials) lacked "methodological rigor" and those studies reported the methods of the research poorly. This type of information gives you the obvious advantage of knowing how much importance you should give the reviewed findings.

Methodological quality: An assessment of the research methods used in a primary study.

The Critical Consumer 9-1

In some systematic reviews and meta-analyses, the authors rate quality by the level of evidence. You need to be aware that identifying the level of evidence for a primary study is not the same as assessing its quality. Primary study quality can be assessed only by examining the methods of the study. If the only entity reported is the level of evidence for each primary study, then you should regard the quality assessment as absent.

Data Extraction

Finally, a planned process of data extraction is important to a meta-analysis. Just as with an experimental study, data extraction for a systematic review is a planned process. This process should be reported as part of the systematic review, preferably in the methods section. As part of the extraction process, the number of people extracting data should be identified, and these should be independent

Table 2. Inclusion and Exclusion Criteria and Outcome Variables for the Included Studies

Author(s)	Quality Score	Stated Inclusion and Exclusion Criteria	Involved Participant or Ankles	Uninvolved Participant or Ankles
Bernier et al[13]	22	Not specified	9	9
Hubbard et al[29]	44	Previous history of unilateral ankle sprain, frequent giving way of the ankle, pain, feelings of instability, and decreased function. No acute ankle sprain within 6 weeks of participation in study, history of surgery or fracture to either lower extremity, or any previous sprain on limb contralateral to the chronically unstable ankle. Control group: free of previous injury or surgery to either lower extremity.	30	30
Kaminski et al[14]	37	Participants (1) experienced at least 1 significant lateral ankle sprain of either right or left ankle, but not both, in which the participant was unable to bear weight or was placed on crutches within last year; (2) had no reported history or fracture to either ankle; (3) sustained at least 1 repeated injury or the experience of feelings of ankle instability or "giving way" in either the right or left ankle but not both; (4) were not undergoing any formal or informal rehabilitation of the unstable ankle; and (5) had no evidence of mechanical instability as assessed by a physician using an anterior drawer test.	21	21
Lentell et al[15]	38	Each participant reported a past history of inversion injury to only 1 ankle, which required protected weight-bearing and/or immobilization. Participant reported no history of fracture to either lower extremity. The involved ankle was reported to be chronically weaker, more painful, and/or less functional than the other at the time of testing. Current subjective complaints were reported to be secondary to the past history of traumatic inversion sprain. No significant trauma reported 3 months before testing. Participant had been full weight-bearing, without a limp, for at least 3 weeks before testing. Participant was currently not undergoing any formal or informal rehabilitation program for the ankle. Participant reported that the functional use of the ankle had plateaued or peaked since the original insult.	42	a
Lentell et al[16]	15	Participant reported a past history of inversion injury to only 1 ankle, which required protected weight-bearing and/or immobilization. Participant reported no history of fracture to either lower extremity. The involved ankle was reported to be chronically weaker, more painful, and/or less functional than the other at the time of testing. Current subjective complaints were reported to be secondary to the past history of traumatic inversion sprain. No significant trauma reported 3 months before testing. Participant had been full weight-bearing, without a limp, for at least 3 weeks before testing. Participant was currently not undergoing any formal or informal rehabilitation program for the ankle. Participant reported that the functional use of the ankle had plateaued or peaked since the original insult.	33	a

Figure 9–5 Quality score reporting. The table shows a reporting of study characteristics including the quality assessment score in the second column. The first column is the study identifier. *(From Arnold, B. L., Linens, S. W., de la Motte, S. J., & Ross, S. E. [2009]. Concentric evertor strength differences and functional ankle instability: A meta-analysis.* Journal of Athletic Training, 44[6], 653-662.)

Construct Validity

1.	Was more than one outcome measure used? (mono-operational bias) E.g., proprioception, strength, balance (dynamic and static conditions would count as separate outcomes), etc.	+1	
2.	Were outcome measures randomly ordered or counterbalanced?	+1	N/A
3.	Were multiple levels of the target outcome variable(s) randomly ordered or counterbalanced? Does not include measures collected simultaneously, e.g., multiple COP excursion measures, EMG w/force, etc.	+1	N/A
4.	Were subjects blinded to the research hypothesis?	+1	
5.	Were data collectors blinded to groups, i.e., unstable and comparison?	+1	

External Validity

6.	Was the population defined (i.e. from where was the sample recruited)?	+1
7.	Were the groups constructed using a representative sampling procedure? (Was it purposively sampled across target groups? Groups may be age, sport, activity level, etc.)	+1
8.	Was more than one criteria used as inclusion criteria? (e.g., # of sprains, time on crutches, immobilization, time since last sprain)	+1
9.	Was a minimum # of sprains required?	+1
10.	Was the number of ankle sprains reported?	+1
11.	Was a minimum # of give-ways required?	+1
12.	Was the number of giving-way episodes reported?	+1
13.	Was mechanical instability measured, eliminated, or included? (manually, arthrometry, or radiographs)	+1
14.	Were acute symptoms excluded?	+1
15.	Was the degree of the initial sprain reported or controlled?	+1
16.	Was the setting described?	+1
17.	Were copers and non-copers included?	+1

Internal Validity

18.	Was the comparison and unstable group equal relative to reported demographics/anthropometrics? (Selection bias) This is "no" if not statistically tested.	+1	
19.	Was/were calibration procedures reported for the variable(s) of interest? (Instrumentation) N/A for surveys, etc.	+1	N/A
20.	Was measurement reliability reported for the variable of interest? (May be referenced to another study or included in current study.)	+1	

Scoring: A = Sum _____
B = 20–N/A _____
A/B*100= _____

Figure 9–6 Primary study quality assessment tool for the ankle: an example of a custom-developed primary study quality assessment tool. The tool was developed for nonrandomized ankle studies. COP, center of pressure; EMG, electromyography; N/A, not applicable. *(From Arnold, B. L., de la Motte, S., Linens, S., & Ross, S. E. [2009]. Ankle instability is associated with balance impairments a meta-analysis.* Medicine and Science in Sports and Exercise, *41[5], 1048-1062.)*

extractors. The typically accepted best practice is three extractors with familiarity with the research topic. For example, for each primary study, the three extractors read the article and identify the data to be used in the systematic review (at least means and standard deviations, but other variables may also be included). Each extractor does this separately, and the results are then compared to make sure all three agree. If all three do not agree, then the discrepancy must be resolved. This resolution process should be clearly described as part of the data extraction process.

Discrepancies among the extractors are usually clerical errors. Occasionally, data are reported in such a way (e.g., only in statistical findings rather than means and standard deviations) that extraction may not be straightforward. Thus, the discrepancy resolution process ensures that the data included in the systematic review are correct. Figure 9–7 is an example of the discrepancy resolution process.

Process of Synthesizing Data

In addition to having an organized process for retrieving and assessing primary studies, systematic reviews synthesize the findings of the primary studies to generate an overall finding. This is done is by calculating an effect size for each study and then presenting the effect sizes in a graphical format.

Effect Sizes

As previously described, the basic concept behind a common form of effect size is that effect size is the difference between the control group and the treatment group on the outcome of interest. For instance, if you want the effect size between a group of patients taking medication for high blood pressure and a control group, the mean blood pressure would be calculated for each group. The absolute value of the difference between those means would produce the **raw mean difference** (Borenstein, Hedges, Higgins, & Rothstein, 2009a). The raw mean difference is the difference between the means of the treatment and control groups. This measure is intuitive and can be used when all subjects in all primary

Raw mean difference: The absolute value of the difference between the means of the treatment and control groups in a particular study.

Data Extraction

For each study, 3 investigators independently extracted means and SDs or other appropriate measures, such as participant n and t values, for the FAI and stable ankle groups (or ankles in studies with contralateral comparisons). We resolved any discrepancies by reexamining the data and agreeing by consensus on the final data to be included. For studies using treatments, we selected only the pretreatment data for inclusion. If pretreatment data were not available, the study was excluded.

Figure 9–7 Data extraction reporting: an example of how the data extraction process may be reported. Note how discrepancies were resolved. FAI, functional ankle instability. (From Arnold, B. L., Linens, S. W., de la Motte, S. J., & Ross, S. E. [2009]. Concentric evertor strength differences and functional ankle instability: A meta-analysis. Journal of Athletic Training, 44[6], 653-662.)

studies are measured on exactly the same scale. However, this is rarely the case. It is more likely that measures across primary studies will be taken on different scales. Balance may be measured as postural sway (i.e., the amount the body sways back and forth) or as time in balance (i.e., how long someone balances on one leg without falling down or touching the other foot down). Postural sway is a distance- or area-based measure, whereas time in balance is based on time. Because of these different measures, primary studies using time in balance cannot be combined with studies measuring postural sway by using the raw mean difference. These measures can be combined using a standardized mean difference. A standardized mean difference is an adjusted raw mean difference, and it allows comparison of measures on different scales and with different units. The basic formula for a standardized mean difference is:

Standardized mean difference: An adjusted raw mean difference that allows comparison of measures on different scales and with different units.

$$d = \frac{\text{Treatment mean} - \text{Control mean}}{\text{Pooled standard deviation}}$$

The pooled standard deviation is calculated by combining all the subjects of the control and treatment groups into one group (i.e., pooling them) and then calculating the standard deviation. More specifically, this formula calculates Cohen's d (or simply d), and is one of the most common effect sizes. An alternative to Cohen's d is Hedge's g or simply g. The effect size g is an adjusted d, and is used when primary studies have small groups, because d can overestimate the effect size when primary studies have small groups (Borenstein et al., 2009a).

Cohen's d and Hedges g are probably the most frequently used effect sizes. However, other effect sizes can be calculated for other types of data. For example, effect sizes can be calculated for odd ratios, risk ratios, and correlations. In the case of correlations, the square of the correlation is the effect size (R^2). Which effect size is used depends on the data. Conveniently, most effect sizes can be converted to the other effect sizes, thereby allowing them to be combined and directly compared.

The key advantage of using effect sizes is that they convey the magnitude of the effect. For d and g, the effect size ranges from zero to infinity, although values higher than 3 are rare. Zero would indicate no effect, and 0.5 to 1 would represent large effect sizes. Effect sizes from 1.5 to 3 are very large and may be valid effect sizes, but they should be viewed suspiciously because they could also be miscalculations.

Effect size also conveys direction. Whether a beneficial effect is represented by a positive or negative effect size depends on whether the beneficial effect increases or decreases the treatment group's outcome measure. Generally, positive effect sizes indicate that the experimental treatment was more effective than the control or standard treatment. Negative effect sizes mean that the standard treatment or control was more effective than the experimental treatment. For example, assume that a set of 30 primary studies comparing strength training with a control is included in a systematic review, with strength being measured by a one-repetition maximum contraction. The effect size d is calculated. In this case, subtracting the control from the treatment group results in a positive effect size. You would interpret the effect size as a beneficial effect (i.e., people in the strength training group became stronger).

Sometimes negative effect size also represents a beneficial effect. Assume that a second systematic review has 30 studies examining the effects of yoga on blood pressure. Because a decline in blood pressure represents a beneficial effect, when the control is subtracted from treatment, the effect size will be negative but still represent a beneficial effect.

Whether a beneficial effect is represented by a positive or negative effect size can be arbitrarily defined by the authors. You must look closely at how the authors have defined a beneficial effect and be aware that negative effect sizes are not necessarily associated with detrimental effects. In the foregoing blood pressure example, the beneficial effect of a decrease in blood pressure was represented by a negative effect size. This is a very intuitive result, but the direction of effect sizes could be reversed so that a decrease in blood pressure (i.e., the beneficial effect) would be represented by a positive effect instead of a negative one. Either way, the beneficial effects would be represented correctly and consistently by magnitude and direction of the effect.

Forest Plot

One of the easiest and fastest ways to interpret a systematic review is to use a **forest plot** (Fig. 9–8), which is the plotting of effect sizes with their confidence intervals. The forest plot is very valuable in summarizing data, especially in systematic reviews that include a large number of primary studies. It also provides you with a method of interpreting the results for yourself. Most systematic reviews provide a forest plot.

When you combine data in a systematic review, the effect size is calculated for every primary study included. Thus, if there are 10 primary studies, there will be 10 effect sizes. These effect sizes are then plotted across the x-axis, and the study, usually by author's name, is plotted on the y-axis. Thus, in one figure, you can see the effect sizes for all the studies. The y-axis is centered on the "no effect" value for the forest plot. For mean differences, this is the actual zero value. However, for some effects sizes, such as odds

Forest plot: A graphic technique showing how different studies that have evaluated a specific condition or treatment have produced independent results.

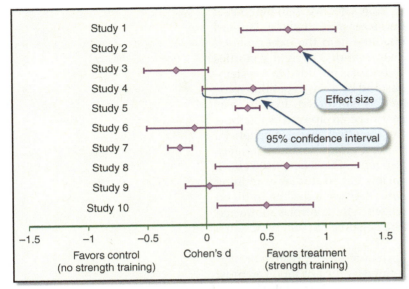

Figure 9–8 Forest plot. Diamonds are the primary study effect sizes. The bars are 95% confidence intervals. Confidence intervals that cross the x-axis zero point indicate that the effect size is not statistically significant.

ratios, the "no effect" point will actually be at the value 1. This is simply a characteristic of the effect size being used, but both should be interpreted as no effect. The 95% confidence interval for each effect size is also displayed on the forest plot.

With the effect size and confidence intervals plotted, you can now visually interpret the results of the systematic review. Figure 9–8 shows data for a fictitious set of strength training studies. You can immediately see that most (seven) of the studies have an effect size that favors the treatment, and three studies favor the control. From this, you could conclude that strength training was effective. However, when the confidence intervals are included in the analysis, a different result emerges. Confidence intervals tell you which of these effect sizes are statistically significant. If a study's confidence interval does not cross the zero point on the forest plot, it is statistically significant, whereas an effect size with a confidence interval that crosses the zero point should be treated as no effect. Based on this rule, you have only five studies with a statistically significant effect for strength training (i.e., studies 1, 2, 5, 8, and 10). One study has a statistically significant effect that supports the control (study 7), and four have no statistically significant effect (studies 3, 4, 6, and 9), thereby making the overall result ambiguous. It could be that the authors of the study did not put sufficient effort into planning the size of their sample, and thus they failed to find a significant difference. Fifty percent of the studies support strength training, and

50% of the studies do not. There is no expectation that the control group would outperform the strength training group, so study 7 is an outlier. This type of result should be viewed suspiciously. It may be an error or may represent something unique about the study that warrants further investigation.

META-ANALYSIS

Closely related to the systematic review is the meta-analysis, which is an extension of the systematic review. Meta-analysis is a statistical analysis of the effect sizes from a systematic review. Systematic reviews are done when there are too few studies for a meta-analysis. As a rule for systematic reviews and meta-analyses, the more studies there are, the better. However, as a consumer you should be aware that when few primary studies exist, meta-analysis results are less trustworthy and are probably not any better than a systematic review. If several primary studies are available, then meta-analysis is preferred. Meta-analyses have the advantage of allowing more quantitative assessment of the primary studies, as well as methods for assessing bias, quality, and several other factors.

Overall Effect Sizes

One of the key advantages of meta-analysis is the ability to generate an overall effect size and an associated confidence interval. The overall effect size is the average effect size of all the included primary studies. This calculation is done using the mathematics of the meta-analysis process and is beyond the scope of this book. However, you can still interpret the overall effect size. Figure 9–9 has the same data as in Figure 9–8, except that the overall effect size has been added with its 95% confidence interval. Using the overall effect size, you should see that the overall effect favors the strength training. However, the effect is small (i.e., near zero), and the confidence interval crosses the zero line, thus indicating that it is not statistically significant. You will recall that previously using only the methods of the systematic review, the results were equivocal or maybe favored the strength training. Now we have a quantity that tells us that when all the evidence is considered, strength training was not effective. It is this ability to compile multiple studies into a single, quantifiable result that is the strength of meta-analysis.

Figure 9–10 presents another situation for the same analysis, except that studies 3, 6, and 7 no longer have negative effect sizes, and the effect size for study 7 is no longer statistically significant. You can also see that the overall effect size is larger, and its confidence interval does not cross the zero line. In this case, your interpretation

Meta-analysis: A form of systematic review that performs a statistical analysis of the effect sizes in a group of studies.

Overall effect size: The average effect size of all the primary studies included in a meta-analysis.

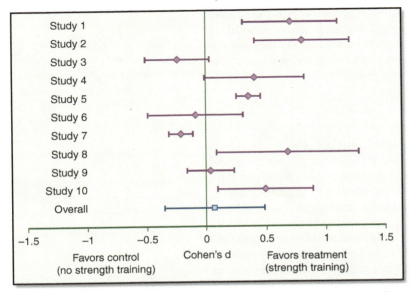

Figure 9–9 Forest plot with the overall effect size included. The data are the same as in Figure 9–8, except that the overall effect size with its 95% confidence interval has been added. Note that the overall effect size is not significant.

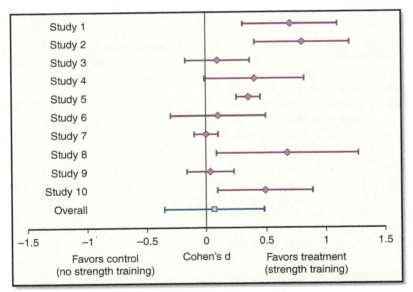

Figure 9–10 Forest plot with significant overall effect size. The data are the same as in Figures 9–8 and 9–9, except the direction of some of the effect sizes have been changed. The result is a larger overall effect size and a smaller 95% confidence interval. In this case, the overall effect size is significant.

would be that the strength training was effective. If you were to interpret these data using vote counting, you would have five studies without, and five with, significant effects. From this, you would probably conclude that the results are equivocal. You would draw the same conclusion if you simply used effect sizes and confidence intervals. However, by combining the effect sizes and confidence intervals of the primary studies into an overall effect size and confidence interval, you can see that the new result supports strength training as effective. Again, this illustrates the strength of meta-analysis in being able to combine apparently conflicting studies into one coherent result.

Fixed Versus Random Effects

When a meta-analysis is performed, the analysis should be reported as either a random effects model or a fixed effect model. The fixed effect model is a statistical model that assumes that the effect sizes of the primary studies represent one true effect size (Borenstein, Hedges, Higgins, & Rothstein, 2009b). The random effects model is a statistical model that assumes that the effect sizes of the primary studies represent a family of effect sizes (Borenstein, Hedges, Higgins, & Rothstein, 2009c). These are statistical procedures, and their mechanics are beyond our scope. However, the different methods require different interpretation of which you should be aware.

Random effects model: A statistical model that assumes that the effect sizes of the primary studies represent a family of effect sizes.

Fixed effect model: A statistical model that assumes that the effect sizes of the primary studies represent one true effect size.

The fixed effect model is used when all the included primary studies are equivalent. This means that the methods (e.g., treatments and measures) are identical, and the population of subjects (e.g., adolescents, retirees, athletes, or obese persons) across studies is the same. In this case, you interpret the overall effect size as the true average effect for the set of studies. For example, assume that you were interested in strength development following strength training or rehabilitation, and you found a meta-analysis that assessed strength development after weight training. If all the primary studies used the same strength test, studied the exact same population (e.g., high school football players), and compared recovery along the same timeline (e.g., before injury to 3 months after injury), then a fixed effect model could be used. However, it is not likely that all these variables would be the same. Most primary studies are not duplicates of other studies. Rather, they are variations of each other, with the goal of asking slightly different questions and progressing the understanding of the problem. Because of this, the fixed effect model is rarely appropriate in meta-analysis, and the random effects model should be used.

When a meta-analysis reports a random effects model, you must interpret the overall effect size differently. It no longer represents a single true effect size, but instead it represents the average effect size for a family of true effects. As such, your expectation for your clients should be that their strength gains will fall somewhere within this range. You may be able to narrow this to a more precise estimate by identifying a primary study within the meta-analysis that best represents your practice. That primary study result would be most representative of your patients or clients.

Bias in Meta-Analysis

As previously indicated, narrative reviews are prone to bias. Systematic reviews attempt to address this bias by applying a specific methodology for finding, including, and evaluating studies. Meta-analysis extends the methods of the systematic review by assessing the potential bias both mathematically and statistically. You can assess whether the bias has a substantial impact on the results of the meta-analysis.

Measures of Bias

There are several methods of assessing bias in the literature, and the three most commonly encountered are presented. Frequently, you will see more than one of these methods within the same meta-analysis. None of the techniques are perfect, and sometimes they contradict each other. However, if two or more of the techniques agree that no bias exists, then you have a much stronger confirmation.

Fail-safe N

Probably the simplest technique for assessing bias is the **fail-safe N** (Rothstein, 2005a). Fail-safe N is a technique whereby the number of primary studies needed to produce a nonsignificant overall effect size is calculated. Fail-safe N was developed to measure publication bias. In other words, how do you know whether there are unpublished research studies with nonsignificant statistical results? You will recall that studies with significant findings are more likely to be published than those with nonsignificant findings. Because of this, it is always possible that other studies are unpublished and could affect the results. For example, assume you found a meta-analysis that examined the effectiveness of anti-inflammatory medication on shoulder tendonitis. In addition, assume that the meta-analysis included 10 primary studies all showing a benefit, but the overall effect size was small. If there were several unpublished studies with no effects and these studies could be included, the new overall result could show no benefit for anti-inflammatory agents.

The fail-safe N procedure calculates the number of possible studies with no benefit that are needed to reduce the overall effect

Fail-safe N: A technique to measure publication bias; it calculates the number of primary studies needed to produce a nonsignificant overall effect size.

size to the point that shows no benefit. In more practical terms, assume that the fail-safe N shows that only three additional primary studies with no benefit are needed to reduce the overall effect size to having no benefit. In this case, you would want to interpret the result cautiously because only a few additional studies could change the result. Conversely, if the fail-safe N indicated that 100 additional studies would be needed to reduce the overall effect size to having no benefit, then you would have much more confidence that the overall effect represented the true findings. Figure 9–11 is an example of how fail-safe N results would be reported in a meta-analysis.

The challenge with fail-safe N is answering the question of how many studies are enough. Certainly, if only two to three studies are needed to reduce the overall effect, then you should consider the overall effect to be weak and the results questionable. However, what about 10, or 30, additional studies? There is no one correct answer to this question. It becomes your judgment to decide where to draw the line.

Funnel Plot

The **funnel plot** is a graphic technique that looks for symmetry in the data (Sterne, Becker, & Egger, 2005). Figure 9–12 is an example of a funnel plot. It takes its name from the shape of diagonal lines on the graph. On the x-axis are the effect sizes for each of the primary studies. On the y-axis is the standard error for each effect size, which is a measure of precision. Every effect size calculated from a primary study is associated with random error. (In the case of the forest plot, this error is represented by the 95% confidence intervals around each study.) Effect sizes plotted higher on the graph are studies with less error, or more precision. This higher precision reflects the number of subjects in each study. A greater number of subjects in a study gives the study more precision. The

Funnel plot: A graphic technique that looks for symmetry in data.

Fail-safe analysis

The fail-safe analysis determined that 707 null effect findings were necessary to lower the cumulative ES to an insignificant level. Specifically, 707 null studies are required to reduce our cumulative effect to a point that various types of ankle trauma would not affect postural control.

Figure 9–11 Fail-safe N: an example of how fail-safe N results would be reported in the literature. ES, effect size. (*From Wikstrom, E. A., Naik, S., Lodha, N., & Cauraugh, J. H. [2010]. Bilateral balance impairments after lateral ankle trauma: A systematic review and meta-analysis. Gait and Posture, 31[4], 407-414.*)

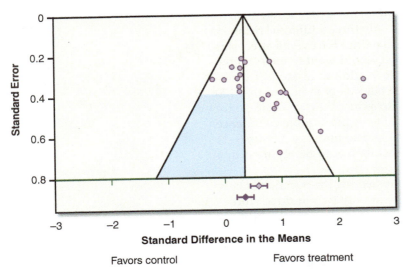

Figure 9-12 Funnel plot. The circles represent effect sizes from primary studies. The diamond is the overall effect size. The width of the diamond represents the 95% confidence interval. The blue region identifies the area where studies are missing. *(Adapted from Arnold, B. L., de la Motte, S., Linens, S., & Ross, S. E. [2009]. Ankle instability is associated with balance impairments: A meta-analysis.* Medicine and Science in Sports and Exercise, *41[5], 1048-1062.)*

diamond below the x-axis is the calculated overall effect size for the included primary studies, and its center is located at the overall effect magnitude. The length of the diamond represents the 95% confidence interval for the overall effect size. The diagonal lines of the funnel represent the expected 95% confidence for each point (i.e., standard error) on the y-axis. When no bias exists, you would expect that the primary study effect sizes would plot uniformly within the funnel. However, you can see that the shaded area is absent of primary study effect sizes. For some reason these studies do not exist. This suggests that bias is present. Missing studies in this section of the funnel plot are expected. The studies that potentially exist in this section are studies with small effect sizes (i.e., close to zero and have larger standard errors and thus, larger confidence intervals). This means these studies are not likely to be statistically significant and may go unpublished.

Looking at the funnel plot, you should be able to see that if studies existed in the shaded area, the overall effect size would be moved toward the zero point, and its confidence interval would enlarge as well. This could move the overall effect size and confidence interval close enough to zero to produce a statistically nonsignificant result. Whether this happens or not cannot be determined from just the funnel plot.

Trim and Fill

Although the funnel plot cannot predict the influence of bias on the overall effect size, this can be determined using a procedure known as **trim and fill**. This mathematical procedure estimates the number of potentially missing studies and their associated effect sizes (Duval, 2005). Figure 9–13 shows the same data, but with the missing studies filled (black circles). You should notice that these filled studies are simply duplicates of studies from the other side of the graph. This technique simply balances both sides of the graph. This is acceptable because theory suggests that the graph should be balanced, and the reason it is not balanced is that statistically nonsignificant studies were never published. On the bottom of the graph, you will notice that a black diamond has been added. This is the adjusted overall effect size and its 95% confidence interval, after the missing studies have been filled. As you can see, this effect size is closer to the zero point, but the 95% confidence interval (the width of the diamond) does not cross the zero point. This means that this adjusted overall effect size would be statistically significant.

The missing studies and the adjusted overall effect size are not real, but rather they are estimates of what could be. Because of

Trim and fill: A mathematical procedure for funnel plots that estimates the number of potentially missing studies and their associated effect sizes.

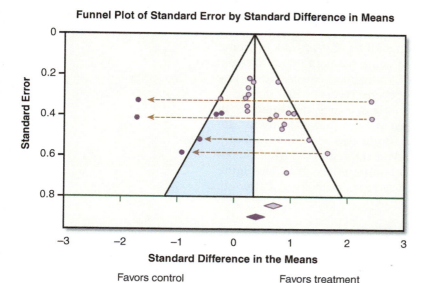

Figure 9–13 Trim and fill. An example of a trim and fill funnel plot. The data are the same as in Figure 9–12. The solid circles represent projected missing studies that are duplicates of actual studies on the right side of the plot. The black diamond represents the adjusted overall effect size after studies have been filled. *(Adapted from Arnold, B. L., de la Motte, S., Linens, S., & Ross, S. E. [2009]. Ankle instability is associated with balance impairments: A meta-analysis.* Medicine and Science in Sports and Exercise, *41[5], 1048-1062.)*

this, you should not interpret the adjusted effect size as the true effect size. Instead, you should interpret it as follows:

1. Addition of the missing studies did not create a nonsignificant effect size. As such, you can believe the treatment really does have a positive benefit.
2. Because the adjusted overall effect size is smaller than the effect size reported (the white diamond), you can believe that the true overall effect size is smaller than the reported overall effect size. In other words, because bias exists, the reported overall effect size probably overestimates the real effect size.

Your expectation for the treatment should be a smaller effect for your patient or client than is reported in the meta-analysis. Keep in mind that the reported effect size is an expected average effect, and each of your patients or clients will likely respond differently.

Subgroup Assessment

In addition to assessing bias, meta-analysis permits other, more complex analyses (Borenstein, Hedges, Higgins, & Rothstein, 2009e). One of those is the assessment of subgroups. For example, you want to know whether exercise has different effects on blood pressure depending on a person's age. Because of this, you would look for a meta-analysis that divides primary studies by the age group of the participant population. In this case, the meta-analysis could divide primary studies into those using participants older than 65 years of age and those younger than 65 years old. By doing this, the authors can make a direct comparison of effect sizes between these two groups of primary studies, and you can determine whether the effects your patients or clients receive will differ based on their age. Figure 9–14 is an example of a subgroup analysis. In this case, the comparison is between fast and slow velocity for isokinetic strength testing of the ankle (indicated in the first column). The arrows mark the group's overall effect size, and the boxes contain the numeric value for the two groups' effect sizes. The figure shows that slower velocities produced greater measured strength at the ankle.

Methodological Quality Assessment in Meta-Analysis

You learned that differing levels of quality could produce bias in systematic reviews and, by extension, in meta-analysis. In Chapter 10, you will learn about different instruments for assessing research quality. These instruments can be included in the meta-analysis to assess whether primary study effect sizes are related to research quality. One of the concerns that can be addressed with meta-analysis is

Pros and Cons 9-2

Assessment of bias is an important part of the systematic review and meta-analysis process. This is especially true in meta-analysis because it can tell you whether the results are likely to change if additional studies are added. However, you should be aware with techniques such as the trim and fill that any filled studies are only *hypothesized* to exist. Maybe they exist, and maybe they do not. Thus, think of the bias assessment as a test of how "bulletproof" the results are. If the projected bias does not meaningfully affect the result, then the result is robust.

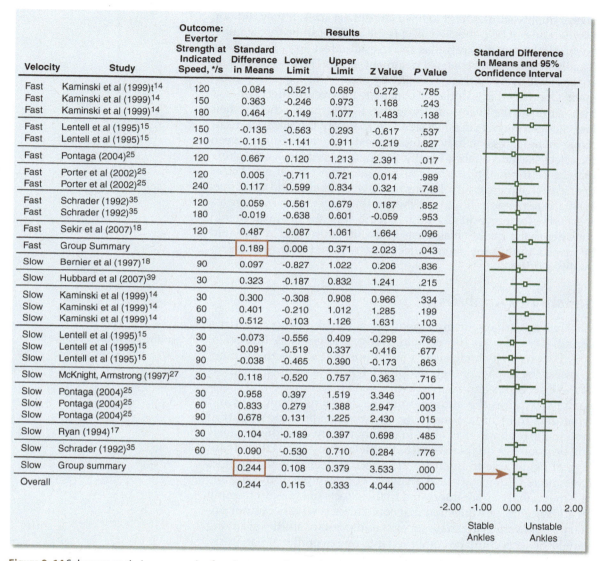

Velocity	Study	Outcome: Evertor Strength at Indicated Speed, °/s	Standard Difference in Means	Lower Limit	Upper Limit	Z Value	P Value
Fast	Kaminski et al (1999)t[14]	120	0.084	-0.521	0.689	0.272	.785
Fast	Kaminski et al (1999)[14]	150	0.363	-0.246	0.973	1.168	.243
Fast	Kaminski et al (1999)[14]	180	0.464	-0.149	1.077	1.483	.138
Fast	Lentell et al (1995)[15]	150	-0.135	-0.563	0.293	-0.617	.537
Fast	Lentell et al (1995)[15]	210	-0.115	-1.141	0.911	-0.219	.827
Fast	Pontaga (2004)[25]	120	0.667	0.120	1.213	2.391	.017
Fast	Porter et al (2002)[25]	120	0.005	-0.711	0.721	0.014	.989
Fast	Porter et al (2002)[25]	240	0.117	-0.599	0.834	0.321	.748
Fast	Schrader (1992)[35]	120	0.059	-0.561	0.679	0.187	.852
Fast	Schrader (1992)[35]	180	-0.019	-0.638	0.601	-0.059	.953
Fast	Sekir et al (2007)[18]	120	0.487	-0.087	1.061	1.664	.096
Fast	Group Summary		0.189	0.006	0.371	2.023	.043
Slow	Bernier et al (1997)[18]	90	0.097	-0.827	1.022	0.206	.836
Slow	Hubbard et al (2007)[39]	30	0.323	-0.187	0.832	1.241	.215
Slow	Kaminski et al (1999)[14]	30	0.300	-0.308	0.908	0.966	.334
Slow	Kaminski et al (1999)[14]	60	0.401	-0.210	1.012	1.285	.199
Slow	Kaminski et al (1999)[14]	90	0.512	-0.103	1.126	1.631	.103
Slow	Lentell et al (1995)[15]	30	-0.073	-0.556	0.409	-0.298	.766
Slow	Lentell et al (1995)[15]	30	-0.091	-0.519	0.337	-0.416	.677
Slow	Lentell et al (1995)[15]	90	-0.038	-0.465	0.390	-0.173	.863
Slow	McKnight, Armstrong (1997)[27]	30	0.118	-0.520	0.757	0.363	.716
Slow	Pontaga (2004)[25]	30	0.958	0.397	1.519	3.346	.001
Slow	Pontaga (2004)[25]	60	0.833	0.279	1.388	2.947	.003
Slow	Pontaga (2004)[25]	90	0.678	0.131	1.225	2.430	.015
Slow	Ryan (1994)[17]	30	0.104	-0.189	0.397	0.698	.485
Slow	Schrader (1992)[35]	60	0.090	-0.530	0.710	0.284	.776
Slow	Group summary		0.244	0.108	0.379	3.533	.000
Overall			0.244	0.115	0.333	4.044	.000

Figure 9–14 Subgroup analysis: an example of a subgroup analysis with both data and the forest plot presented. The data are for effect sizes from fast and slow (labeled in the first column) isokinetic strength assessments. The boxes and corresponding arrows highlight the overall effect sizes for the fast and slow subgroups. *(From Arnold, B. L., Linens, S. W., de la Motte, S. J., & Ross, S. E. [2009]. Concentric evertor strength differences and functional ankle instability: A meta-analysis.* Journal of Athletic Training, 44[6], 653-662.)

whether poorer-quality studies substantially influence the overall effect size. Because of publication bias, primary studies with fewer subjects tend not to be published unless they are statistically significant. To be statistically significant, these smaller studies must have large effect sizes. It is often the case that smaller studies tend to be of poorer quality. Putting these together, it is also often the case that poorer quality studies tend to have large effect sizes. If they did not, they would not be published. The result of this can be that smaller, lower-quality studies can bias the overall effect size. This bias is usually in favor of a beneficial treatment result. Thus, a good meta-analysis will evaluate this possibility by performing a quality assessment. One way this is done is to calculate the overall effect size and then eliminate the lower-quality studies to determine whether their loss changes the overall effect size. Alternatively, the statistical technique meta-regression may be used to test the relationship between the effect size and quality. Ideally, the meta-regression would show that the better-quality studies are associated with larger effect sizes or at least that there is no relationship between quality and effect size. What the regression should not show is that larger effect sizes are associated with poorer-quality studies. If this were the case, you should consider that a quality bias exists in the literature, and you should be suspicious that any overall effect may be biased in favor of lower-quality studies.

Sensitivity Analysis

Another advantage of meta-analysis is the ability to conduct a **sensitivity analysis** (Borenstein, Hedges, Higgins, & Rothstein, 2009d). Sensitivity analysis is a technique that allows the authors to assess the impact of their decisions. It is a test of the robustness of their decisions and results. Every systematic review and meta-analysis requires the authors to make decisions about how and what data to include. Sensitivity analyses can be done as part of systematic reviews. However, in systematic reviews, this analysis will be done in a qualitative fashion. Meta-analysis has the advantage of being able to quantify the effect of decisions the authors have made with a statistical analysis. For example, if the authors of a meta-analysis are interested in the effects of strength training on adolescents, one question that could arise is whether or not primary studies studying male subjects and primary studies studying female subjects could be combined into one overall meta-analysis. One way to handle this would be to select only one group to include. A second way would be to include both in separate, subordinate meta-analyses within the larger meta-analysis. The third way would be to include both groups into one overall meta-analysis and then conduct a sensitivity analysis. The third option could be done by simply conducting subgroup analyses for male and female subjects. If the subgroup analysis showed no difference between the male and female subjects, then the decision to combine them is justified. In this case, the sensitivity analysis is not mechanically different from a subgroup analysis, except in the intent of the authors of the meta-analysis. Had the authors started with the intent

Sensitivity analysis: A technique that allows authors to assess the impact of their decisions on how and what data to include in a study.

to compare male and female subjects, then it would be classified as a subgroup analysis. However, because their intent was to look at strength training in adolescents, they chose to combine male and female subjects and then test the robustness of the decision.

Sensitivity analyses can be conducted on a variety of questions (Borenstein et al., 2009d). The strength training example is an example of testing inclusion and exclusion criteria. Another question could be, "What is the effect on the results if a fixed effect model is completed instead of a random-effects model?" Almost any decision the authors have made is amenable to a sensitivity analysis. As the reader of a meta-analysis, you must decide whether the sensitivity analysis changes the results in a meaningful way. You must also be alert to whether the authors have ignored performing a sensitivity analysis on an important question. In that case, you may want to view the meta-analysis as less credible.

Retention Questions 9-2

1. How are inclusion and exclusion criteria used in systematic reviews?
2. What are four components of searching and assessing data for a systematic review?
3. What is an effect size?
4. What is an overall effect size?

SUMMARY

Narrative reviews are common throughout the clinical literature. They are useful for obtaining a quick snapshot of the literature or, when done by an expert, providing a specific point of view on a topic. However, they can be prone to several different types of bias. Narrative reviews have been increasingly replaced by the systematic review. The advantage of systematic reviews is that they are hypothesis driven and use methodologies that correspond to the rigor of experimental studies. When a systematic review assembles enough data from primary studies, it can be extended to include a meta-analysis. Meta-analysis is not a separate type of review. It is a statistical extension of the systematic review and permits the authors to do a quantitative assessment of the results. Both types can help you determine whether the results of multiple studies can provide a meaningful result that may translate to your patients or clients.

CRITICAL THINKING QUESTIONS

1. Given the choice between a historical review and an expert review, which would better serve you as a practitioner?
2. Given a choice among a narrative review, a systematic review, and a systematic review with meta-analysis, which would best inform your practice?
3. Of the forms of bias in reviews, which most concerns you as a practitioner?
4. Using the evidence-based pyramid, where would you place the narrative review and systematic review?

◼ TRUST AND APPLY

McKeon, P. O., & Hertel, J. (2008). Systematic review of postural control and lateral ankle instability, part II: Is balance training clinically effective? *Journal of Athletic Training, 43*(3), 305-315.

Locate the foregoing article, and using this article address the following questions:

1. Identify the search steps.
   a. Did the research steps follow a logical sequence?
   b. Could you replicate the search on your own?
2. What were the inclusion and exclusion criteria?
3. How was quality assessed?
   a. Was this an appropriate method for assessing quality?
4. Was a sensitivity analysis completed?
   a. If so, what decision was being tested?
   b. If not, what decision would you like to see tested?
5. If this article had included a meta-analysis, what other components would you expect to see?

◼ RESEARCH SCAVENGER HUNT

Using a research topic of your own, find a systematic review or meta-analysis and answer the following questions:

1. What was the stated hypothesis for the systematic review?
2. What were the inclusion criteria for primary studies? Do these criteria address a patient or client population that is important to you? Does that make a difference?
3. How was the quality assessment performed? Were the included primary studies of good quality? How does this affect your opinion of the review's results?
4. How was bias assessed? How does the effect size change as the result of bias? How does this change your interpretation of the results?

◼ REFERENCES

Arnold, B. L., de la Motte, S., Linens, S., & Ross, S. E. (2009). Ankle instability is associated with balance impairments: a meta-analysis. *Medicine and Science in Sports and Exercise, 41*(5), 1048-1062.

Arnold, B. L., Linens, S. W., de la Motte, S. J., & Ross, S. E. (2009). Concentric evertor strength differences and functional ankle instability: A meta-analysis. *Journal of Athletic Training, 44*(6), 653-662.

Borenstein, M., Hedges, V., Higgins, J. P. T., & Rothstein, H. R. (2009a). Effect sizes based on means. In *Introduction to meta-analysis* (pp. 21-32). Chichester, United Kingdom: John Wiley and Sons.

Borenstein, M., Hedges, V., Higgins, J. P. T., & Rothstein, H. R. (2009b). Fixed-effect model. In *Introduction to meta-analysis* (pp. 63-68). Chichester, United Kingdom: John Wiley and Sons.

Borenstein, M., Hedges, V., Higgins, J. P. T., & Rothstein, H. R. (2009c). Random-effects model. In *Introduction to meta-analysis* (pp. 69-76). Chichester, United Kingdom: John Wiley and Sons.

Borenstein, M., Hedges, V., Higgins, J. P. T., & Rothstein, H. R. (2009d). Reporting the results of a meta-analysis. In *Introduction to meta-analysis* (pp. 365-370). Chichester, United Kingdom: John Wiley and Sons.

Borenstein, M., Hedges, V., Higgins, J. P. T., & Rothstein, H. R. (2009e). Subgroup analysis. In *Introduction to meta-analysis* (pp. 149-186). Chichester, United Kingdom: John Wiley and Sons.

Borenstein, M., Hedges, V., Higgins, J. P. T., & Rothstein, H. R. (2009f). Vote counting—a new name for an old problem. In *Introduction to meta-analysis* (pp. 251-255). Chichester, United Kingdom: John Wiley and Sons.

Duval, S. (2005). The trim and fill method. In H. R. Rothstein, A. J. Sutton, & M. Borenstein (Eds.), *Publication bias in meta-analysis: Prevention, assessment, and adjustments* (pp. 127-144). Chichister, United Kingdom: John Wiley and Sons.

Higgins, J. P. T., Altman, D. G., & Sterne, J. A. C. (2011). Assessing the risk of bias in included studies. In J. P. T. Higgins & S. Green (Eds.), *Cochrane handbook for sysematic reviews of inerventions version 5.1.0.* Available from http://handbook.cochrane.org/chapter_8/8_assessing_risk_of_bias_in_included_studies.htm

Hopewell, S., Clarke, M., & Mallett, S. (2005). Grey literature and systematic reviews. In H. R. Rothstein, A. J. Sutton, & M. Borenstein (Eds.), *Publication bias in meta-analysis: Prevention, assessment, and adjustments* (pp. 49-72). Chichister, United Kingdom: John Wiley and Sons.

Internation Committee of Medical Journal Editors. (2014). Overlapping publications. Available from http://www.icmje.org/recommendations/browse/publishing-and-editorial-issues/overlapping-publications.html

Posadzki, P., Cramer, H., Kuzdzal, A., Lee, M. S., & Ernst, E. (2014). Yoga for hypertension: A systematic review of randomized clinical trials. *Complementary Therapies in Medicine, 22*(3), 511-522.

Rothstein, H. R. (2005a). Fail-safe N or file-drawer number. In H. R. Rothstein, A. J. Sutton, & M. Borenstein (Eds.), *Publication bias in meta-analysis: Prevention, assessment, and adjustments* (pp. 111-125). Chichister, United Kingdom: John Wiley and Sons.

Rothstein, H. R. (2005b). Publication bias in meta-analysis. In H. R. Rothstein, A. J. Sutton & M. Borenstein (Eds.), *Publication bias in meta-analysis: Prevention, assessment, and adjustments* (pp. 1-7). Chichister, United Kingdom: John Wiley and Sons.

Sterne, J. A. C., Becker, B. J., & Egger, M. (2005). The funnel plot. In H. R. Rothstein, A. J. Sutton, & M. Borenstein (Eds.), *Publication bias in meta-analysis: Prevention, assessment, and adjustments* (pp. 75-98). Chichister, United Kingdom: John Wiley and Sons.

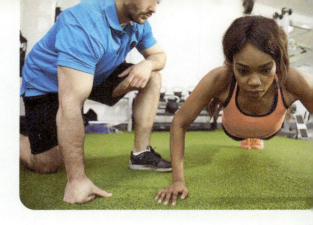

Evaluating Research Quality

Christopher R. Harnish, PhD, ACSM EP-C EIM, CSCS, FMSc
Assistant Professor, Department of Health & Human Performance, Ferrum College,
Ferrum, Virginia

Where Have You Been?

In Chapter 9, an emphasis was placed on discriminating among the differences in various forms of research synthesis, namely, reviews and meta-analyses. Many of the key components that make up high-quality research, as well as components that can diminish overall findings, such as moderator variables, will become the backbone for assessing and using emerging research in evidence-based medicine.

Where Are You Going?

The purpose of Chapter 10 is to provide guidelines for discerning quality (good) research from lesser research. We review the scientific method and discuss how it not only drives new research but also can help you evaluate research quality and integrate it into practice. In addition, this chapter provides insight into where and how to source quality research in a more condensed location to accommodate a busy professional environment. Finally, the chapter concludes by offering specific exercises that will help apply the material covered within this chapter.

Key Terms

Centre for Evidence-Based Medicine (CEBM)

Cochrane reviews

Consolidated Standards of Reporting Trials (CONSORT)

Meta-analysis of Observational Studies in Epidemiology (MOOSE)

Null hypothesis

Peer-review process

Peer-reviewed journal

Physiotherapy Evidence Database (PEDro)

Preferred Reporting Items for Systematic Reviews and Meta-Analyses (PRISMA)

Primary source

Scientific method

Secondary source

Strength of Recommendation Taxonomy (SORT)

■ RESEARCH AND THE SCIENTIFIC METHOD

Research is a broad, sometimes misleading term because many people assume that if it is called research, then it must be vetted in some way. However, research is defined as much by its process as it is by the results it yields. To understand what research is, one must be familiar with, and use, the scientific method, a set of basic principles, elaborated by Isaac Newton (1999), that outline specific instructions for investigating observations, acquiring evidence, and then integrating that evidence into the current body of knowledge. The scientific method is at the heart of evidence-based medicine. In a broad sense, research is *what* we do to answer questions, and the scientific method is *how* we do it. Science-based medicine seeks to build on previous knowledge and relies on the accumulation of objective quantifiable data, in lieu of subjective and easily biased qualified interpretation. When evaluating research quality, it is best to remember these key aspects of the scientific method (Newton, 1999):

Scientific method: A set of basic principles that outline the means for investigating observations, acquiring evidence, and then integrating that evidence into the current body of knowledge.

1. Formulate a question or a need based on an observed problem or occurrence.
2. Devise a clear hypothesis of what is happening.
3. Speculate an outcome based on the developed hypothesis.
4. Develop testing methodology that is clear and that can be replicated given the necessary resources.
5. Use appropriate analyses to test the hypotheses, including appropriate statistics.
6. Interpret the results, and develop conclusions that are in line with, but do not exceed, the findings.
7. Possibly formulate new questions.

As you consider research and its quality, it is important to keep the scientific method in the back of your mind. Poor-quality research often falls short in one or more of the foregoing areas. Moreover, no single study is considered definitive. A research question and hypothesis must be developed, tested, and then confirmed. The more repeated validation that occurs, the more likely it will be the hypothesis is actually true; more on hypothesis testing and validation will be covered later in this chapter. As you read the remainder of the chapter, consider each part of the research method and how you may apply it in your own practice.

Science: Method Not Madness

Health, fitness, and medical practitioners must be wise consumers of emerging research. Thus, understanding both the scientific research method and the subsequent peer-review process (see Box 10-1) will help professionals better recognize not just good and bad research, but also superior, more definitive research (and sources) from satisfactory studies. When taken as a whole, validated research builds a compelling case that defends itself over time. The following subsections describe salient considerations when making your evaluations.

Not All Questions Are Good

Students are typically advised that there is no such thing as a bad question. This is not the rule in research, however. Many poor studies are poor for this very reason; start a study with a bad question, and you can only go down from there. The most obvious bad question is one that is either trivial or irrelevant, or the answer is already known. For example, asking whether regular exercise reduces the risk of cardiovascular disease is broad, and its answer is well supported. A more appropriate question would be one that asks whether a specific exercise duration or intensity is more or less effective at reducing a specific aspect of cardiovascular disease. Table 10–1 summarizes common characteristics of a poor research question.

As a professional, however, you will need to determine quickly whether a question should be asked and whether the hypotheses

Table 10–1 Common Characteristics of a Poor Research Question	
Question Weakness	**Example**
Trivial, broad, or easily answered	A student wishes to study the air composition of two nearby towns and their impact on exercise performance. A researcher wishes to examine the effect a class of drugs has on health and well-being.
Hypothesis strongly supported by previous research	A researcher is interested in whether a low-calorie diet will be effective for weight loss.
Cannot be quantified	How does a particular food additive affect the taste of cough syrup?
Cannot be tested	A company wants to know whether a new cancer drug increases life span.
Impossible to study under control	A doctor wants to study the effect of a complimentary physical examination on residents in a low-income neighborhood.

Adapted from Park, H. M., in http://www.iuj.ac.jp/faculty/kucc625/writing/bad_question.pdf

are supported by what is known. One quick and effective way to evaluate the research question, as well as the hypotheses, is to read the introduction. A well-written introduction will lead the reader to an obvious problem or hole in the research knowledge. If the researchers' questions do not align with what is needed, or if the problem seems vague, answering it will be difficult. The **peer-review process** (Box 10–1), which relies on an independent evaluation of work by a group of competent persons within a similar field of study, is an effective means for eliminating poorly designed studies, which often start with a poor question.

Peer-review process: A process by which a group of competent persons within a similar field of study independently evaluates the body of work.

Hypotheses Are Tested, Not Proven

A good hypothesis is a natural extension of the research question and literature. The most common errors made with hypotheses are in understanding how it fits within the framework of a study and what the results of a study actually tell us. One common mistake made about research and hypothesis testing is that the objective is

---

Box 10–1   Peer Review: A Jury of Our Peers

At the heart of scientific research and publication is peer review. Understanding how the peer-review process works in the publication of quality research provides any practitioner an appreciation of its importance. Evaluation of research quality begins with identifying whether unbiased peer review took place before publication. Research presented without peer review should be viewed with extreme caution, if at all, because it often lacks scientific rigor, by missing one or more of the criteria of the scientific method. Without peer review, there was no evaluation of the merits of the research or determination of whether the study was conducted in a safe, controlled manner. The authors publishing the study may have clear conflicts of interest that could have biased the results or their interpretation. In short, peer review acts as a multilevel system of checks. Research conducted at medical or educational facilities must pass an institutional review board of peers to conduct the research, and then other professionals at a journal typically review a manuscript blinded to authors, to allow for unbiased evaluation and editing of the research before publication. This process may mean rejection of poorly designed studies. Finally, after publication, the research continues through peer review as other professionals such as you read and evaluate it, thus ultimately determining whether the research will stand the test of time. Although imperfect, peer review provides for an organized, balanced assessment of research quality.

to prove something true, when in fact we are actually attempting to cast doubt on what is known. In general terms, a research hypothesis is developed with the objective of rejecting the **null hypothesis**, which is considered the currently accepted position in which no specific relationship exists between two variables. In this respect, we never actually prove anything; rather, we reject the accepted view or fail to reject it. It is for this reason that research methods must be replicable and results should be validated. The more times a finding is validated, the greater the weight of the findings and the less likely it will be that the results were a chance finding.

Methodology: How You Did It Matters

Probably the most difficult, not to mention least read, section of a research paper is the methods section. However, skipping over the methods section entirely can often blind you to obvious or not so obvious problems. One would assume that the peer-review process would identify major flaws in methodology, and it largely does. However, many studies may abridge their methods, or they may have used slightly different clinical techniques or inappropriate statistical methods. Thus, both the scientific method and the subsequent peer-review process (see Box 10–1) provide a specific framework for developing a question, testing that question, and then evaluating both the testing process and answers generated even after publication. In most cases, minor methodological issues typically have minimal impact on overall results. Each professional should consider how these differences would affect his or her own practice outcomes in judging the results. Some questions to consider are as follows:

- Do the researchers clearly identify the population?
- Is the sample size large enough to test the hypothesis?
- Does the study use a control group or any type of control method to identify within-group changes?
- Are other confounding variables controlled for or addressed?
- Are the methods descriptions written thoroughly enough for the study to be replicated?
- Are the test methods valid and accepted within common practice?
- Are equipment, supplies, and other pertinent details listed with enough information to allow the reader to determine what would be needed?
- Are the statistical analyses clearly described and appropriate for the hypotheses and groups?

Although this is not an exhaustive list, it should provide you with the ability to spot egregious errors or methods that may be modified from common practice. This last point is important if you intend to implement a method into practice.

Null hypothesis: The assumption or currently accepted position in which no specific relationship exists between two variables.

Connections 10-1
The choice of independent and dependent variables, as well as study population impact the overall quality of research and how it applies to the clinical question you are asking. For example, studying an intervention in a healthy, or otherwise normal, population is unlikely to result in a change in a dependent variable, leading to potentially erroneous conclusions on treatment efficacy.

◼ WHAT IS A RESULT WORTH?

Being able to read and understand results is essential to evaluating the quality of research. One primary reason is that it is common for an author to interpret data differently, intentionally or not, from what the results suggest. An educated reader can, and should, judge a paper based on the merit of its results, not the discussion and conclusions sections of the paper (Litman, 2012). One should also note whether results are presented accurately, using the correct units. Important questions to ask when reviewing the results section include the following:

- Have the authors included results for all their hypotheses?
- Are results provided for other data collected?
- Did the authors present measures of dispersion (spread) such as standard deviations or standard error? A large dispersion in subject characteristics can affect significance, but it may also skew data or indicate an outlier within the subject pool. It is also preferred that authors report p values and other statistics for both significant and nonsignificant values.
- Are figures and tables cited and properly titled?

The results section of a paper should be clear and tightly written, without providing interpretation of any results. Results are simply a study's outcome measures, absent why they may have occurred. For many research papers, the results section may not be particularly long, and it may include several summary figures and tables.

Interpreting data and data trends, however, is where research results often become obscured by the overreliance on statistical significance (i.e., p values). Simply achieving a difference may or may not be meaningful for a number of reasons, not the least of which is the *effect size,* a measure of the impact or strength of a particular outcome. For example, a large sample size can provide enough power to detect tiny differences in divorce rates between couples meeting online versus offline, but it may hold little actual meaning. In fact, the p value was originally intended to be only part of a larger organic process that included both numerical calculations and subjective insight to draw conclusions (Nuzzo, 2014). Although a full discussion of these issues is beyond the scope of this chapter, you should consider how much weight authors place on their p values and their overall conclusions. Making broad conclusions over a handful of significant p values with small effect sizes often indicates conclusions that exceed the evidence. Similarly, interpretation of p values by using adjectives such as "nearly" significant, or "highly" significant is generally frowned on by researchers; a p value is one threshold that, when crossed, indicates that a meaningful and real difference exists.

Researchers have proposed more robust interpretive options to accompany p value significance levels. Batterham and Hopkins

(2006) proposed magnitude-based inferences, which use confidence intervals (CIs) put into the context of three or more levels of magnitude. For instance, levels could be labelled as harmful, trivial, beneficial, or unclear (if the confidence interval spans all other levels). Although few papers currently use it, this presentation technique could make it far easier to make treatment decisions from individual clinical trials. In lieu of this, it is important to consider how *consistent* a result is (i.e., all subjects improve or worsen versus only half), as well as the relevance of a "significant" finding in clinical practice. In such cases, reviews, meta-analyses, and position statements (all discussed later) can consolidate research into more appropriate applications.

Discussions: Do Not Let Results Get Lost in the Interpretation

Discussions are often the most exciting and informative sections of research papers. A quality research paper effectively summarizes its major findings within the first paragraph and subsequently interprets and integrates these findings into the existing body of knowledge. Every discussion should address each result reported, preferably in order of hypotheses or major findings. Throughout the discussion, the authors should integrate previous publications to support their arguments and strengthen their conclusions. Occasionally, however, discussions can misinterpret the findings of a study to come to misleading, or more commonly, overly important conclusions. This makes reviewing and understanding the results even more critical. Overall conclusions should reflect the breadth and depth of results and provide a final message to consider, including possible future research directions.

EVIDENCE-BASED MEDICINE

"Evidence based medicine is the conscientious, explicit, and judicious use of current best evidence in making decisions about the care of individual patients." (Sackett, Rosenberg, Gray, Haynes, & Richardson, 1996)

Up to this point, the chapter has centered on identifying qualities that create a good research paper. As for many practitioners, however, your time may be too limited to locate individual papers or findings, let alone assess them in detail. The remainder of the chapter discusses what evidenced-based medicine or practice is, why it is important, and the resources available to maintain your edge with the latest research.

Traditional medicine has relied heavily on textbook training and experience of the health-care provider. Unfortunately, rapid

---

Retention Questions 10-1

1. What are the key aspects of the scientific method? *Describe each.*
2. How could an overemphasis on significance level (i.e., p-values) affect the interpretation of the results of an intervention study?

advances in treatments, mounting health-care costs, and the growth of Internet-based information make such an approach far from optimal. To address these and other issues, evidence-based practices were gradually developed to incorporate emerging research and treatment strategies into modern medical practice. Evidence-based medicine aims to incorporate epidemiological evidence with systematic reviews of randomized controlled trials (RCTs) to achieve treatment strategies that are based on objective evidence. Evidence-based medicine is strongly contrasted by medical decisions based solely, or in part, by personal beliefs or a small group of opinions. One need only watch mainstream media reports to witness the impacts of laypersons' beliefs on their own health and those of the larger society. Therefore, it is essential that health-care professionals base their decisions on the preponderance of the scientific evidence.

Evidence-based medicine relies on quality research to drive improved health, medical, and professional decisions. It attempts to integrate the art often found in traditional clinical practice with quantitative evidence, to promote more objective reasoning and decision-making. Moreover, evidence-based medicine is influenced by both the patient and by the clinician and is distinguished by the following aspects (Melnyk & Fineout-Overholt, 2011):

- Effective use of clinical data to integrate patient information, test results, and contemporary research
- Quality record keeping to monitor treatment efficacy
- Critical reasoning ability to promote review and rating of current practices
- Ability to use effective treatments based on the available resources in a cost-effective manner

Most major organizations involved in collating and disseminating research collections and reviews (e.g., the Cochrane Collaboration) adhere to the principles of evidence-based medicine outlined earlier and as such make for good sources of information. Evidence-based medicine relies on employing a hierarchy of evidence based on research design, controls, quality, validation, and consensus. Several organizations have developed databases and a set of standardized criteria to evaluate a given research study critically, whereas others rely on a set of guidelines to evaluate a variety of research types across disciplines. Before discussing many of the leading sources of information, the reader should understand the hierarchy of evidence used for evaluating evidence-based medicine research. Box 10–2 reviews the seven levels of research, as outlined by Melnyk and Fineout-Overholt (2011), in which level I represents the most compelling evidence. Conceptually, the hierarchy is often thought of as a pyramid built on evidence of increasing strength.

> **Box 10–2** **Hierarchy for Well-Designed, High-Quality Research in Evidence-Based Medicine and Practice**
>
> **Level I**
> Evidence from systematic reviews of randomized controlled trials or evidence-based medicine guidelines based on systematic reviews of randomized controlled trials
>
> **Level II**
> Evidence from well-designed randomized controlled trials
>
> **Level III**
> Evidence from quasiexperimental nonrandomized controlled trials
>
> **Level IV**
> Evidence from case-control or cohort studies
>
> **Level V**
> Evidence from systematic reviews of descriptive or qualitative studies
>
> **Level VI**
> Evidence from a descriptive or qualitative study
>
> **Level VII**
> Evidence from authoritative opinions, reports from expert committees, or position stands

Based on the different levels of evidence, systematic reviews and meta-analyses are typically viewed as the strongest evidence. A high-quality systematic review or meta-analysis helps summarize the current state of research by using only the highest standards of inclusion. Such reviews outline *inclusion* and *exclusion* criteria for their reviews and analyses; inclusion criteria outline specific measurements or data that were measured, whereas exclusion criteria are used to eliminate studies that are either of poor quality, lack specific control variables or groups, or use methodology that is incorrect or not comparable to that of other studies. In addition, studies are often excluded when insufficient quantifiable data are presented in the publication. This last factor is particularly important for meta-analyses, which aim to combine similar smaller studies into one, larger pool of data, thereby improving statistical power. Finally, both systematic reviews and meta-analyses are ultimately used to draw more meaningful *overall conclusions* than could be considered from one single large study.

Although **peer-reviewed journals** (academic journals featuring original works that are vetted by expert peers in a particular field of study) are major sources for *research studies* (levels II to VI),

Peer-reviewed journal: An academic journal that features original works that are evaluated by expert peers in a particular field of study.

The Critical Consumer 10-1

Refer to the following article as an initial source:

Born, D. P., Sperlich, B., & Holmberg, H. C. (2013) Bringing light into the dark: Effects of compression clothing on performance and recovery. *International Journal of Sports Physiology and Performance*, 8(1), 4-18.

Review the foregoing article, and then consider the role that advertising and media play in how research is presented to the public regarding compression garments. Compare and contrast media and advertising claims with actual findings of research. Do the media portray research accurately? Research is often cited with ambiguity and blanket phrases such as "clinically proven." As an evidence-based professional, it is important to recognize that the media typically choose the most relevant and advantageous findings or portray anecdotal reports as research. However, as outlined in Box 10-2, anecdotal reports largely fall outside any quality standards, and multiple anecdotal reports do not equate with data. Be prepared to dig deeply into claimed "research." As a case in point, many health supplements combine multiple ingredients that may have been shown to be efficacious individually and often at much higher doses. However, the effects of the combinations and dosages within the product are often unknown.

many journals also include editorials by experts (Sackett et al. [1996] is an example of an editorial), invited opinions, letters to the editor, book reviews, and *review articles*. These review articles are typically not the same as a systematic review, as outlined earlier, and they typically review the overall literature qualitatively. Although such reviews may be prone to bias conclusions, they offer a broad summary of an area and a useful reference list. For most journals, however, most material present is considered *controlled research*, which follows the scientific method to answer a specific question. In this respect, an original research project is conceived, developed, implemented, and reported by the authors, thereby making it a **primary source**. Most primary sources are empirical studies and may be published in peer-reviewed journals or presented at conferences. In contrast, a **secondary source** is a report or paper written about one or more primary sources. Review papers fall into this category, conference symposia and tutorials can also be secondary sources.

Primary source: The original source for an idea or research results. Often synonymous with a primary study but may refer to a narrative or systematic review.

Secondary source: Report or paper written about one or more primary sources.

Weighing the Evidence

With the advent of evidence-based medicine, many organizations now provide resources for a range of professionals to find and review prevetted, high-quality research confidently. Many of these organizations and sites typically outline their criteria for inclusion and the threshold that individual and combined studies must achieve to be listed. Others provide resources for the professional to use to assess research more easily. The following are descriptions of the leading organizations across disciplines.

Centre for Evidence-Based Medicine

www.cebm.net

The **Centre for Evidence-Based Medicine (CEBM)** at Oxford University in the United Kingdom has positioned itself as the new leader in development, education, and promotion of evidence-based medicine. The Centre does this by establishing a multilevel platform for data collation, dissemination, and application of evidence-based medicine to allow health-care professionals to maintain the highest standards in their field. The Centre for Evidence-Based Medicine provides multiple resources, including workshops, as well as an extensive website (Fig. 10–1). Like the Cochrane reviews, the Centre provides areas of research across a broad range of disciplines. The Centre for

Centre for Evidence Based Medicine (CEBM): An organization dedicated to the development, education, and promotion of evidence-based medicine that has established a multilevel platform for data collation, dissemination, and application of evidence-based medicine.

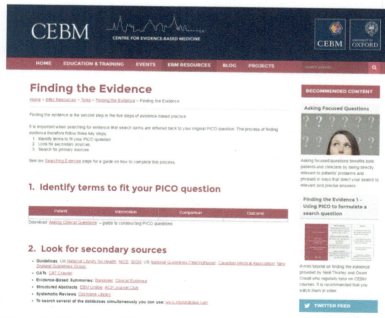

Figure 10–1 The Centre for Evidence-Based Medicine (CEBM) provides many evidence-based medicine resources that help users through all steps of the process of searching, evaluating, and applying research. *(Courtesy of the Centre for Evidence-Based Medicine, University of Oxford, Oxford, United Kingdom: www.cebm.org.)*

Evidence-Based Medicine is an excellent starting point for professionals new to the application of evidence-based medicine.

> *Best for* anyone seeking multiple options for research review, evidence-based medicine learning tools, and more.

Cochrane Reviews

www.cochrane.org

Named for Archie Cochrane, a British epidemiologist and an early proponent of evidence-based medicine and randomized controlled trials for the use of guiding health-care practice, the Cochrane reviews are some of the best-known and most widely respected disseminators of evidence-based medicine. The Cochrane reviews are considered the most reliable and respected research and are published online in the *Cochrane Library*.

The hallmark of evidence-based medicine is the systematic review. Each Cochrane review is assembled by a team of experts to address a distinct health-care question or problem. The team compiles all *primary sources* that meet specific criteria and then evaluates the evidence as a whole to ascertain whether there is conclusive evidence or consensus regarding treatment. Moreover, unlike other published reviews and analyses, Cochrane reviews are periodically updated to provide the best, most relevant evidence on which to base clinical decisions. The online Cochrane Library is easy to search and manage, and it provides a convenient list of the top 50 reviews (Fig. 10–2).

> *Best for* the busy professional who is comfortable relying on scientific consensus of the latest evidence-based medicine.

Cochrane reviews: A database of systematic reviews and meta-analyses that summarize and interpret the results of medical research; published online in the Cochrane Library.

Consolidated Standards of Reporting Trials

www.consort-statement.org

Consolidated Standards of Reporting Trials (CONSORT) is a group of initiatives developed by the CONSORT group. This diverse group of professionals developed and periodically updates the statement, currently CONSORT 2010 (Schulz, Altman, Moher, 2010), and is a 25-item checklist (Fig. 10–3), as well as flow chart, which diagrams a participant's progress throughout a trial. The checklist serves as a criterion measure for professionals to use to rate the design, analysis, and conclusions of a randomized controlled trial. The CONSORT website provides extensive information and additional resources for persons interested in evaluating randomized controlled trials, as well as designing and reporting their own studies.

> *Best for* the researcher interested in producing the best possible randomized controlled trial or the reviewer or professional wanting a concise and clear method for evaluating randomized controlled trials.

Consolidated Standards of Reporting Trials (CONSORT): A group of initiatives developed by the group by this name to alleviate the problems that arise from inadequate reporting of randomized controlled trials. This group developed and updates the CONSORT 2010 statement, a 25-item checklist, and a flow chart that diagrams a participant's progress throughout a trial.

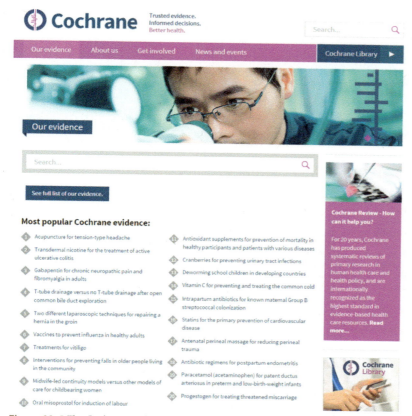

Figure 10–2 The Cochrane website has an extensive search function, a list of popular Cochrane evidence, and a comprehensive, sortable list of all published evidence. *(Courtesy of Cochrane, London, United Kingdom: www.cochrane.org.)*

Meta-analysis of Observational Studies in Epidemiology

As opposed to databases, working groups, or consortiums, the **Meta-analysis of Observational Studies in Epidemiology (MOOSE)** is a set of guidelines developed by 27 leading experts on how to report, evaluate, and rate meta-analyses and other studies effectively in epidemiology, as the name implies (Stroup et al., 2000). The guidelines were developed at a workshop, from which a checklist, similar to that devised for CONSORT, was developed to guide researchers, authors, reviewers, and editors on the publication of studies. The paper, published by the *Journal of the American Medical Association,* is available online (Stroup et al., 2000).

Best for a researcher, reviewer, or editor looking for a checklist resource in addition to CONSORT 2010.

Meta-analysis of Observational Studies in Epidemiology (MOOSE): A set of guidelines developed by 27 leading experts on how to report, evaluate, and rate meta-analyses and other studies in epidemiology effectively; it was developed to guide researchers, authors, reviewers, and editors on the publication of studies.

CONSORT 2010 checklist of information to include when reporting a randomised trial*

Section/Topic	Item No	Checklist item	Reported on page No
Title and abstract			
	1a	Identification as a randomised trial in the title	_____
	1b	Structured summary of trial design, methods, results, and conclusions (for specific guidance see CONSORT for abstracts)	_____
Introduction			
Background and objectives	2a	Scientific background and explanation of rationale	_____
	2b	Specific objectives or hypotheses	_____
Methods			
Trial design	3a	Description of trial design (such as parallel, factorial) including allocation ratio	_____
	3b	Important changes to methods after trial commencement (such as eligibility criteria), with reasons	_____
Participants	4a	Eligibility criteria for participants	_____
	4b	Settings and locations where the data were collected	_____
Interventions	5	The interventions for each group with sufficient details to allow replication, including how and when they were actually administered	_____
Outcomes	6a	Completely defined pre-specified primary and secondary outcome measures, including how and when they were assessed	_____
	6b	Any changes to trial outcomes after the trial commenced, with reasons	_____
Sample size	7a	How sample size was determined	_____
	7b	When applicable, explanation of any interim analyses and stopping guidelines	_____
Randomisation:			
Sequence generation	8a	Method used to generate the random allocation sequence	_____
	8b	Type of randomisation; details of any restriction (such as blocking and block size)	_____
Allocation concealment mechanism	9	Mechanism used to implement the random allocation sequence (such as sequentially numbered containers), describing any steps taken to conceal the sequence until interventions were assigned	_____
Implementation	10	Who generated the random allocation sequence, who enrolled participants, and who assigned participants to interventions	_____
Blinding	11a	If done, who was blinded after assignment to interventions (for example, participants, care providers, those assessing outcomes) and how	_____

	11b	If relevant, description of the similarity of interventions	_____
Statistical methods	12a	Statistical methods used to compare groups for primary and secondary outcomes	_____
	12b	Methods for additional analyses, such as subgroup analyses and adjusted analyses	_____
Results			
Participant flow (a diagram is strongly recommended)	13a	For each group, the numbers of participants who were randomly assigned, received intended treatment, and were analysed for the primary outcome	_____
	13b	For each group, losses and exclusions after randomisation, together with reasons	_____
Recruitment	14a	Dates defining the periods of recruitment and follow-up	_____
	14b	Why the trial ended or was stopped	_____
Baseline data	15	A table showing baseline demographic and clinical characteristics for each group	_____
Numbers analysed	16	For each group, number of participants (denominator) included in each analysis and whether the analysis was by original assigned groups	_____
Outcomes and estimation	17a	For each primary and secondary outcome, results for each group, and the estimated effect size and its precision (such as 95% confidence interval)	_____
	17b	For binary outcomes, presentation of both absolute and relative effect sizes is recommended	_____
Ancillary analyses	18	Results of any other analyses performed, including subgroup analyses and adjusted analyses, distinguishing pre-specified from exploratory	_____
Harms	19	All important harms or unintended effects in each group (for specific guidance see CONSORT for harms)	_____
Discussion			
Limitations	20	Trial limitations, addressing sources of potential bias, imprecision, and, if relevant, multiplicity of analyses	_____
Generalisability	21	Generalisability (external validity, applicability) of the trial findings	_____
Interpretation	22	Interpretation consistent with results, balancing benefits and harms, and considering other relevant evidence	_____
Other information			
Registration	23	Registration number and name of trial registry	_____
Protocol	24	Where the full trial protocol can be accessed, if available	_____
Funding	25	Sources of funding and other support (such as supply of drugs), role of funders	_____

*We strongly recommend reading this statement in conjunction with the CONSORT 2010 Explanation and Elaboration for important clarifications on all the items. If relevant, we also recommend reading CONSORT extensions for cluster randomised trials, non-inferiority and equivalence trials, non-pharmacological treatments, herbal interventions, and pragmatic trials. Additional extensions are forthcoming: for those and for up to date references relevant to this checklist, see www.consort-statement.org.

Figure 10–3 The Consolidated Standards of Reporting Trials (CONSORT) checklist was developed to aid in understanding and assessing the quality and validity of a randomized controlled study. *(Courtesy of the Consolidated Standards of Reporting Trials: www.consort-statement.org.)*

Physiotherapy Evidence Database

www.pedro.org.au

Physiotherapy Evidence Database (PEDro) is a free database of nearly 30,000 randomized controlled trials, systematic reviews, and physiotherapeutic (physical therapy) guidelines. Similar to CONSORT, every trial listed is independently reviewed and rated using an objective 11-question (PEDro) scale that allows users conveniently to assess the validity and efficacy of incorporating findings into practice (Fig. 10–4).

> ***Best for*** anyone, including the health-care practitioner, looking for easily accessible research information, as well as an overall score assessment for applicability, the latter of which can help direct persons who are deciding whether a study is worth reading more thoroughly.

Physiotherapy Evidence Database (PEDro): A database that catalogs systematic reviews and clinical trials in the field of physical therapy and that are focused on rehabilitation. It is maintained by the Centre for Evidence-Based Physiotherapy at the George Institute for Global Health at the University of Sydney in Australia.

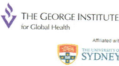

Figure 10–4 The Physiotherapy Evidence Database of the George Institute for Global Health (PEDro) evidence database can be searched using a variety of methods and may be limited to results that meet a minimum quality score. *(Courtesy of the Physiotherapy Evidence Database, George Institute for Global Health, University of Sydney, Sydney, Australia: www.pedro.org.au.)*

Preferred Reporting Items for Systematic Reviews and Meta-Analyses

www.prisma-statement.org

Preferred Reporting Items for Systematic Reviews and Meta-Analyses (PRISMA) is a set of minimum standards to aid authors in the reporting of evidence-based systematic reviews and meta-analyses. Although the traditional focus has been on randomized controlled trials, PRISMA can also be used for other research. Similar to CONSORT 2010, the PRISMA Statement consists of a checklist of 27 items and a flow chart (Fig. 10–5) (Maher, 2009).

Best for adding another resource for evaluating research for a variety of studies.

Preferred Reporting Items for Systematic Reviews and Meta-Analyses (PRISMA): A set of minimum standards to aid authors in the reporting of items in evidence-based systematic reviews and meta-analyses.

 PRISMA 2009 Checklist

Section/topic	#	Checklist item	Reported on page #
TITLE			
Title	1	Identify the report as a systematic review, meta-analysis, or both.	
ABSTRACT			
Structured summary	2	Provide a structured summary including, as applicable: background; objectives; data sources; study eligibility criteria, participants, and interventions; study appraisal and synthesis methods; results; limitations; conclusions and implications of key findings; systematic review registration number.	
INTRODUCTION			
Rationale	3	Describe the rationale for the review in the context of what is already known.	
Objectives	4	Provide an explicit statement of questions being addressed with reference to participants, interventions, comparisons, outcomes, and study design (PICOS).	
METHODS			
Protocol and registration	5	Indicate if a review protocol exists, if and where it can be accessed (e.g., Web address), and, if available, provide registration information including registration number.	
Eligibility criteria	6	Specify study characteristics (e.g., PICOS, length of follow-up) and report characteristics (e.g., years considered, language, publication status) used as criteria for eligibility, giving rationale.	
Information sources	7	Describe all information sources (e.g., databases with dates of coverage, contact with study authors to identify additional studies) in the search and date last searched.	
Search	8	Present full electronic search strategy for at least one database, including any limits used, such that it could be repeated.	
Study selection	9	State the process for selecting studies (i.e., screening, eligibility, included in systematic review, and, if applicable, included in the meta-analysis).	
Data collection process	10	Describe method of data extraction from reports (e.g., piloted forms, independently, in duplicate) and any processes for obtaining and confirming data from investigators.	
Data items	11	List and define all variables for which data were sought (e.g., PICOS, funding sources) and any assumptions and simplifications made.	
Risk of bias in individual studies	12	Describe methods used for assessing risk of bias of individual studies (including specification of whether this was done at the study or outcome level), and how this information is to be used in any data synthesis.	
Summary measures	13	State the principal summary measures (e.g., risk ratio, difference in means).	
Synthesis of results	14	Describe the methods of handling data and combining results of studies, if done, including measures of consistency (e.g., I^2) for each meta-analysis.	

Page 1 of 2

Figure 10–5 The Preferred Reporting Items for Systematic Reviews and Meta-Analyses (PRISMA) checklist is a 27-item checklist that helps improve the reporting of systematic reviews and meta-analyses. *(Courtesy of the Preferred Reporting Items for Systematic Reviews and Meta-Analyses, Ottawa Hospital Research Institute, Ottawa, Canada, and University of Oxford, Oxford, United Kingdom: www.prisma-statement.org.)*

PRISMA 2009 Checklist

Section/topic	#	Checklist item	Reported on page #
Risk of bias across studies	15	Specify any assessment of risk of bias that may affect the cumulative evidence (e.g., publication bias, selective reporting within studies).	
Additional analyses	16	Describe methods of additional analyses (e.g., sensitivity or subgroup analyses, meta-regression), if done, indicating which were pre-specified.	
RESULTS			
Study selection	17	Give numbers of studies screened, assessed for eligibility, and included in the review, with reasons for exclusions at each stage, ideally with a flow diagram.	
Study characteristics	18	For each study, present characteristics for which data were extracted (e.g., study size, PICOS, follow-up period) and provide the citations.	
Risk of bias within studies	19	Present data on risk of bias of each study and, if available, any outcome level assessment (see item 12).	
Results of individual studies	20	For all outcomes considered (benefits or harms), present, for each study: (a) simple summary data for each intervention group (b) effect estimates and confidence intervals, ideally with a forest plot.	
Synthesis of results	21	Present results of each meta-analysis done, including confidence intervals and measures of consistency.	
Risk of bias across studies	22	Present results of any assessment of risk of bias across studies (see Item 15).	
Additional analysis	23	Give results of additional analyses, if done (e.g., sensitivity or subgroup analyses, meta-regression [see Item 16]).	
DISCUSSION			
Summary of evidence	24	Summarize the main findings including the strength of evidence for each main outcome; consider their relevance to key groups (e.g., healthcare providers, users, and policy makers).	
Limitations	25	Discuss limitations at study and outcome level (e.g., risk of bias), and at review-level (e.g., incomplete retrieval of identified research, reporting bias).	
Conclusions	26	Provide a general interpretation of the results in the context of other evidence, and implications for future research.	
FUNDING			
Funding	27	Describe sources of funding for the systematic review and other support (e.g., supply of data); role of funders for the systematic review.	

From: Moher D, Liberati A, Tetzlaff J, Altman DG, The PRISMA Group (2009). Preferred Reporting Items for Systematic Reviews and Meta-Analyses: The PRISMA Statement. PLoS Med 6(6): e1000097. doi:10.1371/journal.pmed1000097

For more information, visit: www.prisma-statement.org.

Page 2 of 2

Figure 10–5—cont'd

Strength of Recommendation Taxonomy

The **strength of recommendation taxonomy (SORT)** (Ebell et al., 2004) is a uniform taxonomy developed for family medicine practice that can be used to assess the quality, quantity, and consistency of evidence across multiple disciplines. Built around outcomes that measure patients' morbidity or mortality, the research is given a grade of A, B, or C. A-level research consists of quality, consistent patient-oriented evidence, whereas B-level research results are inconsistent or limited in quality. A level of C is given for consensus opinions, common practice, disease-based outcomes, or case reports. Consistent use of the strength of recommendation taxonomy or similar taxonomies allows authors and readers to translate research into practice more effectively (Table 10–2).

Best for researchers and practitioners to evaluate and translate research into practice consistently and easily.

Strength of recommendation taxonomy (SORT): A method used to address the quality, quantity, and consistency of study evidence, by emphasizing the use of patient-oriented outcomes. Authors are allowed to rate individual studies or bodies of evidence. The taxonomy rates studies using the following letter grade scale: an A-level recommendation is based on consistent and good-quality patient-oriented evidence; a B-level recommendation is based on inconsistent or limited-quality patient-oriented evidence; and a C-level recommendation is based on consensus, usual practice, opinion, disease-oriented evidence, or case series for studies of diagnosis, treatment, prevention, or screening.

Table 10–2	Examples of How to Apply the Strength of Recommendation Taxonomy in Practice
Example 1	Although a number of observational studies (level of evidence 2) suggested a cardiovascular benefit from vitamin E, a large, well-designed, randomized trial with a diverse patient population (level of evidence 1) showed the opposite. The strength of recommendation against routine, long-term use of vitamin E to prevent heart disease, based on the best available evidence, should be A.
Example 2	A Cochrane review finds seven clinical trials that are consistent in their support of a mechanical intervention for low back pain, but the trials were poorly designed (i.e., unblinded, nonrandomized, or with allocation to groups unconcealed). In this case, the strength of recommendation in favor of these mechanical interventions is B (consistent but lower-quality clinical trials).
Example 3	A meta-analysis finds nine high-quality clinical trials of the use of a new drug in the treatment of pulmonary fibrosis. Two of the studies find harm, two find no benefit, and five show some benefit. The strength of recommendation in favor of this drug would be B (inconsistent results of good-quality, randomized controlled trials).
Example 4	A new drug increases the forced expiratory volume in 1 second and peak flow rate in patients with an acute asthma exacerbation. Data on symptom improvement are lacking. The strength of recommendation in favor of using this drug is C (disease-oriented evidence only).

Copyright © 2004 by the American Academy of Family Physicians.

Pros and Cons 10-1

Refer to Box 10–2, and review the different levels of research. Consider how each of these levels fits into the spectrum of evidence-based medicine. Is it practical, or even feasible, for all research to be conducted as level I or II? Similarly, are levels VI and VII of any meaningful value to the practitioner? In your own words, explain why or why not.

Consider one the greatest limiting factors for research, which is funding. Although it would be ideal to have large-scale, well-controlled studies, it is not feasible for several reasons, including a full understanding of the problem or treatment. Many large studies are built on years of smaller interventions that are easier to fund and to implement. These lower-level studies, including case-control studies and anecdotal qualitative reports, help identify both problems and fixes, as well as eliminate unfeasible interventions. A well-controlled randomized controlled trial depends on correctly identifying study groups and variables to study.

Retention Questions 10-2

1. Describe what evidence-based medicine is and is not. What distinguishes it from traditional medical approaches?
2. Briefly define each level of research quality, and provide an example for each.
3. Explain the difference between primary and secondary sources.
4. Choose a topic of interest, and locate a recent *randomized controlled trial* or *meta-analysis* from one of the websites listed in this chapter.

◼ SUMMARY

Evidence-based medicine has become integral to the best practices in health care. At the heart of evidence-based medicine is the scientific method, which drives the formulation of quality research questions and hypotheses. To test a hypothesis, however, sound methodologies must be used to achieve valid and reliable results, which are interpreted appropriately. As scientific research studies (particularly randomized controlled trials) have become more common, the need to rate the quality of these studies and organize them for easy access has grown increasingly important. Fortunately, several organizations have developed guidelines for evaluating research (e.g., Consolidated Standards of Reporting Trials, Meta-analysis of Observational Studies in Epidemiology, and the strength of recommendation taxonomy), whereas others collate high-quality research for dissemination, including the Centre for Evidence-Based Medicine, the Cochrane reviews, and the Physiotherapy Evidence Database. Despite these resources, evaluation and application of quality research will ultimately require the involvement of the entire clinical practice to cultivate a culture of collaboration and inquiry and to identify the highest-quality research to apply.

◼ TRUST AND APPLY

Locate the following article:

Bicici, S., Karatas, N., & Baltaci, G. (2012). Effect of athletic taping and kinesiotaping® on measurements of functional performance in basketball players with chronic inversion ankle sprains. *International Journal of Sports Physical Therapy, 7*(2), 154-166.

1. Evaluate the foregoing article by using the most appropriate rating checklist outlined in this chapter.

2. Based on your rating assessment, answer the following questions:
   a. Does this research appear valid, reliable, and applicable?
   b. Does kinesiology (KT) taping appear to have a clinically significant application in practice? How?
   c. How would you use the findings of this research in your own practice?

3. Refer back to the scientific method. Find a recent original research paper (not a review) of interest. Evaluate it using the seven aspects of the scientific method, and note the areas that fall short.

RESEARCH SCAVENGER HUNT

1. Use one or more of the websites reviewed in the section "Weighing the Evidence."

2. Springboard from the article you chose in Retention Questions 10-2, and locate a systematic review or meta-analysis on the area of treatment relating to that earlier article. For example, if you located a research paper on the effect of icing after a specific acute injury, locate a paper on an overall review of the use of ice.

3. You may wish to evaluate the paper using any of the rating systems.

4. Based on your evaluation, answer the following questions:

   A. What were the overall findings for this area or intervention?

   B. What questions or concerns remain regarding this area?

   C. Do the findings warrant its use or discontinuation in practice?

   D. Regarding this area, how has the media influenced the intervention or practice in question? For example, the media portrays KT tape (KT Health, American Fork, UT) as clinically proven to work and often cites anecdotal reports to back up claims. Does this actually constitute evidence?

   E. Has there been follow-up research since this paper was published?

REFERENCES

Batterham, A. M., & Hopkins, W. G. (2006). Making meaningful inferences about magnitudes. *International Journal of Sports Physiology and Performance, 1*, 50-57.

Ebell, M. H., Siwek, J., Weiss, B. D., Woolf, S. H., Susman, J., Ewigman, B., & Bowman, M. (2004). Strength of recommendation taxonomy (SORT): A patient-centered approach to grading evidence in the medical literature. *American Family Physician, 69*, 549-557.

Litman, T. (2012). *Evaluating research quality* (pp. 1-20). Victoria, BC, Canada: Victoria Transport Policy Institute.

Maher, C. (2009). PRISMA: Helping to deliver information that physical therapists need. *Physical Therapy, 89*(9), 870-872.

Melnyk, B. M., & Fineout-Overholt, E. (2011). Steps zero, one, two: Getting started. In *Evidence-based practice* (2nd ed.). Philadelphia: Wolters Kluwer Health Lippincott Williams & Wilkins.

Newton, I. (1999). Newton's rules for the study of natural philosophy. pp 794-796. In I. B. Cohen, A. Whitman, & J. Bundenz, trans. *The Principia: Mathematical principles of natural philosophy* (pp. 794-796). Oakland, CA: University of California Press.

Nuzzo, R. (2014). Statistical errors: P values, the 'gold standard' of statistical validity, are not as reliable as many scientists assume. *Nature, 513*, 150-152.

Sackett, D. L., Rosenberg, W. M., Gray, J. A. Haynes, R. B., & Richardson, W. S. (1996). Evidence based medicine: What it is and what it isn't. *BMJ, 312*, 71-72.

Schulz, K. F., Altman, D. G., & Moher, D. (2010). CONSORT 2010 statement: Updated guidelines for reporting parallel group randomised trials. *BMJ, 340*, 698-702.

Stroup, D. F., Berlin, J. A., Morton, S. C., Olkin, I., Williamson, G. D., Rennie, D., Moher, D., Becker, B. J., Sipe, T. A., & Thacker, S. B.. (2000). Meta-analysis of observational studies in epidemiology: A proposal for reporting. *JAMA, 283*(15), 2008-2012.

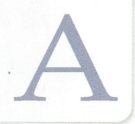

Selected Journals

ATHLETIC TRAINING

Athletic Training & Sports Health Care: The Journal for the Practicing Clinician
International Journal of Athletic Therapy & Training
Journal of Athletic Training
Journal of Sport Rehabilitation
Physiotherapy

BIOMECHANICS AND KINESIOLOGY

Applied Bionics and Biomechanics
Clinical Biomechanics
Gait & Posture
Human Movement Science
Journal of Applied Biomechanics
Journal of Biomechanics
Journal of Electromyography and Kinesiology
Journal of Human Kinetics
Sports Biomechanics

EXERCISE SCIENCE

ACSM's Health and Fitness Journal
Aerospace Medicine and Human Performance
Archives of Exercise in Health and Disease
Biology of Sport
European Journal of Sport Science
Exercise and Sport Sciences Reviews

Journal of Sports Sciences
Journal of Strength and Conditioning Research
Measurement in Physical Education and Exercise Science
NSCA Coach
Pediatric Exercise Science
Personal Training Quarterly
Research Quarterly for Exercise and Sport
Science & Sports
Strength and Conditioning Journal
Training and Conditioning
TSAC Report

■ MEDICAL AND GENERAL SCIENCE

American Family Physician
American Heart Journal
American Journal of Cardiology
American Journal of Hypertension
American Journal of Industrial Medicine
Archives of Internal Medicine
Arthritis and Rheumatism
Arthritis Care and Research
BMC Musculoskeletal Disorders
BMJ
Cancer
Clinical Therapeutics
Complementary Therapies in Medicine
Controlled Clinical Trials
Diabetes
Diabetes Care
Diabetes and Metabolism
Health Technology Assessment
Hypertension
International Journal of Eating Disorders
International Journal of Obesity
JAMA
Journal of General Internal Medicine
Journal of the American College of Cardiology
Lancet
Medical Care
Nature
New England Journal of Medicine
Obesity Research
Pain
Quality of Life Research
Science
Social Science and Medicine

■ NUTRITION

American Journal of Clinical Nutrition
Annals of Nutrition and Metabolism
Annual Review of Nutrition
Clinical Journal of Sports Medicine
European Journal of Clinical Nutrition
International Journal of Sport Nutrition
International Journal of Sport Nutrition and Exercise Metabolism
Journal of the International Society of Sports Nutrition
Journal of Nutrition

■ ORTHOPEDICS

Acta Orthopaedica Scandinavica
Clinical Orthopaedics and Related Research
Current Opinion in Orthopedics
Foot and Ankle Clinics
Foot & Ankle International
Hand Clinics
International Orthopaedics
Journal of Shoulder and Elbow Surgery
Knee Surgery, Sports Traumatology, Arthroscopy
Orthopaedic Clinicsof North America
Orthopedics
Orthopedics Today
Spine Journal
Techniques in Orthopaedics
The Knee

■ PHYSICAL THERAPY

Journal of Orthopaedic and Sports Physical Therapy
Pediatric Physical Therapy
Physical Therapy
Physical Therapy in Sport
Physical Therapy Reviews

■ PHYSIOLOGY

Acta Physiologica Scandinavica
American Journal of Physiology
Annual Review of Physiology
Applied Psychological Measurement
Canadian Journal of Applied Physiology

Canadian Journal of Physiology and Pharmacology
European Journal of Applied Physiology
Experimental Physiology
Journal of Applied Physiology
Journal of Clinical Exercise Physiology
Journal of Exercise Physiology
Journal of Physiology
Physiological Reviews
International Journal of Sports Physiology and Performance

PSYCHOLOGY

American Psychologist
International Journal of Sport Psychology
Journal of Applied Psychology
Journal of Applied Sport Psychology
Journal of Clinical Psychology
Journal of Clinical Sport Psychology
Journal of Sport & Exercise Psychology
Psychology of Sport and Exercise
The Sport Psychologist

PUBLIC HEALTH

American Journal of Epidemiology
American Journal of Health Promotion
American Journal of Public Health
Annual Review of Public Health
International Journal of Epidemiology
Journal of Aging and Physical Activity
Journal of Clinical Epidemiology
Journal of Epidemiology and Community Health
Journal of Physical Activity and Health

REHABILITATION

Archives of Physical Medicine and Rehabilitation
Journal of Back and Musculoskeletal Rehabilitation
Physical Medicine and Rehabilitation Clinics

SPORTS MEDICINE

American Journal of Sports Medicine
British Journal of Sports Medicine

Clinical Journal of Sport Medicine
Clinical Journal of Sports Medicine
Clinics in Sports Medicine
Current Sports Medicine Reports
International Journal of Sports Medicine
Journal of Science and Medicine in Sport
Journal of Sport Sciences
Journal of Sports Medicine and Physical Fitness
Medicine and Science in Sports and Exercise
Operative Techniques in Sports Medicine
Physician and Sportsmedicine
Research in Sports Medicine
Sports Health: A Multidisciplinary Approach
Sports Medicine
Sports Medicine and Arthroscopy Review
Sports Medicine, Training, and Rehabilitation

B

Professional Organization Research-Based Stands and Statements

Many professional organizations release research-based stands and consensus statements that include evidence-based recommendations for the profession. The following is a current list of examples from two professional organizations. Full text of these position stands, position statements, and consensus statements can be found on each organization's website.

Some professional organizations, such as the National Athletic Trainers' Association, are now providing a category of evidence, based on the strength of recommendation taxonomy (SORT), for each recommendation contained within the statements.

■ AMERICAN COLLEGE OF SPORTS MEDICINE POSITION STANDS

www.acsm.org/public-information/ position-stands

Quantity and Quality of Exercise for Developing and Maintaining Cardiorespiratory, Musculoskeletal, and Neuromotor Fitness in Apparently Healthy Adults: Guidance for Prescribing Exercise (July 2011)

Exercise and Type 2 Diabetes: American College of Sports Medicine and the American Diabetes Association: Joint Position Statement (December 2010)

Exercise and Physical Activity for Older Adults (July 2009)

Nutrition and Athletic Performance (March 2009)

Progression Models in Resistance Training for Healthy Adults (March 2009)

Appropriate Physical Activity Intervention Strategies for Weight Loss and Prevention of Weight Regain for Adults (February 2009)

The Female Athlete Triad (October 2007)

Exercise and Acute Cardiovascular Events: Placing the Risks Into Perspective (May 2007)

Exertional Heat Illness During Training and Competition (March 2007)

Exercise and Fluid Replacement (February 2007)

Prevention of Cold Injuries During Exercise (November 2006)

Physical Activity and Bone Health (November 2004)

Exercise and Hypertension (March 2004)

Joint Position Statement: Automated External Defibrillators (AEDs) in Health/Fitness Facilities (March 2002)

American Heart Association (AHA)/American College of Sports Medicine (ACSM) Joint Position Statement: Recommendations for Cardiovascular Screening, Staffing, and Emergency Policies at Health/Fitness Facilities (June 1998)

Weight Loss in Wrestlers (October 1996)

The Use of Blood Doping as an Ergogenic Aid (October 1996)

Exercise for Patients With Coronary Artery Disease (March 1994)

The Use of Anabolic-Androgenic Steroids in Sports (October 1987)

■ NATIONAL ATHLETIC TRAINERS' ASSOCIATION POSITION STATEMENTS

www.nata.org/position-statements

Management of Sport Concussion (March 2014)

Preparticipation Physical Examinations and Disqualifying Conditions (February 2014)

Conservative Management and Prevention of Ankle Sprains in Athletes (August 2013)

Lightning Safety for Athletics and Recreation (March 2013)

Evaluation of Dietary Supplements for Performance Nutrition (February 2013)

Anabolic-Androgenic Steroids (September 2012)

National Athletic Trainers' Association Position Statement: Preventing Sudden Death in Sports (February 2012)

National Athletic Trainers' Association Position Statement: Safe Weight Loss and Maintenance Practices in Sport and Exercise (June 2011)

Pediatric Overuse Injuries (April 2011)

National Athletic Trainers' Association: Skin Disease (August 2010)

Acute Management of the Cervical Spine–Injured Athlete (June 2009)

Environmental Cold Injuries (December 2008)

Preventing, Detecting, and Managing Disordered Eating in Athletes (February 2008)

Management of the Athlete With Type 1 Diabetes Mellitus (December 2007)

Management of Asthma in Athletes (September 2005)

Management of Sport-Related Concussion (September 2004)

Head Down Contact and Spearing in Tackle Football (March 2004)

Exertional Heat Illnesses (September 2002)

Emergency Planning in Athletics (March 2002)

Fluid Replacement for Athletes (June 2000)

■ NATIONAL ATHLETIC TRAINERS' ASSOCIATION CONSENSUS STATEMENTS

www.nata.org/consensus-statements

Interassociation Recommendations for Developing a Plan to Recognize and Refer Student-Athletes With Psychological Concerns at the Secondary School Level: A Consensus Statement (March 2015)

Inter-Association Consensus Statement on Best Practices for Sports Medicine Management for Secondary Schools and Colleges (January 2014)

Inter-Association Recommendations in Developing a Plan for Recognition and Referral of Student-Athletes With Psychological Concerns at the Collegiate Level (October 2013)

Inter-Association Task Force for Preventing Sudden Death in Secondary School Athletics (July 2013)

Inter-Association Task Force for Preventing Sudden Death in Collegiate Conditioning Sessions: Best Practices Recommendations (August 2012)

Preseason Heat-Acclimatization Guidelines for Secondary School Athletics (June 2009)

Sickle Cell Trait and the Athlete (June 2007)

Inter-Association Recommendations on Emergency Preparedness and Management of Sudden Cardiac Arrest in High School and College Athletic Programs (March 2007)

Inter-Association Task Force on Exertional Heat Illnesses (June 2003)

Managing Prescriptions and Non-Prescription Medication in the Athletic Training Facility Appropriate Medical Care for Secondary School-Age Athletes (February 2003)

The Disablement Continuum

◾ THE DISABLEMENT CONTINUUM

As explained in Chapter 3, Saad Nagi proposed the original disablement model in 1965 (Nagi, 1965), with the intent to characterize disease across a continuum of dysfunction, rather than limit it to a description of the disease process (see Fig. 3–1). Before the development of the World Health Organization (WHO) model, several other models were developed. Each was designed to improve on the Nagi model or address disablement from a different perspective.

One of the limitations of Nagi's model is that it did not recognize the impact of societal factors, such as the availability of elevators or handicap ramps, on normal function for disabled persons. The National Center for Medical Rehabilitation Research (NCMRR) took Nagi's model further and developed a disablement model that breaks disablement down into five components including societal limitations on activities of daily living (National Advisory Board for Medical Rehabilitation Research, 1993).

In addition to the Nagi and National Center for Medical Rehabilitation Research models are three other disablement models in the literature:

1. The revised National Center for Medical Rehabilitation Research model
2. The World Health Organization model
3. The Institute of Medicine (IOM) model

The first two models are evolutions of the Nagi model and were developed as understanding of disablement evolved. The third model developed to accommodate the needs of the field of rehabilitation engineering more effectively.

The National Center for Medical Rehabilitation Research Model

The National Center for Medical Rehabilitation Research model (National Advisory Board for Medical Rehabilitation Research, 1993) divides disablement into five distinct components and includes Nagi's original dimensions in addition to societal limitations (Appendix Fig. C–1) (Snyder et al., 2008). The advantage of this division is that it aids clinicians' understanding of what they are treating and facilitates a better therapy model to improve health across the entire spectrum.

Pathophysiology

Pathophysiology refers to damage at the cellular level. All disease or injury involves some type of damage or alteration in physiology at the cellular level. For example, a heart attack results in death of cardiac tissue, and high blood pressure causes damage to the blood vessels. Alternatively, a knee meniscal cartilage tear results in some amount of tissue tearing damage.

At this level, diagnosis requires some type of medical test to assess the damage. For a heart attack, this could be an electrocardiogram or coronary angiogram. For the meniscus tear, a magnetic resonance image would be needed to visualize the damage.

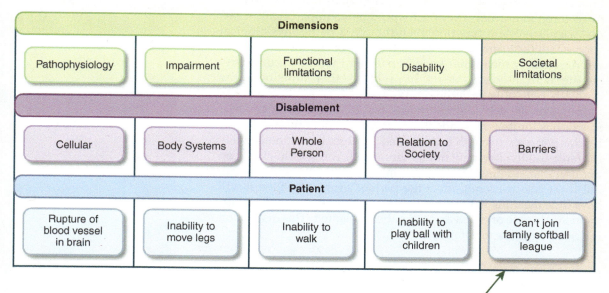

Appendix Figure C–1 The Nagi model extended to the National Center for Medical Rehabilitation Research (NCMRR) model. *(From Snyder, A. R., Parsons, J. T., Valovich McLeod, T. C., Bay, R. C., Michener, L. A., & Sauers, E. L. [2008]. Using disablement models and clinical outcomes assessment to enable evidence-based athletic training practice, part I: Disablement models.* Journal of Athletic Training, *43[3], 428-436.)*

These types of tests are outside the scope of the practice of most allied health practitioners and exercise scientists. These tests do not relate directly to the functional status of the patient. They are useful in diagnosing disease and maybe the severity of the pathological process, but they do not inform clinicians of the patient's functional status. They also do not assess the function of the organ system, for which other tests are required.

Impairment

Impairment is the second level of the disablement continuum, representing the function of the body's organ systems. Whereas pathophysiology refers to tissue damage, impairment refers to the inability of the system to perform. For example, in the case of heart attack, function may be measured by a cardiac stress test. The stress test would reveal that the heart is not functioning normally. Similarly, damage to the knee's meniscus may result in a restriction on pain-free range of motion or a loss in strength.

At first, you may think that pathophysiology and impairment are connected, but they are not. For example, a minor heart attack would produce some tissue damage to the heart that would be detectable by medical tests. However, assuming a very mild heart attack and appropriate rehabilitation, overall heart function could be restored to normal. The effect would be no impairment in cardiovascular system function even though a pathophysiological state exists (i.e., cardiac scar tissue). A tear of the meniscus does not necessarily mean that knee impairment would occur. Many people with meniscus tears have knees that function quite normally with only periodic symptoms.

Impairment such as strength loss at a joint does not mean that function is limited. It means that strength is not at normal levels. If your patient's strength is decreased enough, limitation is likely to result, but the two may not be connected. You should also keep in mind that strength loss may be important to you as a clinician, but if the loss does not affect the patient's function, then it will have little meaning to the patient. Thus, many measures of impairment are disease oriented and not patient oriented. This distinction is discussed in more detail later.

Functional Limitations

Functional limitations are limitations resulting from some pathological process or disease that affects a person at the whole body level. For example, a meniscus tear (i.e., pathophysiology) may result in sufficient inflammation at the joint (more pathophysiology) that pain and weakness result (i.e., joint impairment). This impairment may then result in a decrease in the patient's ability to run or even walk normally (i.e., functional limitation). The heart attack would result in cardiac muscle death (i.e., pathophysiology). This could lead to decreased cardiovascular function (i.e., impairment). Increased impairment of the cardiovascular system could result in an inability to walk long distances or climb stairs (i.e., functional limitation). These functional limitations are manifested in the patient's daily life beyond pain, fatigue, or range of motion by limiting the ability to perform simple daily tasks such as housework or even dressing.

Functional limitations are about the performance of the individual person, not the performance of the organs or organ systems. At this level of disablement, the disease or injury has a direct impact on things that are important to the patient. Thus, as you consider your practice's impact on patients and clients, you should also consider including treatments that will improve functional limitations.

Disability

The next level of the continuum is disability. *Disability* is interference by a disease or pathological process with a person's role in society. In general, roles may include being an employee, parent, homemaker, athlete, and so forth. These general roles break down into more specific roles such as carpenter, triathletes, and so forth.

One example would be a firefighter who sustained a meniscus tear (pathophysiology). His knee has some pain and swelling that restriction the knee's movement (impairment). As a result, he cannot climb ladders and has difficulty getting into his fire truck (functional limitation). Furthermore, because he cannot climb, he is on leave until the knee heals; thus, he is unable to fulfill his role as a firefighter (disability).

It is important to understand that disability is not restricted to work roles. It can also include roles outside of work. For example, maybe the firefighter is also a scoutmaster. Because of his knee injury, he is unable to hike trails, thus restricting his role as scoutmaster and resulting in further disability. As suggested earlier, roles can be any type of societal interaction, including but not limited to other roles such as parenthood. If an injury prevents your patient from participating in his or her normal life, the patient is disabled. It also includes social activities such as going to the movies.

Disability often manifests as a decrease in quality of life. People who cannot participate in their normal life activities often feel that their life is less fulfilling. Thus, as a clinician, be mindful that your treatments should not just focus on restoring functional limitations or impairments. Rather, they should have the additional goal of improving disability and quality of life. Keep this in mind when searching the literature for evidence. Include quality of life outcomes in addition to outcomes focusing on impairment or functional limitations in your view of evidence as you form your clinical question (as noted in Chapter 2).

Societal Limitations

Societal limitations are those limitations placed on an individual person by society. These may include limitations such as social prejudices, but they most typically involve physical barriers. Examples of accommodations for physical barriers include wheelchair ramps, elevators, adaptations to automobiles, and similar accommodations. In the sporting world, this could also include modifications to games to allow for wheelchair basketball, balls that chirp to allow blind persons to play soccer, and modifications to weightlifting equipment to allow its use by wheelchair bound persons, among others.

As a clinician, these limitations may be beyond your control because they may be public policy decisions. However, they may affect your direction in terms of patient access or how exercise is modified to accommodate level of disability. Even if societal limitations do not have a direct effect on your evidence-based practice, some awareness is needed to understand the goals of treatment for the lower three levels of disability.

The Updated National Center for Medical Rehabilitation Research Model

The National Center for Medical Rehabilitation Research disablement model described earlier was updated in 2006 (National Center for Medical Rehabilitation Research, 2006). The new model is shown in Appendix Figure C–2. As you can see, only four levels of disablement are presented, and disability is replaced with roles. This is a fundamental refocusing of the model to emphasize the importance of a person's ability to participate in his or her selected roles.

The other major change in the model is the addition of influences. These influences are the factors that act as barriers to or facilitators of persons' movement from one level to the next. In other words, the change requires clinicians to focus on those aspects that move patients to the next level of disability. Thus, your focus should be seeking evidence to support treatments that affect these influences across the whole spectrum of disablement.

The Critical Consumer A-1

Much of medical research has historically focused on the pathophysiology and impairment levels of the disease. It has also been the case that improvements in patients' physiology or impairment are accepted as proof that the treatment or therapy has worked. Although science directed at these dimensions is very worthwhile and is establishing the foundation for future research, it is important to recognize that these dimensions do not capture qualities that are necessarily important to the patient. Improvement from the patients' perspective begins at the functional limitation and disability levels of the continuum. Thus, for a treatment to be effective it must go beyond improving the patients' physiology.

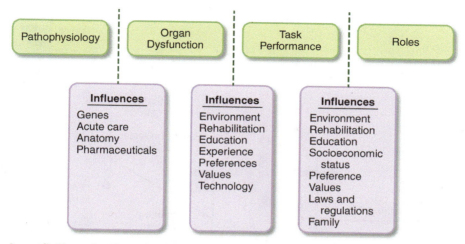

Appendix Figure C–2 The updated National Center for Medical Rehabilitation Research (NCMRR) model. *(From National Center for Medical Rehabilitation Research. [2006].* Report to the NACHHD Council. *Washington, DC: U.S. Department of Health and Human Services.)*

The World Health Organization Model

As discussed in Chapter 3, the World Health Organization constructed the International Classification of Function (World Health Organization, 2002). This model differs structurally from the other models in that it is a two-part model (see Fig. 3–2). The first part of the model focuses on the first four levels of the previous models: *pathophysiology, impairment, functional limitations,* and *disability,* which become *health condition, body functions and structure, activity,* and *participation* in the International Classification of Function, respectively. The second part of the model focuses on personal and environmental aspects of disablement. Predominantly, this second part relates to societal limitations (including physical access) of the previous models. However, it also recognizes that individual personal experiences also affect a person's level of disablement. The advantage of this model is that it structurally separates those factors that the practitioner can influence from those that the individual person and society influences. However, that does not mean that the clinician cannot or should not try to influence aspects of the model's second part.

Institute of Medicine Model

The Institute of Medicine also developed a model that in many ways is simpler (Committee on Assessing Rehabilitation Science and Engineering, 1997). This model (Appendix Fig. C–3) has a

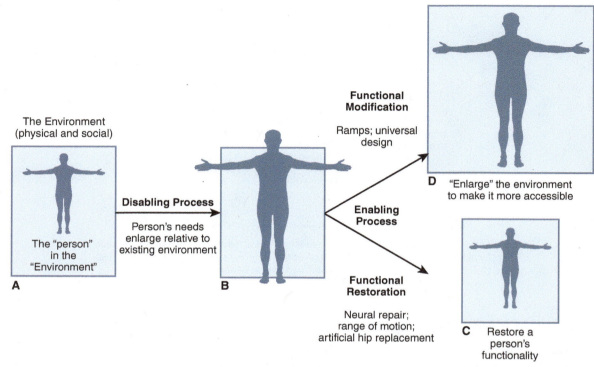

The Environment
(physical and social)

The "person"
in the
"Environment"

A

Disabling Process

Person's needs
enlarge relative to
existing environment

B

**Functional
Modification**

Ramps; universal
design

D "Enlarge" the environment
to make it more accessible

**Enabling
Process**

**Functional
Restoration**

Neural repair;
range of motion;
artificial hip replacement

C Restore a
person's
functionality

Appendix Figure C–3 The Institute of Medicine model of disability. *(From Committee on Assessing Rehabilitation Science and Engineering, Division of Health Sciences Policy, Institute of Medicine. [1997]. Enabling America: Assessing the role of rehabilitation science and engineering [E. N. Brandt & A. M. Pope, Eds.]. Washington, DC: National Academy Press.)*

strong focus on biomedical engineering. Nevertheless, the model's conceptual simplicity makes it useful. The model starts with the idea that, as people, our needs fit within our social and physical "environment." Through the disabling process, our needs expand relative to our environment. Fitting needs back into the environment becomes a challenge. Two general methods or enabling processes for this are proposed by the model. The first is to expand the environment to meet the new needs. This is done by engineering, including the building of ramps, devices, or other appliances (e.g., prosthetics). The second method is functional restoration (e.g., rehabilitation, medical treatment). This process brings the individual patient's needs back into the environment. As you may imagine, both of these processes are frequently used together. A patient with hip arthritis may have his or her hip replaced to restore normal function. Similarly, the patient may make certain environmental adjustments (e.g., using access ramps instead of stairs) to navigate his or her physical environment. Both approaches would contribute to bringing the individual patient's needs back inside the environment.

SELECTING A DISABLEMENT MODEL

As a research consumer, it is not necessary for you to pick a model you prefer. The researcher will usually have done that as part of the research. Although the researcher may not directly state the model, you can infer it from the outcomes measured. What is important as the consumer is to realize that these models have evolved over time, and that not all the models contain all the same elements. It also means the available research may not address all elements of a model.

Instead of choosing a model, you should use these models to identify components that are relevant to you and your patients or clients. For example, studies on pathophysiology are not likely to have practical meaning to your patients or clients. Focusing on this type of research may not benefit your practice. Instead, you may want to focus on those dimensions of the models that more directly relate to your patients (e.g., functional limitations and disability). Once you have decided which dimensions of these models best fit your practice, this should lead you to the appropriate outcomes. The outcomes fit into the dimensions. In other words, the outcomes you choose to focus on depend on which dimensions you select from the models. Appendix Figure C–4 shows the Nagi, National Center for Medical Rehabilitation Research, and International Classification of Functioning, Disability, and Health models applied to four different patient's cases.

Extending the Model to Human Performance

The previous discussion focused on applying the disability models to a person with a disease. However, there is no reason that it cannot be applied to human performance. Using the first National Center for Medical Rehabilitation Research model, the same principles apply in each category, although different names would be more appropriate for the first four. For example, pathophysiology could be changed to "tissue development." This could be represented by strength training producing muscle hypertrophy. Impairment could be changed to "performance development" and be represented by measurable strength gains. Functional limitations could be changed to "functional improvements" and be represented by improvements in running speed, throwing distance, and so forth. Finally, disability could be renamed "achievement" and could mean becoming a member of an athletic team.

The point of the previous examples is not to create a new model to be applied to human performance. Rather, it is hoped that it will provide you with a new framework by which to think about human performance evidence. By now, you should understand

Dimension	Nagi Model					
Dimension	Pathophysiology	Impairment	Function Limitations	Disability		
	NCMRR Model					
Dimension	Pathophysiology	Impairment	Functional Limitations	Disability	Societal Limitations	
	ICF Model					
Dimension	Health Condition	Body Structure and Function	Activity	Participation	Environmental Factors	Personal Factors
Level of disability	Disorder or Disease	Body Systems	Whole Person	Person's Relation to Society	Legal/social, Attitudes, Climate, Architecture Terrain	Gender, Age, SES, Education
20-year-old collegiate pitcher	Rotator Cuff Impingement	Restricted range of motion and pain with movement	Inability to throw ball	Cannot continue to pitch for team	Coach sidelines pitcher resulting in a sense of alienation from the team.	Athlete elects to quit team rather than sit out and pursue rehabilitation.
55-year-old office worker	Diabetes	Early stages of proximal neuropathy with muscle weakness in both legs, pain	Difficulty moving from sitting to standing without assistance	Missing work due to associated pain	Employer unwilling to modify job to meet employees needs.	Age may continue to contribute to additional diabetes complications.
12-year-old soccer player	Tibial apophysitis	Knee pain	Inability to run	Unable to compete in soccer league	Physician limits participation on team.	Realizing that the condition will resolve with time the athlete elects to stay on team.
50-year-old part-time warehouse worker	Knee osteoarthritis	Knee pain and limited range of motion	Inability to walk or stand for long periods without antiinflammatory medication.	Unable to be employed in warehouse.	As a part-time employee, lacks health-care insurance.	Limited income prevents purchasing over-the-counter pain medications.

Appendix Figure C–4 The Nagi, National Center for Medical Rehabilitation Research (NCMRR), and International Classification of Functioning, Disability, and Health (ICF) models as applied to four different patient examples. Note which dimensions best fit your practice.

that human performance has multiple levels. Thus, as you begin searching for evidence to support your practice, you should consider which of these levels you are trying to influence. For example, strength gain for strength gain's sake may not meet the true goal of strength training, at least from the point of view of an athlete interested in improved performance.

■ DISABLEMENT SUMMARY

Each of the previous models has their strength and weaknesses. The point of presenting them is to familiarize you with different ways to think about disablement. It is not necessary for you do identify the best model. It may be appropriate for you to consider each model and then select one that best meets your needs. Perhaps the most important point of these models is that injury and illness should not be thought of just as the disease or pathological process. Rather, you should be mindful that there is a spectrum of disablement. With it is a variety of measures used to assess all levels of disablement. As you search for evidence, you should be mindful of these different levels and associated outcomes.

REFERENCES

Committee on Assessing Rehabilitation Science and Engineering, Division of Health Sciences Policy, Institute of Medicine. (1997). *Enabling America: Assessing the role of rehabilitation science and engineering* (E. N. Brandt & A. M. Pope, Eds.). Washington, DC: National Academy Press.

Nagi, S. (1965). Some conceptual issues in disability and rehabilitation. In M. Sussman (Ed.), *Sociology and rehabilitation* (pp. 100-113). Washington, DC: American Sociological Association.

National Advisory Board for Medical Rehabilitation Research. (1993). *Research plan for the national center for medical rehabilitation research.* (NIH Publication No. 93-3509). Washington, DC: U.S. Department of Health and Human Services.

National Center for Medical Rehabilitation Research. (2006). *Report to the NACHHD Council.* Washington, DC: U.S. Department of Health and Human Services.

Snyder, A. R., Parsons, J. T., Valovich McLeod, T. C., Bay, R. C., Michener, L. A., & Sauers, E. L. (2008). Using disablement models and clinical outcomes assessment to enable evidence-based athletic training practice, part I: Disablement models. *Journal of Athletic Training, 43*(4), 428-436.

World Health Organization. (2002). *Towards a common language for functioning, disability, and health: ICF the International Classification of Functioning, Disability, and Health.* Geneva: World Health Organization.

A

Absolute risk reduction (ARR): A measure of the change in risk of an experimental treatment in relation to a control treatment. It is calculated by subtracting the experimental event rate from the control event rate.

Accuracy: A measure of how much systematic error is in an assessment or how well a set of measures is centered on the true score.

Active comparator arm: The clinical trial arm in which the participants receive the standard, clinically effective treatment (sometimes identified as the comparison group). One of the five typical treatment arms used in clinical trials.

Administration burden: The time, complexity, work force needed, and cost required to score a questionnaire.

Administration time: The time it takes the client or patient to complete a questionnaire.

Adverse effects: One of a group of five types of questions that can be asked as part of a clinical trial. Adverse effects (side effects) document adverse events encountered during the course of the trial. These types of questions are typically unplanned because adverse advents cannot usually be predicted.

Adverse event: Any injury or otherwise adverse outcome to the health of a participant that happens during a clinical study or within a certain time period after the study is over.

Agent: A factor whose presence, excessive presence, or relative absence is essential for the occurrence of a disease.

Ancillary questions: One of a group of five types of questions that can be asked as part of a clinical trial. Ancillary questions are not specifically planned but can be addressed with the study data. These are often considered substudies within the main study.

Applicability: The relevance of the clinical evidence to the specific client you are treating.

Area under the curve (AUC): An accuracy measure of a clinical test that takes into account all cutoff scores in your investigation and provides the probability that the test result will positively identify a condition.

Attributable risk: The percentage of instances of an illness that can be accounted for by a particular risk factor. Also called attributable fraction.

B

Bias: A measure of inaccuracy or any effect or interference that produces results that systematically depart from the true value.

Biological gradient: The systematic relationship between a proposed cause and altered rates of disease, injury, or death.

Block randomization: A process of assigning individual subjects to study groups. The researcher divides individual subjects into subgroups called blocks and then randomly assigns individual subjects within each block to treatment conditions.

Boolean operator: A connecting symbol or word, such as AND or OR, that allows a computer user to include or exclude items from a text search.

Boolean search: Performing a text search by using Boolean operators to include or exclude items, thereby making the search results more precise.

C

Case-control study: A study that compares subjects with the disease (cases) with those absent of the disease (control) and tests for differences between those two groups.

Ceiling effect: A measurement error indicating that the outcome scale range is too narrow, and very high data points cluster at the top end of the scale.

Centre for Evidence-Based Medicine (CEBM): An organization dedicated to the development, education, and promotion of evidence-based medicine that has established a multilevel platform for data collation, dissemination, and application of evidence-based medicine.

Citation bias: The tendency for studies with statistically significant results to be cited more often than those without statistically significant results.

Clinical relevance: How well results from clinical evidence apply to your typical circumstances, such as your clients, setting, and available treatments.

Clinician-based outcomes: Measures that are collected by a clinician; data and information that cannot be provided by the patient without the involvement of the clinician.

Cochrane Library: A collection of databases that contain Cochrane reviews, clinical trials, and other types of relevant research. The collection is maintained by the Cochrane Collaboration and is updated regularly.

Cochrane reviews: A database of systematic reviews and meta-analyses that summarize and interpret the results of medical research and are published online in the Cochrane Library.

Coherence: The association between a proposed cause and the known biology and natural history of a disease.

Comparison: One element of the PICO (patients, intervention, comparison, and outcome) format that is used to create a specific clinical question before beginning to search the research literature. Comparison refers to what is being compared in the clinical question.

Concurrent validity: A form of criterion validity: the degree to which two measuring devices or methods agree with each other.

Confidence interval (CI): The range of values within which the true value of a parameter is expected to lie. The confidence interval shows whether results are statistically significant and the magnitude of measurement error.

Confounder: An extraneous variable that affects the outcomes that are being studied such that the test results do not reflect the actual relationship between the outcomes that are under investigation. It is a variable that the researcher fails to control or eliminate such that it damages the internal validity of an experiment. Also called confounding variable or third variable.

Consistency of association: The requirement that a proposed cause produces similar effects across different conditions.

Consolidated Standards of Reporting Trials (CONSORT): A group of initiatives developed by the CONSORT group to alleviate the problems that arise from inadequate reporting of randomized controlled trials. The CONSORT group developed and updates the CONSORT 2010 statement, a 25-item checklist, and a flow chart that diagrams a participant's progress throughout a trial.

Construct: An abstraction that is created by researchers to conceptualize a variable they wish to test but that is not directly observable, such as quality of life.

Construct validity: A form of criterion validity: the degree to which a test accurately measures or quantifies the intended construct.

Control group: In a true experimental design, the group (arm) that receives no treatment or receives standard treatment. This group can be compared with the treatment or experimental group. Also called a control.

Control event rate (CER): The rate at which events occur in the no treatment arm, or control group, of a study.

Convergent validity: A form of construct validity: the degree to which two measures of constructs that theoretically should be related are actually related.

Criterion validity: A measure of how well an outcome estimates a target value or gold standard measure.

Critically appraised paper (CAP): A professional summary of a single research study.

Critically appraised topic (CAT): A professional summary, typically focused on a clinical question, of a small number of research studies (three to five). The critically appraised topic is typically shorter and less rigorous than the systematic review.

Cross-sectional design: A study design in which the relationship between health outcomes and other factors of interest are examined, within a defined population, at one particular time period.

Cumulative incidence: The risk of developing a disease over a defined period.

Cutoff score: The value of each data point on a receiver operating characteristic curve that is used to determine the presence or absence of a condition.

D

DARE: The Database of Abstracts of Reviews and Effects. This database contains abstracts of systematic reviews that have been assessed for quality by using a specific set of criteria. The database is maintained and regularly updated by the Centre for Reviews Dissemination in the United Kingdom.

Dependent variable: In a research study, the outcome that is measured.

Dimension-specific outcomes: Outcomes that assess one specific aspect of health status.

Direct causal association: A cause-and-effect relationship in which one event is the direct cause of a second event.

Disablement continuum: The range of factors that contribute to or detract from health and normal function of the individual person.

Disablement models: Structured representations or frameworks of the disablement continuum that identify the components of disablement and the interactions among them.

Disease-specific outcomes: Measures of patients' function in relation to a specific disease.

Disease-oriented evidence (DOE): Measures that focus on the qualities or aspects of the disease and are collected by the clinician to help with the understanding of the current state of the disease.

Disease-oriented outcome: Measures that assess qualities that are related to a disease, such as blood pressure and bone density.

Divergent validity: A form of construct validity: the degree to which the new instrument is correlated to another instrument with dissimilar attributes or qualities.

Double blind: A method of conducting a study in which neither the participants receiving treatment nor the researchers know whether the participants are in the control group or the experimental group. Double-blind studies attempt to eliminate observer and subject bias.

Duplication bias: The tendency to duplicate publication of study results, such as the initial publication in conference proceedings or abstracts, followed by publication as a full journal manuscript.

E

Effect modification: A cause-and-effect relationship in which the effect of one exposure on disease risk is modified by the presence of another exposure.

Effect size: The magnitude of the difference between the control group and the treatment group on the dependent variable or outcome of interest.

Effectiveness: A positive result for a treatment under normal, real-world conditions.

Efficacy: A positive result for a treatment under ideal, experimentally controlled conditions.

Environment: All the external conditions and influences affecting the life and development of an individual entity.

Epidemiological triad: The traditional model of disease causation, which includes three components: agent, host, and environment.

Epidemiology: The study of the occurrence of health-related events and their determinants in human populations.

Equivalency study: A clinical investigation in which two distinct treatments are compared against each other to identify whether one treatment is as effective as another and has fewer drawbacks.

Evidence-based medicine (EBM): Medicine that is based on data, rather than anecdote, intuition, or belief.

Evidence-based practice (EBP): The practice of applying research findings to professional practice.

Experimental arm: The clinical trial arm in which the participants receive the experimental treatment. One of five typical treatment arms used in clinical trials.

Experimental event rate (EER): The rate at which events occur in the experimental arm, or experimental group, of a study.

Experimental group: In a clinical investigation, a group that receives a treatment that is different from that of the control group.

Experimental research: Method of research in which the researcher manipulates variables. An experiment classically conducts tests on two randomly assigned groups, a control group and an experimental group, and compares the different outcomes of the tests for each group. Also called true experimental design.

Expert review: A narrative review written by an expert in the field.

External validity: The degree to which the results of a study can be generalized to other groups of subjects, settings, treatments, or outcomes.

F

Face validity: A form of criterion validity: the degree to which an outcome measures what it is intended to measure; the degree to which a measurement is logical, reasonable, or acceptable.

Factorial design: A clinical study in which four treatment arms are used: the control arm, treatment arm A, treatment arm B, and treatment arm AB. In the case of the treatment AB arm, participants receive both treatments.

Fail-safe N: A technique to measure publication bias. It calculates the number of primary studies needed to produce a nonsignificant overall effect size.

False-negative rate: The percentage of persons who do have the attribute or disease but receive negative test results. The notation used for false-negative rate is $1 -$ sensitivity.

False-negative score: A score that indicates the number of persons who actually have the condition but receive negative results on a clinical test.

False-positive rate: The percentage of persons who do not have the attribute or disease but receive positive test results. The notation used for false-positive rate is $1 -$ specificity.

False-positive score: The number of persons who do not have the condition but receive positive results on a clinical test.

Fixed effect model: A statistical model that assumes that the effect sizes of the primary studies represent one true effect size.

Floor effect: A measurement error indicating that the measurement scale range is too narrow, and very low data points cluster at the bottom end of the scale.

Forest plot: A graphic technique showing how different studies that have evaluated a specific condition or treatment have produced independent results.

Funnel plot: A graphic technique that looks for symmetry in data.

G

General adverse event: Any adverse event that is reported to, or observed by, clinicians during a clinical study.

Generic outcomes: Measures that assess a very broad range of aspects of health status.

Global rating of change: Measures that ask patients whether they are better, are about the same, or are worse across some period of time.

Group allocation design: A process of assigning groups to study arms. The researcher randomly assigns intact groups, such as communities, schools, and so forth, to treatment conditions.

H

Historical control design: A clinical study that compares a treatment arm against a set of control participants who were observed at some time in the past or for whom data are available through a database.

Historical review: A narrative review with the implied purpose of reviewing all the existing literature on a topic.

Host: A person or other living organism that is infected by an infectious agent.

I

Incidence: A measure of the number of new cases of disease or injury during a defined period of time, divided by the product of the number of persons monitored during the same time period. Also called incidence rate.

Included study population: The participants included in the primary studies.

Independent variable: In a research study, the variable that the research controls.

Indirect casual association: A cause-and-effect relationship in which one event may be associated with a third event, which is really the causal event.

Information bias: Bias resulting from errors in classification of risk status or disease status.

Intent-to-treat analysis: A clinical trial in which data from all participants are included, even if the participants failed to complete the study or comply with the treatment protocol.

Internal consistency: A form of reliability typically used to determine the consistency of individual items within a questionnaire.

Internal validity: The degree to which a researcher controls or eliminates all extraneous variables, including cofounders, of a study.

Interpretability: The ability to assign qualitative meaning to a quantitative score.

Intersession reliability: An alternative form of test-retest reliability in which measures are collected at two different time points.

Interval data: Data on a scale of measurement in which the intervals between points on the scale are fixed and equal. One of the four basic types of data, which include nominal, ordinal, interval, and ratio.

Intervention: One element of the PICO (patients, intervention, comparison, and outcome) format that is used to create a specific clinical question before beginning to search research literature. Intervention refers to treatments that are applied to patients or clients in the clinical question.

Intrasession reliability: An alternative form of test-retest reliability with relatively little time passing between each measure.

L

Language bias: The tendency for authors to exclude studies that are not published in their native language.

Levels of evidence: Indicators, by category, of the strength of research.

Likelihood ratio: The percentage of persons with a condition for a certain test result compared with the percentage of persons without a condition for the same test result.

M

Mean: A calculated measure of central tendency that is the average of all the scores.

Measurement error: The difference between the true value of something that is being measured and the value that is actually obtained by measurement.

Median: A measure of central tendency that is the middle number in a sorted list.

Meta-analysis: A form of systematic review that performs a statistical analysis of the effect sizes in a group of studies.

Meta-analysis of Observational Studies in Epidemiology (MOOSE): A set of guidelines developed by 27 leading experts on how to report, evaluate, and rate meta-analyses and other studies effectively in epidemiology. It was developed to guide researchers, authors, reviewers, and editors on the publication of studies.

Methodological quality: An assessment of the research methods used in a primary study.

Minimal detectable change: The minimum amount of change between data points that must exist to ensure that the change was not the result of measurement error.

Minimal important difference: The smallest amount of change in an outcome that represents an important change to the patient.

Minimal clinical important difference (MCID): The smallest amount of change in an outcome that represents an important change to the clinician and maybe to the patient.

Mode: The measure of central tendency that represents the value occurring most frequently.

N

Narrative review: Any review that collects, organizes, and synthesizes primary references without using inclusion or selection criteria.

Natural history: One of a group of five types of questions that can be asked as part of a clinical trial. Natural history questions address the origins, evolutions, and interrelationships of a disease. These questions are addressed by the no intervention arm of the trial.

Negative likelihood ratio: A comparison of the false-negative rate (the probability of a person who has the attribute or disease but tests negative) with the true-negative rate (the probability of a person who does not have the attribute or disease but tests negative). The notation used for the false-negative rate is 1 – sensitivity.

Negative posttest probability: The probability of having the condition given a negative test result. It is computed as 1 minus the value of the negative predictive value.

Negative predictive value: The probability that a person with a negative test result does not have a given condition.

No intervention arm: The clinical trial arm in which the participants receive no treatment (sometimes identified as the control group). One of five typical treatment arms used in clinical trials.

Nominal data: Categorically discrete data. One of the four basic types of data, which include nominal, ordinal, interval, and ratio.

Nonrandomized concurrent control: Studies in which participants are not randomly assigned to a control group or an experimental group. Also called nonequivalent control group designs.

Null hypothesis: The assumption or currently accepted position in which no specific relationship exists between two variables.

Number needed to harm (NNH): The number of people needed to be treated so that one person experiences an adverse effect or harm.

Number needed to treat (NNT): The number of people needed to be treated so that one person experiences a benefit.

O

Odds ratio (OR): The probability that an event will occur in a group compared with the probability that an event will not occur in another group, a close approximation of the relative risk. Also called cross-product ratio.

Ordinal data: Data that have a rank order, but that order is arbitrary. One of the four basic types of data, which include nominal, ordinal, interval, and ratio.

Outcome: One element of the PICO (patients, intervention, comparison, and outcome) format that is used to create a specific clinical question before beginning research. Outcome refers to aspects of a patient's health or fitness that are expected to change in response to an intervention in the clinical question.

Overall effect size: The average effect size of all the primary studies included in a meta-analysis.

P

Patient-based outcome: Measures that the patients complete for themselves. This type of measure tends to be surveys or questionnaires.

Patient-oriented evidence that matters (POEM): Measures that directly assess the patient's health status, including risk of dying, quality of life, loss of function, life span, and so forth.

Patient-oriented measures: Measures that assess qualities that are related to the whole patient, such as mortality and quality of life, with the goal of emphasizing changes that patients easily understand.

Patients: One element of the PICO (patients, intervention, comparison, and outcome) format that is used to create a specific clinical question before beginning research. Patients refers to the person or group you are trying to treat or serve in the clinical question.

PEDro: The Physiotherapy Evidence Database (PEDro). This database catalogs systematic reviews and clinical trials in the field of physical therapy and that are focused on rehabilitation. It is maintained by the Centre for Evidence-Based Physiotherapy at the George Institute for Global Health at the University of Sydney in Australia.

Peer-review process: A process in which a group of competent persons within a similar field of study independently evaluates the body of work.

Peer-reviewed journal: An academic journal that features original works that are evaluated by expert peers in a particular field of study.

Per protocol analysis: A clinical trial in which data from only those participants who complete the trial and comply with the treatment protocol are included. This is in contrast to the intent-to-treat analysis.

Persistence: The length of time the disease or injury remains exposed to risk or mitigating factors.

Phase I trial: A clinical trial in which a treatment is tested on humans for the first time. Before a phase I trial, the treatment has been studied in animals, and the results have demonstrated promise for treatment in humans. Phase I trials tend to enroll a small number of individual subjects and focus on biological mechanisms. The type of outcome measure is often disease oriented and scientist or clinician based.

Phase II trial: A clinical trial in which an efficacy study is performed to determine whether a given treatment works at all. Phase II trials are typically small (hundreds of patients) and use a randomized control. These types of trials are often thought of as laboratory trials involving humans.

Phase III trial: A clinical trial in which an effectiveness study is performed. Phase III trials often involve thousands of patients and use a randomized control.

Phase IV trial: A clinical trial in which a monitoring study is performed. These trials are conducted to determine whether the effectiveness and safety of the treatment are maintained. These studies often are long-term studies and serve to identify safety issues and the effectiveness of the intervention.

Physiotherapy Evidence Database (PEDro): *See* PEDro.

Placebo arm: The clinical trial arm in which the participants receive a fake drug or medication in the form of a similar-appearing, inert substance. One of five typical treatment arms used in clinical trials.

Plausibility: The ability to explain the association between death and disease and a proposed cause.

Population attributable fraction (PAF): The proportion of cases in a population that occurred in a subgroup having the risk factor of interest.

Positive likelihood ratio: A comparison of the true-positive rate (the probability that a person who has the attribute or disease will test positive) with the false-positive rate (the probability that a person who does not have the attribute or disease will test negative).

Positive posttest probability: *See* Positive predictive value.

Positive predictive value: The probability that a person with a positive test result actually has a given condition. It is computed as the percentage of true-positive scores in all persons with and without the condition who have positive test results.

Precision: A measurement's variability as a result of random error, measured by the standard error of the measure.

Predictive validity: A form of criterion validity: the degree to which a test measurement accurately predicts a future event.

Preferred Reporting Items for Systematic Reviews and Meta-Analyses (PRISMA): A set of minimum standards to aid authors in the reporting of items in evidence-based systematic reviews and meta-analyses.

Prevalence: A proportional measure of the number of cases of a disease or injury, present in a specified population, at a specified time period.

Primary question: One of a group of five types of questions that can be asked as part of a clinical trial. The primary question is the specific question that the study is designed to answer.

Primary reference: *See* Primary source.

Primary source: The original source for an idea or research results. Often synonymous with a primary study but may refer to a narrative or systematic review.

Primary study: Research study in which researchers directly recruit and collect data on subjects.

Prospective cohort design: A longitudinal study that follows a group of similar individual subjects (cohorts), who differ with respect to certain factors under study, to determine how these factors affect rates of a particular outcome. Also called a prospective cohort study (PCS).

Publication bias: The tendency of professional journals to publish studies that report statistically significant results more often than studies that report statistically nonsignificant results.

PubMed: A database that includes MEDLINE as its primary subset. It contains articles indexed from a broad range of medical and nursing journals, life science journals, and textbooks. The database is maintained by the National Center for Biotechnology Information (NCBI), part of the U.S. National Library of Medicine.

Q

Quasiexperimental research: Method of research similar to experimental research except without the random assignment to groups. Also called quasiexperimental design.

R

Random assignment: A method used to place subjects in groups (after they have been selected to participate in a study) based on a random process, rather than based on some personal characteristics or by personal choice. The intent of random assignment is to create equal groups.

Random effects model: A statistical model that assumes that the effect sizes of the primary studies represent a family of effect sizes.

Random error: Errors in measurement caused by factors that vary from one measurement to another.

Random sampling: A method of randomly selecting subjects from the population to participate in a study.

Randomized controlled trial: A study design that consists of a treatment and a control group and in which the participants are randomly assigned to each group. Considered the "true" experimental design.

Ratio data: Interval data with an absolute zero point. One of the four basic types of data, which include nominal, ordinal, interval, and ratio.

Raw mean difference: The absolute value of the difference between the means of the treatment and control groups in a particular study.

Readability: The reading level of a questionnaire or the ease with which it is understood.

Receiver operating characteristic (ROC) curve: A graphic way to represent the positive likelihood ratio values for each point in a data set; the sensitivity of a test divided by the false-positive rate (1 – specificity).

Region-specific outcomes: Measures that are limited to a specific area of the body.

Relative risk (RR): The ratio of the rate in a population subgroup exposed to an agent that is believed to cause a disease, injury, or death to the rate in a population subgroup not exposed.

Responsiveness: An outcome's ability to change when it is expected to change.

S

Sampling error: The difference between two sample means of the same population. The formula is:

$$SE = \frac{\text{Sample standard deviation}}{\sqrt{\text{Number of subjects in the sample}}}$$

Science Citation Index: A database of articles that allows a researcher to identify which later articles cite any particular earlier article, or the articles of any particular author, or which articles are cited most frequently.

Scientific method: A set of basic principles that outline the means for investigating observations, acquiring evidence, and then integrating that evidence into the current body of knowledge.

Secondary association: A cause-and-effect relationship in which two events are very common and therefore associated, but not in a causal fashion. Also called a noncausal association.

Secondary question: One of a group of five types of questions that can be asked as part of a clinical trial. The secondary questions are questions that are not the main reason for the study and focus on assessing different dependent measures from the primary question.

Secondary source: Reports or papers written about one or more primary sources.

Secondary study: Reviews and syntheses of existing primary studies.

Selection bias: Bias caused by choosing the individual subjects or groups to take part in a study, such as when only certain subjects from a community are enrolled in a study when broader representation is desired.

Sensitivity: The percentage of people who have a positive test result and, in fact, have the condition tested for; true-positive test results divided by the sum of positive and negative test results for a condition.

Sensitivity analysis: A technique that allows authors to assess the impact of their decisions on what data to include in a study and how to include it.

Serious adverse event: An adverse event that threatens life or results in permanent or long-term disability, hospitalization, birth defect, or congenital abnormality.

Sham arm: The clinical trial arm in which the participants receive a fake treatment or therapy that does not include the key components necessary to make the treatment effective. One of five typical treatment arms used in clinical trials.

Simple randomization: A process of randomly assigning individual subjects to study groups as they enroll, typically by using a random numbers table.

Single blind: A method of conducting a study in which either the participants receiving treatment or the clinicians providing care know whether the participants are in the control group or the experimental group. Single-blind studies attempt to eliminate observer or subject bias, depending on which group is "blinded."

Specificity: The percentage of people who have a negative test result and, in fact, do not have the condition tested for; true-negative test results divided by the total sum of negative and positive test results for noncondition.

Specificity of association: The requirement that the pattern of reduced risk seen with increasing levels of an agent must remain in the presence and in the absence of other potential causes of the disease.

Standard deviation (SD): The average deviation of scores around a group mean. Also the square root of variance.

Standard error of the mean (SE): The mathematical estimate of the sampling error.

Standard error of the measure (SEM): The mathematical estimate of random (measurement) error.

Standardized mean difference: An adjusted raw mean difference that allows comparison of measures on different scales and with different units.

Statistically meaningful association: The requirement that an association is not likely to be explainable by random or chance observation.

Stratified randomization: A process of assigning individual subjects to study groups in which the researcher creates groups for a specific purpose, such as some preexisting factor (e.g., sex), and then randomly assigns individual subjects from the groups to a treatment group.

Strength of recommendation: A letter grade assigned to groups of existing studies that address an important clinical problem by using patient-oriented measures. Grades are assigned based on the quality, quantity, and consistency of available data by using the strength of recommendation taxonomy (SORT).

Strength of recommendation taxonomy (SORT): A method used to address the quality, quantity, and consistency of study evidence by emphasizing the use of patient-oriented outcomes. Authors are allowed to rate individual studies or bodies of evidence. The taxonomy rates studies using a letter grade scale in which an A-level recommendation is based on consistent and good-quality patient-oriented evidence; a B-level recommendation is based on inconsistent or limited-quality patient-oriented evidence; and a C-level recommendation is based on consensus, usual practice, opinion, disease-oriented evidence, or case series for studies of diagnosis, treatment, prevention, or screening.

Study arm: In a clinical trial, each group or subgroup of participants receiving experimental treatment or no treatment.

Summary scales: One or two questions about general health or disability that assess the overall health of an individual subject.

Systematic review: A review that follows a preplanned methodology for searching and choosing existing research studies and a synthesis of those research study results into a single research finding.

T

Temporality: The timing between the proposed cause and lower rates of disease or injury.

Test-retest reliability: The measure of the ability of a test to produce consistent results when it is used multiple times under nearly identical conditions.

Threat: Any factor that potentially confuses or confounds the results of research.

Trim and fill: A mathematical procedure for funnel plots that estimates the number of potentially missing studies and their associated effect sizes.

TRIP: Turning Research into Practice (TRIP), a search engine that organizes results so that stronger, more relevant, and more recent sources, based on their rank on the evidence pyramid, are presented near the top of the search results.

Triple blind: A method of conducting a study in which the participants receiving treatment, the clinicians providing care, and a data monitoring board do not know whether the participants are in the control group or the experimental group.

True-negative rate: The percentage of persons who do not have the attribute or disease who receive negative test results. The term used for the true-negative rate is specificity.

True-negative score: The number of persons who do not have the condition and receive negative results on a clinical test.

True-positive rate: The percentage of persons who do have the attribute or disease who receive positive test results. The term used for the true-positive rate is sensitivity.

True-positive score: The number of persons who actually have the condition and receive positive results on a clinical test.

V

Validity: The degree to which data or results of a study are correct or true; a measure of a study's ability to establish what it intended to establish.

Variance: A measure of variability of a group of scores around the group mean. Also the average squared deviation of scores around a group mean.

Vote counting: A method of narrative review that by simply counts the number of studies with statistically significant results in favor of a new treatment and compares that number with the number of studies with statistically significant results in favor of the alternative treatment or control group.

W

Web of causation: An interrelationship of multiple factors that contribute to the occurrence of a disease or injury.

Withdrawal study: A clinical trial in which patients receiving treatment are withdrawn from the treatment or the treatment dose is decreased.

Y

Youden index: A method of summarizing the performance of a clinical test. Computed by adding the sensitivity and specificity values and then subtracting the number 1, the value ranges from 0 to 1. A value of 1 indicates a perfect test; a value of 0 indicates a useless test.

INDEX

Page numbers followed by "f" denote figures. Page numbers followed by "t" denote tables. Page numbers followed by "b" denote boxes.